Essentials of Human Parasitology

Judith S. Heelan, PhD

Director of Microbiology, Memorial Hospital of Rhode Island

Clinical Associate Professor of Pathology and Laboratory Medicine, Brown Medical School

Adjunct Professor, University of Rhode Island and Community College of Rhode Island

Frances W. Ingersoll, MS, CLS (NCA)

Technical Specialist in Microbiology, St. Joseph Health Services—Fatima Hospital

Adjunct Professor, University of Rhode Island and Community College of Rhode Island

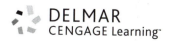

DELMAR
CENGAGE Learning

Australia • Brazil • Japan • Korea • Mexico • Singapore • Spain • United Kingdom • United States

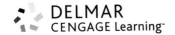
DELMAR
CENGAGE Learning™

Essentials of Human Parasitology
Judith Heelan, Frances Ingersoll

Business Unit Director: William Brottmiller

Executive Editor: Cathy L. Esperti

Development Editor: Darcy M. Scelsi

Executive Marketing Manager:
   Dawn F. Gerrain

Production Editor: Mary Colleen Liburdi

Illustrator: Argosy Publishing

Cover Design: William Finnerty

For product information and technology assistance, contact us at
Cengage Learning Customer & Sales Support, 1-800-354-9706

For permission to use material from this text or product,
submit all requests online at **www.cengage.com/permissions**
Further permissions questions can be emailed to
permissionrequest@cengage.com

ISBN-13: 978-0-7668-1284-0

ISBN-10: 0-7668-1284-7

Delmar
Executive Woods
5 Maxwell Drive
Clifton Park, NY 12065
USA

Cengage Learning is a leading provider of customized learning solutions with office locations around the globe, including Singapore, the United Kingdom, Australia, Mexico, Brazil, and Japan. Locate your local office at **international.cengage.com/region**

Cengage Learning products are represented in Canada by Nelson Education, Ltd.

For your lifelong learning solutions, visit **delmar.cengage.com**

Visit our corporate website at **www.cengage.com**

PREFACE

INTRODUCTION

This text presents basic descriptions of parasites commonly found to cause human disease. The book was written to provide information for a one-semester course in medical parasitology to address the needs of students in the health science fields, especially in the area of clinical laboratory science (medical technologists and medical laboratory technicians). However, the text might also be used by nursing students and biology majors, as well as by students in other allied health fields, such as respiratory therapy and physical therapy. The authors sought to provide the clear, concise, practical, and clinically relevant information necessary to gain an understanding of the pathogenesis of parasitic infections and to be able to diagnose these infections in the laboratory, without including the voluminous amounts of extraneous material often found in textbooks on medical parasitology. Critical thinking skills are developed by the inclusion of multiple choice questions and case studies in each chapter. The student should have some knowledge of biology as a prerequisite to taking this course.

In recent years, the field of medical parasitology has expanded with the recognition of new and emerging parasites, especially in the immunocompromised host. Additionally, increased travel has necessitated a global approach to the diagnosis of "exotic" diseases, not commonly seen in the United States in years past. This text has attempted to include both the "old" parasites, which have been recognized for many years, as well as the "new" parasites mentioned above. The authors have purposely omitted parasites that are rarely encountered in this country, and have limited discussion to protozoa and helminths (worms) that are known to parasitize humans.

In addition to conventional microscopic methods, this text also includes a discussion of non-traditional methods of parasite detection, using immunological and molecular techniques that have been introduced during the past few years. These methods are frequently more sensitive and allow the laboratory worker to more quickly diagnose parasitic infections, thereby increasing cost-effectiveness and improving patient care.

TEXT ORGANIZATION

The textbook *Essentials of Human Parasitology* consists of fourteen chapters divided into three sections. Parasites are divided into the two broad groups, protozoa and helminths.

Part I begins with an introduction (Chapter One), which provides an overview of medical parasitology and commonly used terms. Chapter Two discusses the collection, preservation, and processing of specimens for the recovery of parasites, and Chapter Three presents current information on immunological techniques available to diagnose parasitic infections. Although this information is mentioned briefly in the laboratory diagnosis of each parasite, this chapter provides more in-depth information on each type of method. A discussion of molecular diagnostic techniques is also included.

Part II consists of seven chapters devoted to the protozoa. Intestinal amebae are discussed in Chapter Four, while the free-living amebae, *Acanthamebae* species and *Naegleria* species, are discussed in Chapter 5. Intestinal and atrial flagellates and ciliates are presented in Chapter Six; blood and tissue flagellates are covered in Chapter Seven (*Leishmania* species) and Chapter Eight (*Trypanosoma* species). The intestinal Sporozoa (coccidia) are presented in Chapter Nine. Blood and tissue Sporozoa (*Plasmodium* species) causing malaria, *Babesia* species, *Toxoplasma* species, and *Pneumocstis* species) are discussed in Chapter Ten.

Part III consists of four chapters on helminths worms. Intestinal nematodes (roundworms) are discussed in Chapter Eleven and blood/body/tissue nematodes are discussed in Chapter Twelve. Trematodes (flukes) are included in Chapter Thirteen, and cestodes (tapeworms) are covered in Chapter Fourteen.

FEATURES

Each chapter in Parts II ad III is organized according to the following outline:

- List of parasites—Parasites are listed sequentially as they appear in the chapters.
- Learning Objectives—Learning objectives are listed to guide the student in mastering information contained in the chapter.
- Key Terms—Key terms are listed alphabetically; pronunciations follow some terms. Key terms are typed in bold and the appropriate definition given when first encountered in the chapter, and also in the "Master Glossary."
- Introduction—The introduction is an overview of material contained in the chapter.
- Name of Parasite
- Morphology—A description of developmental forms of the parasite which may be detected in human specimens is given. Figures and diagrams usually accompany these descriptions. Color photographs of selected parasites can be found in the full color insert.
- Life Cycle—The reproduction and development of the parasite in the relevant host is described and often illustrated.
- Transmission and Pathogenesis—Modes of transmission of infection and pathogenesis of infection are described.
- Laboratory Diagnosis—methods used in the laboratory to detect and identify each parasite are described.
- Treatment and Prevention—The treatment (if any) of choice is given, along with means of prevention of infection.
- Summary—One or two paragraphs summarize important points found in the chapter.
- Review Questions—Multiple choice review questions based on the chapter material are provided to reinforce principles covered in the chapter.
- Case Studies—Clinical findings and parasite descriptions are provided and the student is challenged to identify the parasite causing the infection. Questions on various aspects of the infection follow each case history.

ANCILLARY MATERIAL

Supplements for *Essentials of Human Parasitology* include a Student Workbook and an Instructor's Manual.

Workbook to Accompany Essentials of Human Parasitology

Each chapter of the workbook begins with learning objectives from the text. Concepts presented in the textbook are reinforced through numerous review questions, including matching columns created using key terms provided in the text, short answer questions, multiple choice questions, and labeling diagrams. Case Studies similar to those provided in the text are also included.

Instructor's Manual to Accompany Essentials of Human Parasitology

This supplement includes a proposed schedule for a 15-week, one-semester course, to fully utilize the material in the text, and also includes answers to the Review Questions and Case Studies found in each chapter. A section called "Instructor's Guide and Teaching Suggestions" addresses each chapter from the text, providing an overview, learning objectives, key terms, and summaries from the text, as well as suggested teaching activities, including the use of handouts, slides, and transparencies. Additional Case Studies and transparency masters are included in this section.

ACKNOWLEDGMENTS

I would like to thank members of the editorial staff of Delmar Publishing for their assistance during the preparation of this textbook, and the reviewers for their comments and suggestions for improvements to the text. In addition, I would like to thank my family, including my husband, Jack, as well as John, Stephanie and Brian, for their encouragement and support.

JSH

I would like to express my appreciation to the reviewers and the editorial staff of Delmar Cengage Learning for their assistance and direction the work leading to the completion of this textbook. Special acknowledgment is given to Andy Crump at the World Health Organization and to the Centers for Disease Control and Prevention for their contribution of images. In addition, I would like to thank my family, Frank and Josh, for their patience and encouragement, and my parents, John and Louise, who will always be my heroes.

FWI

ABOUT THE AUTHORS

Judith S. Heelan, PhD earned her MS and PhD degrees from the University of Rhode Island, Kingston, RI. and is a registered Medical Technologist (ASCP). She is Director of Microbiology at Memorial Hospital of Rhode Island, Pawtucket, and Clinical Associate Professor of Pathology and Laboratory Medicine at Brown Medical School. She is also an adjunct professor at the University of Rhode Island and the Community College of Rhode Island. In addition to writing journal articles and poster presentations, she was a contributor to the Delmar publication, *Essentials of Diagnostic Microbiology,* and the *Medical Dictionary for Health Related Professionals.* Her research interests include rapid methods in microbiology, and antibiotic resistance.

Frances W. Ingersoll, MS, CLS (NCA) is currently Technical Specialist for the Microbiology Laboratory at St. Joseph Health Services—Fatima Hospital in North Providence. She earned her undergraduate degree in Microbiology at the University of Rhode Island and Master of Science at the University of Massachusetts Dartmouth. She is a certified Medical Technologist and has served as a staff microbiologist, Program Director of a Medical Technology Program, Full Time Visiting Lecturer at the University of Massachusetts Dartmouth, and Technical Specialist in Microbiology. She is also an adjunct professor at the University of Rhode Island and the Community College of Rhode Island. In addition to published articles, she has co-authored the Delmar publication *The Study Guide to Essentials of Diagnostic Microbiology.*

CONTENTS

Introduction; Specimen Collection, Preservation and Processing; Immunodiagnostic Techniques

CHAPTER ONE
Introduction

OUTLINE

DEFINITION OF A PARASITE

IMPORTANCE OF MEDICAL PARASITOLOGY

PARASITES IN THE IMMUNOCOMPROMISED HOST

CLASSIFICATION AND DESCRIPTION OF PARASITES OF MEDICAL SIGNIFICANCE
Phylum Sarcomastigophora
Phylum Ciliophora
Phylum Apicomplexa

Phylum Microspora
Phylum Aschelminthes
Phylum Platyhelminthes

CHARACTERISTICS USED IN THE IDENTIFICATION OF PARASITES
Identification of Protozoa
Identification of Helminths

ARTIFACTS WHICH MAY BE CONFUSED WITH PARASITES

LEARNING OBJECTIVES

After reading and studying this chapter, the student should be able to:

- Define parasite.
- Recognize the importance of Medical Parasitology, especially with regard to the immunocompromised patient.
- Classify and describe parasites having medical significance for humans.

- List and describe characteristics used to identify protozoan and helminthic parasites involved in human infection.
- Appreciate the similarity of artifacts to parasites, detailing characteristics used to distinguish among them.
- Understand the organization and format of this textbook.

KEY TERMS

Aschelminthes
   (ASH-hel-min-thes)
Apicomplexa
   (APE-ee-com-PLEKS-a)
Chromatin (KRO-ma-tin)
Chromatoid bodies (KRO-ma-
   toyd BOD-ees)
Cilia (SIL-ee-a)
Ciliophora (SIL-ee-OF-o-ra)

Commensals (ko-MEN-sals)
Cysts (SISTS)
Definitive host
   (dee-FIN-i-tiv HOST)
Endemic (en-DEM-ik)
Flagella (fla-JEL-a)
Hermaphroditic
   (her-MAF-ro-DIT-ik)

Intermediate host
   (in-ter-MEE-dee-at HOST)
Karyosome (KAR-ee-o-som)
Mastigophora
   (MAS-tig-OF-or-a)
Microspora (MY-kro-SPOR-a)
Miracidium (MIR-a-SID-ee-um)
Oncosphere (ON-ko-sfer)
Parasite (PAR-a-site)

(continues)

KEY TERMS (continued)

Pseudopods (SOO-doe-pods)	Sarcodina (SAR-ko-DI-na)	Trophozoites
Platyhelminthes	Sarcomastigophora	(TRO-fo-ZO-ites)
(PLAY-tee-hel-min-thes)	(SAR-ko-MAS-tig-OF-or-a)	

DEFINITION OF A PARASITE

A **parasite** is a live organism living in, or on, and having some metabolic dependence on another organism known as a host. A **definitive host** is one in which the parasite reaches sexual maturity and where the adult form of the parasite usually resides, or in which sexual stages of reproduction occur. An **intermediate host** is one in which the immature or larval form usually resides, or in which the parasite undergoes asexual reproduction. A parasite may directly invade a definitive host, or it may have a complex life cycle involving one or more intermediate hosts. A parasite may be a pathogen, causing disease in a host, or it may be nonpathogenic, causing no harm. Many of these nonpathogenic parasites of humans are **commensals**, and are not known to produce human disease. Pathogenic parasites may cause illnesses ranging from asymptomatic infections, to mild gastrointestinal disease to life-threatening systemic infections.

IMPORTANCE OF MEDICAL PARASITOLOGY

Medical Parasitology has assumed greater importance in recent years in the United States because of the increase in travel among Americans, as well as the increased number of immigrants entering the United States. These individuals are often from areas where parasitic diseases are **endemic**, which means that the parasite is present in these areas at all times. Travelers to foreign countries may acquire parasitic diseases in endemic regions and bring them back to their own countries.

It is imperative that physicians are knowledgeable about parasitic diseases, and that microbiologists be skilled in the diagnosis of causative agents. Collection of appropriate specimens for analysis is essential for the rapid diagnosis of parasitic diseases. Collection of specimens for the recovery of parasites is addressed in Chapter 2.

PARASITES IN THE IMMUNOCOMPROMISED HOST

The large number of individuals who are immunocompromised by diseases, such as the acquired immunodeficiency syndrome (AIDS), enhances the need to accurately diagnose parasitic diseases since these infections are frequently more severe in these patients. Increasing numbers of transplant patients, as well as cancer patients being treated with chemotherapy, and patients receiving steroids, are especially vulnerable to infections with certain parasites. Parasites known to cause mild to moderately serious infections in healthy individuals, but particularly serious infections in the immunocompromised host, include the protozoans *Toxoplasma gondii, Pneumocystis carinii, Cryptosporidium parvum, Isospora belli, Cyclospora cayetanensis,* species of *Microsporidia,* and the helminth *Strongyloides stercoralis.* The most important indicator of whether a person will be affected by a parasite is his general health status.

CLASSIFICATION AND DESCRIPTION OF PARASITES OF MEDICAL SIGNIFICANCE

Parasitic protozoans of medical significance to humans are found in the phyla **Sarcomastigophora** (amebae and flagellates), **Ciliophora** (ciliates), **Apicomplexa** (protozoans with complex life cycles), and **Microspora** (tiny intracellular parasites). Helminths (worms) are found in the phyla **Platyhelminthes** (flatworms), and **Aschelminthes** (roundworms). Parasites in the phyla Acanthocephala (thorny-headed worms) and Arthropoda (arthropods) are less frequently encountered in the United States, and will not be discussed in this text.

Phylum Sarcomastigophora

This phylum is divided into two subphyla, **Sarcodina** or amebae and **Mastigophora** or flagellates. The amebae move by means of cytoplasmic protrusions called **pseudopods** (false feet); flagellates move by means of whiplike appendages known as **flagella**. Asexual reproduction is common among members of this phylum. Although most amebae and flagellates are free-living and harmless, several members of this group of protozoans are intestinal and tissue pathogens. *Entamoeba histolytica* causes amebic dysentery, but may also cause extra-intestinal infections. Other intestinal amebae are usually considered to be nonpathogenic. *Naegleria* and *Acanthamoeba* are free-living amebae, which may be involved in human infection. Intestinal flagellates include the pathogens, *Giardia lamblia* and *Dientamoeba fragilis*.

The tissue flagellates are found in the genus *Leishmania*, and in the genus *Trypanosoma*.

Phylum Ciliophora

These protozoans move by means of **cilia**, thread-like extensions which are shorter, and more numerous than flagella, and which arise from small basal granules. Most ciliates are free-living and nonpathogenic. The sole human pathogen in this phylum is *Balantidium coli,* which is the largest intestinal protozoan known to infect man. This rare parasite may cause severe intestinal disease.

Phylum Apicomplexa

This phylum, class Sporozoa, consists of protozoans usually having complex life cycles with alternating sexual and asexual generations. Pathogens include the Coccidia, parasites found in the intestinal mucosa and classified in the genera *Cryptosporidium, Isospora, Cyclospora,* and *Sarcocystis,* found in tissues. Blood and tissue protozoans in this phylum include agents causing malaria in the genus *Plasmodium,* as well as agents in the genus *Babesia.*

The tissue parasites *Pneumocystis carinii* and *Toxoplasma gondii* are also included in this phylum, although recent evidence supports the reclassification of the former organism as a fungus.

Phylum Microspora

These tiny intracellular parasites cause infections in a variety of vertebrates and invertebrates; only a small number of genera are known to infect humans. Immunocompetent individuals are rarely infected. Infections have been recognized in immunocompromised individuals, especially in those patients suffering from the acquired immunodeficiency syndrome (AIDS). Parasites most often isolated from humans are found in the genera *Encephalitozoon, Enterocytozoon, Pleistophora, Nosema,* and *Microsporidia.*

Phylum Aschelminthes

Roundworms (nematodes) are found in the class Nematoda, and have round, elongated bodies with coiled tails. The sexes are separate, with the male usually being smaller than the female. Although most nematodes are free-living, some species are parasitic for humans. The life cycles of some nematodes involve intermediate as well as definitive hosts. Intestinal roundworms known to infect humans include *Enterobius vermicularis, Ascaris lumbricoides, Trichuris trichiura,* the hookworms, *Ancylostoma duodenale* and *Necator americanus,* and *Strongyloides stercoralis.* Tissue-dwelling nematodes, including *Trichinella spiralis,* and filariae, such as *Wuchereria bancrofti,* are described separately in this text.

Phylum Platyhelminthes

These helminths are called flatworms, because of the flattened shape of the adult worm. Most flatworms are **hermaphroditic**, having both male and female reproductive structures in a single organism. Flatworms are found in the classes Trematoda (flukes) and Cestoda (tapeworms).

The flukes have leaf-shaped bodies and often attach to their hosts by means of suckers. Most flukes have complex life cycles. Flukes that are parasitic for man may infect the intestine, liver, lung, or circulatory system of the human host. Trematodes have complex life cycles, with at least one intermediate host. The most common trematodes which infect humans include *Fasciolopsis buski, Fasciola hepatica, Clonorchis sinensis, Paragonimus westermani,* and the schistosomes.

Tapeworms have elongated, ribbonlike bodies, consisting of a scolex, an organelle of attachment, anteriorly, a neck region, and segments called proglottids. Most cestodes have complex life cycles, requiring intermediate hosts. Adult tapeworms reside in the small intestine. Tapeworms commonly found in humans include *Diphyllobothrium latum, Taenia* species, *Hymenolepis species,* and *Echinococcus granulosis.*

Table 1–1 lists the parasites belonging to each of the preceding phyla.

CHARACTERISTICS USED IN THE IDENTIFICATION OF PARASITES

The identification of parasites is usually made by detecting protozoan **trophozoites** (the motile, actively feeding multiplying form) or **cysts** (the dormant, non-feeding resistant stage), or the ova (eggs), larvae, or adult forms of helminths. Microscopic examination of fecal specimens, blood, body fluid, or biopsy material is the traditional procedure used to diagnose

TABLE 1–1 ► Classification of Pathogenic and Commensal Parasites Found in Humans

PHYLUM	PARASITE
PROTOZOA	
Sarcomastigophora	
Subphylum Sarcodina	*Entamoeba histolytica*
	E. hartmanni
	E. coli
	Endolimax nana
	Iodamoeba butschlei
	Blastocystis hominis (uncertain classification)
	Naegleria fowleri
	Acanthamoeba species
Subphylum Mastigophora	*Giardia lamblia*
	Chilomastix mesnili
	Enteromonas hominis
	Retortamonas intestinalis
	Trichomonas hominis
	Dientamoeba fragilis
	Trichomonas vaginalis
	Trichomonas tenax
	Leishmania species
	Trypanosoma species
Ciliophora	*Balantidium coli*
Apicomplexa	
Coccidia	*Cryptosporidium parvum*
	Isospora belli
	Cyclospora cayetanensis
	Sarcocystis species
	Toxoplasma gondii
	Plasmodium species
	Babesia microti
	Pneumocystis carinii (uncertain classification)
Microspora	*Encephalitozoon*
	Enterocytozoon
	Pleistophora
	Nosema
	Microsporidia
HELMINTHS	
Aschelminthes	
Class Nematoda	
Intestinal	*Enterobius vermicularis*
	Ascaris lumbricoides
	Trichuris trichiura
	Ancylostoma duodenale
	Necator duodenale
	Strongyloides stercoralis
Blood/Tissue	*Trichinella spiralis*
	Wuchereria bancrofti
	Dracunculus medinensis
	Brugia species
	Loa loa
	Onchocerca volvulus
	Mansonella species
	Dirofilaria immitis
Platyhelminthes	
Class Trematoda	*Fasciolopsis buski*
	Heterophyes heterophyes
	Metagonimus yokogawai
	Fasciola hepatica
	Clonorchis sinensis
	Paragonimus westermani
	Schistosoma species
Class Cestoda	*Diphyllobothrium latum*
	Taenia species
	Hymenolepis species
	Dipylidium caninum
	Echinococcus species
	Multiceps species

parasitic infections, although serological methods may sometimes be useful.

Identification of Protozoa

The identification of intestinal protozoan parasites is based on the detection of characteristic cysts and trophozoites in stool specimens. Typical trophozoite and cyst stages of an ameba, a flagellate, and a ciliate are demonstrated in Figure 1–1. The presence of various developmental stages of fecal parasites is related to the type of stool specimen obtained from the patient. Watery or liquid stools are more apt to contain large numbers of trophozoites, while cysts usually predominate in formed or solid stools. Semi-formed fecal material may contain both cysts and trophozoites.

Motility is most often seen when trophozoites are detected in liquid stool specimens. One of the most important determinations in identifying protozoans is the accurate measurement of the size of the trophozoite or cyst on a permanently stained smear. A calibrated ocular micrometer is essential for this purpose.

Nuclei must be carefully counted and described, since the number and morphological appearance of protozoan nuclei are characteristic for each species of parasite. Although most trophozoites have only one nucleus, the number varies in cysts. Other important morphological traits include the presence or absence of peripheral nuclear **chromatin**, which consists of DNA, and the size and location of the **karyosome**, a small mass of chromatin material found in the nuclei of certain protozoa.

The appearance of the cytoplasm in cysts and trophozoites is helpful in the identification of the parasite. Glycogen and **chromatoid bodies** may be seen in cysts. Chromatoid bodies are usually rodlike structures of RNA, with rounded or jagged ends, depending on the parasite. Although several members of the phylum Apicomplexa (*Cryptosporidium parvum*, *Isospora belli*, and *Cyclospora cayetanensis*) stain pink using the modified acid-fast technique, they may be differentiated by size, and by the autofluorescent nature of the latter parasite.

Blood protozoans may be recognized by examination of thick and thin blood films. Blood is concentrated in a small area on thick blood films, while a thin layer of blood is spread on a glass slide to prepare a thin film. Erythrocytes remain intact in thin smears, but are lysed during the staining procedure on thick smears. Although thick smears, with a greater concentration of blood, are preferred for making a rapid diagnosis of infection, thin smears provide more typical morphological characteristics of the parasite. Thick and thin blood films are recommended for the diagnosis of

	Entamoeba histolytica (ameba)	*Giardia lamblia* (flagellate)	*Balantidium coli* (ciliate)

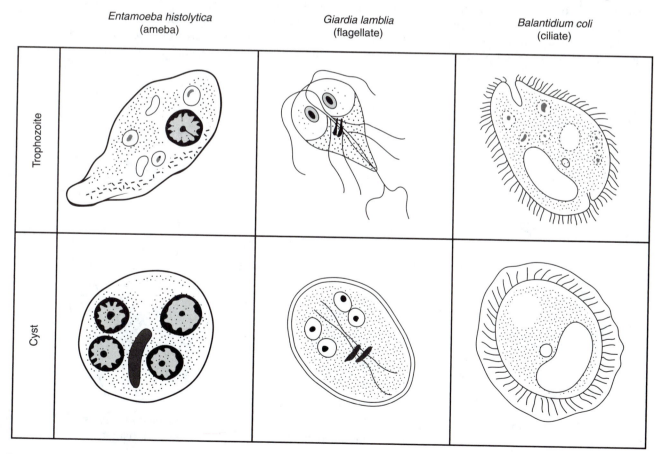

FIG 1–1 Trophozoites and Cysts of Intestinal Protozoa

malaria. Malarial parasites are identified by recognition of various stages of ring forms, trophozoites, schizonts, merozoites, and gametocytes seen in blood. A diagnosis of babesiosis or trypanosomiasis is made by identification of typical morphologic stages of the parasite in blood smears. Leishmaniasis is usually diagnosed by the identification of characteristic stages in tissue specimens. Toxoplasmosis may be diagnosed histologically or serologically. The presence of cysts in respiratory specimens may be used to diagnose *Pneumocystis carinii* pneumonia (PCP). Characteristic features of tissue protozoa are demonstrated in Figure 1–2.

Identification of Helminths

Diagnostic stages of helminths found in feces include ova (eggs), larvae, proglottids, and, occasionally, adult worms. Adult nematodes are rarely found in stool specimens. Exceptions are the pinworm (*Enterobius vermicularis*) and *Ascaris*. Adult trematodes are not found in feces, but proglottids may be found in some cestode infections. Ova are usually seen. Typical ova of a nematode, a trematode, and a cestode are demonstrated in Figure 1–3.

Characteristic eggs produced by nematodes, trematodes, and cestodes are most frequently used to make a diagnosis of infection with these parasites. Gravid proglottids of cestodes may rupture, releasing eggs. Eggs produced by a particular species of helminth are usually the same size and shape, and have the same stage of development when passed in feces. Charac-

teristics used most frequently to identify helminth eggs include size, shape, appearance of the eggshell, and stage of development.

A calibrated ocular micrometer is necessary to accurately determine measurements of helminth eggs. The size of these eggs ranges from 25 to 90 micrometers in length. The shape of the egg varies from spherical or round to oval. Infertile eggs may have a shape different from fertile eggs. Eggshells may be clear or colored (bile stains appear yellowish or brownish), and may be thick or thin. The eggs of *Ascaris*, *Enterobius*, and *Trichuris* are thick; those of the hookworms (*Necator* and *Ancylostoma*) are thin.

Modifications of the eggshell are characteristic of certain species. Knobs and spines are characteristic of certain species of trematodes.

The stage of development of the parasite within the eggs is characteristic for the species. Embryonated and unembryonated eggs may be found in feces. Development of the embryo may occur in the environment. Trematode eggs may contain an embryo known as a **miracidium**. A cestode egg usually contains a six-hooked larva called an **oncosphere**. Unfertilized eggs of *Ascaris lumbricoides* usually contain unorganized masses of globular material.

No ova of *Strongyloides stercoralis* are passed in stool specimens; larvae constitute the diagnostic stage found in feces. These are the only nematode larvae usually found in fecal specimens. However, hookworm larvae may occasionally be present if the specimen is allowed to stand at room temperature for more than

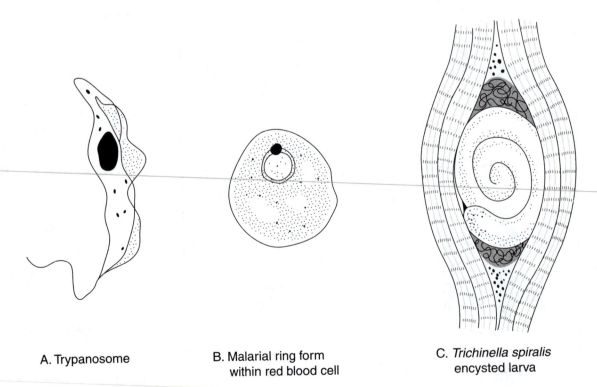

A. Trypanosome

B. Malarial ring form within red blood cell

C. *Trichinella spiralis* encysted larva

FIG 1–2 Characteristic Features of Tissue Parasites

Ascaris lumbricoides	Fasciolopsis buski	Taenia saginata
(Nematode)	(Trematode)	(Cestode)

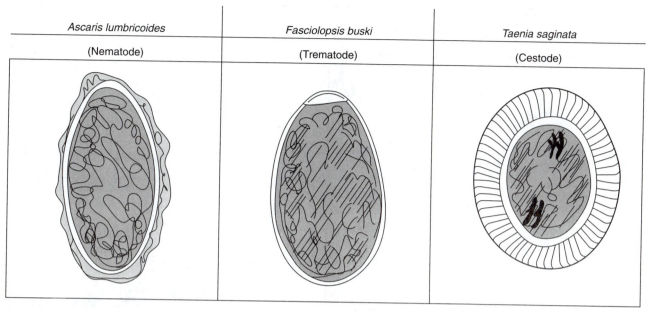

FIG 1–3 Helminth Ova

a day. Distinguishing between these two parasites may be difficult.

Infection with filarial nematodes is usually detected by demonstrating the presence of microfilariae in blood or skin. Recognition of characteristic morphologic types may allow more specific identification of the parasite.

Immunoassays for parasite antigens and antibodies produced in response to parasitic infections, although mentioned briefly in chapters devoted to specific parasites, will be discussed in more detail in Chapter 3.

ARTIFACTS WHICH MAY BE CONFUSED WITH PARASITES

Artifacts may cause confusion by being identified as human parasites (Figure 1–4). Yeast cells may resemble protozoan cysts or helminth eggs, but lack internal structure, and may be observed as budding forms. Pollen grains and vegetable cells may be mistaken for helminth eggs. Striations in the pollen grain wall may be confused with those found in the eggs of *Taenia* species. These structures generally are irregular and vary in size.

Starch granules may be confused with protozoan cysts, but are very refractile. Plant hairs and undigested food fibers may be mistaken for nematode larvae. Internal structure is usually lacking in these artifacts, which have thick, refractile walls. Polymorphonuclear leukocytic neutrophils may resemble amebic cysts, but usually have more irregular, poorly defined borders. The nuclei of these white blood cells are larger in proportion to the cytoplasm than are nuclei in amebic

cysts, lack peripheral nuclear chromatin, and may be linked by strands of chromatin.

SUMMARY

Medical Parasitology has assumed great importance in recent years with the increase in travel of Americans to foreign countries, where parasitic diseases are endemic, and the increased immigration of individuals from such foreign countries into the United States. Opportunistic parasitic diseases have become more problematic also among immunocompromised individuals resulting from the spread of AIDS, the increased numbers of cancer patients receiving chemotherapy, and the frequency of organ transplantation.

The most common members of the subphylum Sarcodina having medical significance for humans are separated in this textbook into intestinal amebae and free-living amebae. Clinically significant members of the subphylum Mastigophora and the phylum Ciliophora are separated into intestinal and atrial flagellates and ciliates, and blood and tissue flagellates. Sporozoans are divided into intestinal, and blood and tissue Sporozoa.

Helminths are included in chapters on intestinal nematodes, blood/body fluid/tissue nematodes, trematodes, and cestodes. Collection of specimens for the recovery of parasites, and immunoassays are discussed in separate chapters.

Characteristics used in the identification of parasites include a variety of developmental stages seen in microscopic preparations of feces, blood, tissues, and other body fluids. Trophozoites and cysts are

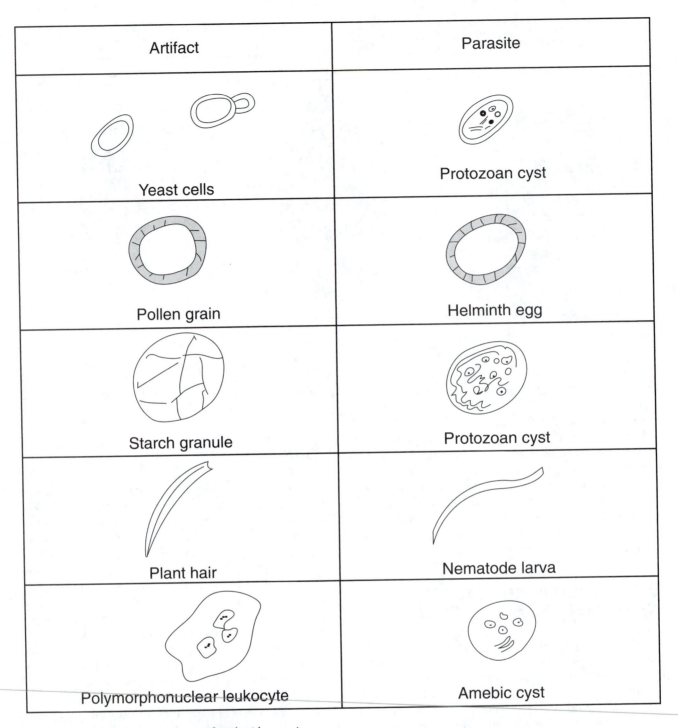

FIG 1–4 Artifacts which may be confused with parasites

characteristic of intestinal protozoa; trophozoites and other morphological forms may be used to identify blood and tissue protozoans. Helminths may be identified by detection of adult forms or larvae, but are most commonly recognized by the presence of their characteristic eggs.

REVIEW QUESTIONS

1. A parasite not known to cause infections in the immunocompromised host is
   a. *Cryptosporidium parvum*
   b. *Strongyloides stercoralis*
   c. *Enterobius vermicularis*
   d. *Toxoplasma gondii*

2. Which of the following protozoans is found in the phylum Apicomplexa?
   a. *Cryptosporidium parvum*
   b. *Strongyloides stercoralis*
   c. *Enterobius vermicularis*
   d. *Entamoeba histolytica*

3. Amebae and flagellates are found in the phylum
   a. Apicomplexa
   b. Ciliophora
   c. Platyhelminthes
   d. Sarcomastigophora

4. Flukes and tapeworms are found in the phylum
   a. Apicomplexa
   b. Ciliophora
   c. Platyhelminthes
   d. Sarcomastigophora

5. Watery or liquid stool specimens are more likely to harbor protozoan
   a. cysts
   b. trophozoites
   c. schizonts
   d. eggs

6. The embryo found in a tremadode egg is called a
   a. miracidium
   b. oncosphere
   c. microfilaria
   d. proglottid

7. The larva of a_____may be confused with the larva of *Strongyloides stercoralis*.
   a. filarial nematode
   b. hookworm
   c. pinworm
   d. tapeworm

8. Striations in a pollen grain may cause confusion with the eggs of
   a. *Strongyloides stercoralis*
   b. pinworm
   c. hookworm
   d. *Taenia* species

9. Thin eggshells are characteristic of
   a. *Ascaris*
   b. *Enterobius*
   c. *Necator*
   d. *Trichuris*

10. Blood and tissue protozoans include all but
    a. *Cryptosporidium*
    b. *Babesia*
    c. *Leishmania*
    d. *Plasmodium* (malaria)

CASE STUDY

A 28-year old male homosexual patient who admitted to having many sexual partners presented to his physician complaining of persistent diarrhea for several months duration. He had also lost 12 pounds during this period. Imodium and other over-the-counter antidiarrheal medications had not relieved his symptoms. Bacterial cultures were negative for enteric pathogens. Routine tests for ova and parasites were negative. No white blood cells were seen in a fecal smear. The stool specimen was negative for *Clostridium difficile* toxin. A modified acid-fast procedure was positive for the causative agent.

(continues)

CASE STUDY (continued)

Questions

1. The sexual history of this patient placed him at risk for infection with which virus?

2. What parasites are known to cause serious disease in patients infected with this virus, and would give positive results using a modified acid-fast procedure?

3. To what phylum do these protozoans belong?

4. How would you distinguish among these agents?

5. How can this infection, and many other diarrheal diseases be prevented?

▶ BIBLIOGRAPHY

Garcia, L.S. & Bruckner, D.A. (1997). *Diagnostic medical parasitology* (3rd ed.). Washington, D.C.: ASM Press.

Koneman, E. W., Allen, S.D., Janda, W.M., Schreckenberger, P.C., & Winn, Jr, W.C. (1997). *Color atlas and textbook of diagnostic microbiology* (5th ed.). Philadelphia: Lippincott.

Markell, E. K., Voge, M. A., & John, D. T. (1992). *Medical parasitology* (7th ed.). Philadelphia: W. B. Saunders.

CHAPTER TWO

Processing Specimens for Recovery of Parasites

OUTLINE

LEARNING OBJECTIVES

After reading and studying this chapter, the student should be able to:

- Describe the proper methods of collection of specimens for recovery of parasites.

- Describe commonly used methods for microscopic examination for parasites.

- Discuss methods used for less commonly encountered parasites.

- Explain procedures to collect and process specimens, other than feces, for the identification of parasites.

- Describe methods used to prepare and stain blood smears for parasites.

KEY TERMS

Biological safety hood
Diurnal periodicity
Formalin
Formalin-ethyl acetate
  sedimentation technique
Nocturnal periodicity
Non-periodic

Occult blood
Occupational Safety and
  Health Administration
  (OSHA)
Ocular micrometer
PVA
Sheather's sugar flotation

Sodium acetate-formalin (SAF)
Stage micrometer
Standard precautions
Zinc sulfate flotation
  technique

INTRODUCTION

Specimens submitted to the laboratory for examination for parasites must be collected properly and transported to the laboratory without delay. Upon receipt, specimens should be processed immediately, or preserved to maintain the quality of the specimen. Improperly collected specimens may lead to the inability to identify parasites or incorrect interpretation of results. Processing of specimens involves a number of standardized procedures used in the routine analysis for ova and parasites (e.g., stool specimen for ova and parasites or O&P), as well as specialized procedures performed only upon request.

COLLECTION AND HANDLING OF FECAL SPECIMENS

Fecal specimens should be collected in clean, wide-mouthed containers with tight fitting lids, and sealed in plastic bags for transport. All specimens should be collected prior to radiological studies using barium or the administration of bismuth, mineral oil or certain antibiotics and antidiarrheal medications that may interfere with the detection and identification of intestinal parasites. If therapy has already begun, stool samples should not be collected until 5–7 days after completion of treatment. Care should be taken to avoid contamination with urine or water, which might harm existing organisms or introduce free-living organisms from the environment.

Acceptable specimens should contain a sufficient amount of material to perform the examination procedures, approximately 5–7 grams of feces (or about the size of a marble). Specimens should always be properly labeled, including the patient's name, identification number, physician's name and the date and time that the specimen was collected.

Safety is always an issue. Specimens should be handled as infectious waste and **standard precautions** (protection against exposure to blood-borne

pathogens) should be observed. Protective clothing (gown and gloves) should always be worn when handling *all* specimens, and processing should be performed in a **biological safety hood**. This is an enclosure in which work can be done on potentially dangerous organisms without risk of acquiring or spreading infection.

If laboratory specimens are to be forwarded to an outside reference laboratory, the package must conform to the United States Postal Service mailing regulations. With the exception of microscope slides, parasitological specimens should be packaged within double mailing containers. Sample containers are placed inside an aluminum screw cap mailing tube which is then stuffed with cotton or absorbent material to prevent breakage and avoid spills. Instruction sheets including the patient information and test requisition can be wrapped around the cylinder. The canister is then placed within an outer cardboard mailer that is addressed for shipping.

Number of Specimens

At least three pre-therapy specimens should be submitted for routine examination for intestinal parasites. Since parasites may be present intermittently, it is recommended that specimens be collected on alternate days. Two of the stool specimens should be collected from normal bowel movements and the third specimen should be collected following the use of a non-oil-based cathartic. *Fleet Phospho-Soda* and magnesium sulfate are very effective. Laxatives are contraindicated for patients with pre-existing diarrhea. When the physician suspects intestinal amebiasis, a total of six specimens may be ordered. If any stool specimen tests positive for parasites, the remaining specimens in the series may be unnecessary.

Post-therapy stool specimens are recommended, particularly for patients who have been treated for intestinal protozoan infections. A series of three specimens should be collected, as above, and examined to confirm the effectiveness of treatment.

Timing of Specimens

As previously mentioned, intestinal parasites may not be shed into the feces in consistent numbers on a daily basis to facilitate adequate recovery and identification. For this reason, a series of three specimens should be submitted, on alternate days if possible, or within no more than a 10 day interval. When a six specimen series is ordered, collection should be completed within no more than 14 days.

A series of three specimens is generally recommended for post-therapy patients, but the timing of these specimens varies with diagnosis. Patients who have been treated for protozoan infections are typically checked 3 to 4 weeks after therapy. A patient treated for helminth infection may be checked 1 to 2 weeks post therapy and checks for *Taenia* may be delayed for 5 to 6 weeks post therapy.

Fresh versus Preserved Specimens

When properly collected and prepared, stool specimens for ova and parasite examination may reveal both protozoa and helminth parasites, if present. It is imperative that stool specimens be transported to the laboratory immediately because the age of the specimen directly influences the recovery of certain organisms.

A freshly passed stool specimen, which is received in the laboratory and examined within 30 minutes of passage, is the ideal specimen for parasite studies. In fact, this type of specimen is mandatory for the recovery of trophozoite forms and flagellates. Unfortunately, a rapid turn around is not always possible and samples must be preserved to maintain parasite integrity.

The decision to use a preservative may be influenced by the time the specimen may be in transit and the existing laboratory workload. The following time limits have been suggested as a guideline. Liquid stool specimens should be examined within 30 minutes of passage or the specimen should be placed in a suitable preservative. If protozoan parasites are suspected, it is important to remember that only trophozoites are typically found in liquid stools. Semi-formed stools (stools having a soft consistency) should be examined within 1 hour of passage or they too should be preserved. Both protozoan trophozoites and cysts can be found in semi-formed specimens. The time limits for the examination of formed stool specimens are not as crucial. It is recommended that these specimens be examined within 24 hours of passage to ensure the recovery of protozoan cysts. In all cases, if the time limits cannot be met, a portion of the specimen should be adequately preserved for later review.

Fecal specimens should never be frozen, incubated, or left at room temperature for extended periods prior to examination. If any of the acceptance criteria are in question, the specimen should be rejected and a new specimen requested.

Several types of fixatives are available for the preservation of specimens. Commercially manufactured two-vial kits, such as the *Parapak Stool System* by Meridian, are particularly useful for outpatient specimen collection. One vial generally contains either 5% or 10% formalin and the other contains **PVA** solution (polyvinyl alcohol resin plus Schaudinn's fixative). Prompt fixation helps to maintain true organism morphology.

Within the clinical laboratory, fresh stool specimens are placed in similar preservatives when samples cannot be processed in a timely fashion. The three most commonly used fixatives are: formalin, PVA, and sodium acetate-formalin (SAF). The advantages and drawbacks of each method will be discussed.

Formalin (an aqueous solution of formaldehyde) is an effective all-purpose fixative for the recovery and long-term preservation of protozoan cysts, helminth eggs and larvae. Two different strength solutions are commonly used — a 5% concentration, which is effective for preserving protozoan cysts, and a 10% concentration, which is recommended for the recovery of helminths. Preparation of formalin is outlined in Figure 2–1. Formalin should be added to the fecal material in a ratio of 3 parts formalin to 1 part feces and mixed thoroughly to ensure good preservation. Specimens preserved in formalin can be routinely used for direct examination, concentration techniques, and monoclonal antibody studies, but are not appropriate for making permanent smears. In addition, formalin does not preserve trophozoites well. Laboratories handling and processing formalin-fixed specimens should always perform procedures in a biological safety hood and follow guidelines developed by the **Occupational Safety and Health Administration (OSHA)**. This federal agency was established to monitor and reduce the occurrence of occupational hazards, injuries, and illnesses.

PVA (polyvinyl alcohol) fixative solution is one of the most commonly used means of preserving protozoan cysts and trophozoites, as well as helminth eggs. The PVA technique utilizes a combination of

Figure 2–1 ▶ **Preparation of 10% Formalin**	
Formaldehyde (USP)	100 ml
Physiologic Saline (0.85% NaCl)	900 ml

Dilute 100 ml of formaldehyde with 900 ml physiologic saline solution.

Schaudinn's fixative and polyvinyl alcohol resin, mixed with stool in a ratio of 3 parts PVA to 1 part stool. The PVA preserved specimen has the advantage of being able to be used for the complete parasite examination: direct exam, concentration techniques, and permanent mounts. In fact, the adhesive nature of the resin glues the specimen onto the slide and allows for the preparation of high quality permanent slides using such stains as trichrome or iron hematoxylin. PVA has a long shelf life, remaining stable at room temperature for months to years and specimens preserved in PVA are allowed to be shipped by regular mail.

One major disadvantage of PVA-Schaudinn's fixative is the presence of large amounts of mercuric compounds in the Schaudinn's fixative (Figure 2–2). These compounds are highly toxic and present a serious health risk if not handled with extreme precautions. Attempts to modify the Schaudinn's formula by substitution of compounds other than mercury have not yet produced the same quality of preservation. Also, specimens preserved in PVA cannot be used for monoclonal antibody studies. Preparation of PVA fixative in the clinical laboratory is cumbersome; however it can be purchased commercially.

Some laboratories have begun using the **Sodium acetate-formalin (SAF)** method of fixation as an alternative to PVA with Schaudinn's because of the concern surrounding the use of mercuric chloride. SAF contains 10% formalin as a fixative plus sodium acetate, which acts as a buffer. It is easy to prepare and store (Figure 2–3), eliminates the use of mercuric compounds, can be used for concentration and permanent smears and does not interfere with monoclonal antibody studies. SAF aids in the recovery of protozoan cysts and trophozoites, helminth eggs and larvae, and intestinal coccidians (such as *Cryptosporidium parvum*).

For those individuals who are used to making permanent smears with PVA, SAF may take some practice. SAF does not have the adhesive quality of the PVA resin. The addition of Meyer's albumin to the microscope slide enhances adhesion. Iron hematoxylin stain provides better results than trichrome stain. Modified

Figure 2–3 ► SAF Fixative

Sodium acetate	1.5 g
Glacial acetic acid	2.0 ml
40% formaldehyde	4.0 ml
Distilled water	92.5 ml

acid-fast stain can be used for the identification of organisms such as *Cryptosporidium* and *Isospora* species.

PROCESSING SPECIMENS

The methods used for processing both fecal and non-fecal specimens for parasite studies are considered "standard processing techniques," combining macroscopic observations (an overall description of the stool specimen) with microscopic examination consisting of direct wet preparations, concentration techniques and permanent stains. All the individual findings and characteristics are considered together for diagnostic purposes.

Macroscopic Examination

Unpreserved stool specimens submitted to the laboratory for parasite studies should first be examined macroscopically to determine the color (Figure 2–4) and consistency (Figure 2–5) of the sample and to screen for the presence of blood, mucus, visible parasites or foreign bodies. As previously stated, freshly passed stool is the specimen of choice for intestinal parasite studies. A gross examination can provide suggestive evidence as to the type of organisms that might be present. If the laboratory protocol allows only for the acceptance of preserved samples, then information pertaining to the color and consistency of the original specimen should be included with the request slip.

Stool consistency is typically graded as formed, soft or liquid depending on moisture content (see Figure 2–5). A watery or liquid stool may suggest the presence of protozoan trophozoites which are almost never found in formed stools. On the other hand, protozoan cysts are rarely seen in liquid samples but are commonly found in formed stools. Helminth eggs and larvae, as well as microsporidian spores and coccidian oocysts may be found in stool of any consistency.

The abnormal color of a stool specimen (Figure 2–4) may be indicative of a gastrointestinal problem (like a GI bleed), ingestion of medication or colored food

Figure 2–2 ► Preparation of Schaudinn's Fixative

2 Parts: Mercuric chloride (HgCl$_2$), saturated aqueous solution
1 Part: 95% ethyl alcohol

This stock solution keeps indefinitely. Immediately before use, add 5 ml of glacial acetic acid to each 100 ml of the stock solution.

Figure 2–4 ▶ Color Range of Fresh Stool Specimens

Color	Possible Cause
Black	Iron or bleeding in the bowel
Dark Brown	Range of normal colors
Brown	Range of normal colors
Pale Brown	Range of normal colors
Reddish Brown	Presence of blood, ingested material
Greenish	Ingested material, rapid transit through the bowel
Clay	Residual barium, biliary obstruction
Other (Blue, red, purple)	Special medications

Figure 2–5 ▶ Terms Used for Macroscopic Exam of Stool

Consistency	Reference
Hard	Cannot be punctured with an applicator stick
Formed	Maintains shape, can be punctured
Semi-formed	Bottom side flattens in the container
Soft	Can be cut with an applicator stick
Mushy	Can be reshaped with an applicator stick
Loose	Stool shapes to the container
Diarrhea	Stool will flow slowly out of the container
Watery	Fluid-like stool pours out of the container

product, or diagnostic procedure (such as a barium enema). A normal stool specimen is brown in color but samples may be received for examination that range in color from black to clay colored. Color should always be noted.

The gross examination of the stool should also include a macroscopic exam of the surface of the specimen for parasites and blood. Adult pinworms, and even *Ascaris,* can sometimes be seen on the surface of a fresh specimen. Tapeworm proglottids may be found on or within the specimen. An applicator stick can be used to separate the specimen for observation. If adult worms or parasite segments are found, the specimen can be washed through a wire screen or gauze with physiologic saline to isolate the organism for identification.

Blood is an abnormal finding in stool but may be present in a variety of forms. Red blood on the surface of formed stool is often a sign of bleeding hemorrhoids. If bloody mucus is found in loose or liquid fecal specimens, it may be suggestive of amebic ulceration in the large intestine or an inflammatory condition of the bowel, most notably ulcerative colitis. Dark colored stool may contain **occult blood** (blood present only in microscopic amounts) which could indicate intestinal bleeding due to parasitic infection or other potential pathologies such as neoplasm or ischemic bowel.

Microscopic Examination

The microscopic portion of the ova and parasite examination (the observations made using a microscope) provides voluminous amounts of information when performed by experienced laboratories using standard procedures. The exam can be divided into three distinct steps: the direct wet mount, the concentration, and the permanent stained smear. There is no all-purpose technique. Each part of the exam provides valuable information that aids in the overall diagnosis. The methods suggested here are chosen from many that are reliable and well proven. Each laboratory must choose those methods that fit its individual needs and work flow.

Calibration of the Microscope

Many of the morphologic characteristics that we attribute to certain parasites relate to size. One cannot accurately determine the size of an organism, in micrometers, without first calibrating the **ocular micrometer** of the microscope. The ocular micrometer is a circular glass disk, engraved with a ruler-like scale, that fits snugly into the eyepiece of the microscope. The scale is generally numbered from 0 to 50. The distance between the lines is an arbitrary value that only has meaning when calibrated for each objective using a **stage micrometer**. The stage micrometer has an exact, known scale with lines measuring 0.01mm apart.

Measurements are made by looking through the oculars and superimposing one scale on the other. The number of divisions on the ocular micrometer (from the zero mark) that coincide exactly with one gradation on the stage micrometer are counted. Figure 2–6 illustrates how the scales will look when they are properly aligned. In this diagram, seven ocular divisions fall within one stage division of 0.01mm. With a simple calculation, it is determined that each division of the ocular scale equates to 0.00143 mm.

Since there are 1000 micrometers in 1 millimeter, each division is 1.43 micrometers (μm) apart. This procedure should be repeated for each objective and performed at least once per year for quality control purposes. A suggested procedure is described in Procedure 2–1.

Direct Wet Mounts

The primary purpose for the direct wet mount, also known as the wet prep, is to detect protozoan trophozoites and their characteristic motility. This procedure is also used as a screening procedure for parasites, prior to performing the concentration technique and the permanent slide. The vast majority of samples that are reviewed are stools, but the direct wet mount is equally applicable to non-fecal specimens, such as aspirates and fluids.

The direct wet mount is prepared by mixing a small amount of material (approximately 2 mg) in a drop of 0.85% (physiologic) saline on a clean, dry microscope slide. The sample should be obtained from different parts of the specimen using a wooden applicator stick and mixed with saline to form a homogeneous suspension. If blood or mucus is present, it should also be examined. As a rule, the mixture should be thin enough to read newsprint through the slide. Some laboratories may prefer to use the larger 2 × 3 inch slides which provide a greater working surface. Place a 22 × 22 mm coverslip over the mixture and scan on low power (100X magnification) using low light. This is accomplished by lowering the condenser and adjusting the iris diaphragm. The entire area of the coverslip should be systematically reviewed. Most parasites tend to appear transparent and refractile. All parasites (protozoan, eggs, and larvae) should be readily visible using low power. Questionable objects may be subject to further investigation using the high dry objective (400x total magnification). The use of an oil immersion lens is not recommended unless the edges of the slide have been sealed with nail polish or a heated paraffin-Vaseline mixture.

The identification of protozoa is better accomplished by adding stain to the wet mount. The stain that is most widely used is a weak iodine solution called Lugol's iodine (Figure 2–7).

A drop of iodine stain can be added to the edge of the coverslip of the wet saline prep or a new smear can be made using the iodine solution. Iodine kills the parasites and enhances the appearance of the nucleus and cytoplasmic structures.

Laboratory policy generally dictates whether or not the direct wet mount will be performed. Many laboratories have abandoned the direct wet mount for cost-effective reasons or because their samples arrive in preservative. Other labs only perform direct wet mounts on liquid or diarrhetic stool, where the odds of recovering protozoan trophozoites is greater. In any case, all findings of intestinal protozoa in direct wet preparations should be confirmed by concentration and/or permanent stained slides. A suggested procedure for the direct wet mount is described in Procedure 2–2.

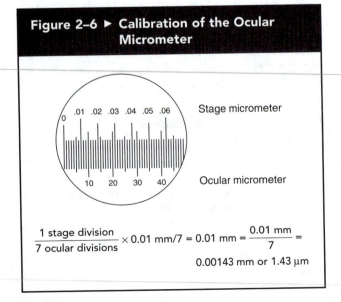

Figure 2–6 ▶ Calibration of the Ocular Micrometer

$$\frac{1 \text{ stage division}}{7 \text{ ocular divisions}} \times 0.01 \text{ mm/7} = 0.01 \text{ mm} = \frac{0.01 \text{ mm}}{7} =$$

0.00143 mm or 1.43 μm

Figure 2–7 ▶ Lugol's Iodine Solution

Distilled water	100 ml
Potassium iodide	10 g
Iodine crystals	5 g

Store in brown glass stoppered bottle in the dark.

PROCEDURE 2–1
Calibration of the Ocular Micrometer

Principle

An ocular micrometer, positioned in the eyepiece of the microscope and properly calibrated, is instrumental for measuring the size of microorganisms in a microscopic field. The distance between the graduations on the ocular micrometer are calibrated for each objective lens using the following procedure.

Materials

Ocular micrometer or eyepiece that contains a micrometer disk
Stage micrometer

Method

1. Insert the ocular micrometer disk into the bottom of the ocular or replace the ocular with one containing an ocular micrometer.
2. Place the stage micrometer on the stage of the microscope and center it over the light source.
3. Using the low power objective (10x), bring the scale of the stage micrometer into focus. Rotate the eyepiece until the ocular scale is parallel to that of the stage micrometer.
4. Superimpose the two scales so that the left edge of the stage micrometer lines up with the left edge of the ocular micrometer scale.

(Figure 2–6) The zero points on each scale should coincide.
5. Without moving the stage, visually follow the scale to the right and locate another line on the micrometer scale that overlaps *exactly* with one on the stage micrometer.
6. Each division of the stage micrometer is exactly 0.01 mm (or 10 micrometers) apart. To calculate the value of each ocular division:

$$\frac{\text{Number of stage divisions}}{\text{Number of ocular divisions}} \times 0.01 \text{ mm} =$$

Value of each ocular division in millimeters
Ocular value in millimeters $\times$ 1000 = Value of each ocular division in micrometers
7. Repeat the procedure for each objective lens. (If the oil immersion lens is being calibrated, place a drop of immersion oil on the stage micrometer.)

Example 1 *(Refer to Figure 2–6)*

$$\frac{1 \text{ stage division}}{7 \text{ ocular divisions}} \times 0.01 \text{ mm} = \frac{0.01 \text{ mm}}{7} =$$

0.00143 mm or 1.43 μm

Example 2

Two divisions on the stage micrometer line up with 15 divisions on the ocular micrometer. What is the value of each ocular division?

$$\text{Each ocular division} = \frac{2 \times 0.01 \text{ mm}}{15} =$$

0.00133 mm or 1.33 μm

Concentration Procedures

Most of the specimens that are received in the clinical laboratory for parasite studies contain some type of debris that can overshadow the presence of parasitic elements. Concentration methods aid in the removal of debris and allow for the detection of even small numbers of parasites in a sample. Concentrated specimens can be examined directly in wet mount and with the addition of iodine.

Two types of procedures are commonly used: sedimentation and flotation. Sedimentation procedures are performed by suspending the fecal material in an aqueous suspending fluid and through centrifugation, heavier protozoa, oocysts, eggs and larvae are separated from the lighter fecal debris. Flotation procedures enhance the separation of parasitic elements by combining the fecal material with solutions of greater specific gravity. The lighter protozoa, oocysts, eggs and larvae float to the top and can be recovered in the surface film. Three specific techniques will be discussed: formalin-ethyl acetate sedimentation, zinc sulfate flotation and Sheather's sugar flotation.

The **formalin-ethyl acetate sedimentation technique** is one of the most widely used O & P concentration methods. The process is easy to perform, inexpensive, and allows for the recovery of all protozoan cysts, helminth eggs and larvae. Protozoan trophozoites and coccidian oocysts are only likely to

PROCEDURE 2–2
Direct Wet Mount

Principle

The direct wet mount is performed to detect motile protozoan trophozoites and to determine cellular morphology.

Materials

Sample material
Clean glass microscope slide
22 × 22 mm coverslip
0.85% NaCl solution
Lugol's iodine solution
Biohazard discard container

Method

Saline Mount

1. Place 1 drop of 0.85% NaCl on a clean, dry, 2 × 3 inch microscope slide.
2. With an applicator stick, transfer a small amount (~2 mg) of fecal sample and emulsify in the saline drop.
3. Place a 22 × 22 mm coverslip (No. 1) over the suspension.

4. Using the low power objective (10X), systematically scan the entire surface area of the coverslip for parasites.
5. The high dry objective (40X) should be used for investigation of suspicious objects.

Iodine Mount

1. An iodine stained mount can be prepared in the above manner, substituting one drop of Lugol's iodine for the saline.
2. A drop of iodine can also be added to the edge of the coverslip of a previously examined saline mount. The iodine will diffuse into the stool-saline mixture, kill the organisms, and stain the cellular elements.

Quality Control

Known positive specimens should be processed to verify the recovery of organisms at least quarterly and the results should be properly recorded.

Expected Results

Motile protozoan trophozoites will demonstrate their characteristic motility in saline wet mounts. Addition of iodine solution will kill the organisms and stain the cellular elements for easier recognition.

---

be seen if they exist in large numbers. Fresh, formalin-fixed, SAF or PVA specimens may be used.

Ethyl acetate is added to an aliquot of saline-washed formalin-fixed sample. The ethyl acetate extracts the debris and fecal fat and, after centrifugation, four distinct layers remain: sediment, formalin, debris, and ethyl acetate. The specimen is then decanted and the concentrated sediment is examined for parasites in wet mounts with and without iodine. A suggested step-by-step procedure for formalin-ethyl acetate concentration is described in Procedure 2–3.

In contrast to the formalin-ethyl acetate technique in which the parasites are more dense than the suspending fluid, flotation methods, such as the **zinc sulfate flotation technique** concentrate lighter potential parasites at the surface of a suspending fluid that has a specific gravity of approximately 1.18 (for fresh stool specimens). When using zinc sulfate flotation, a loopful of the surface fluid is used to make wet mounts with and without iodine.

Zinc sulfate flotation has the advantage of effectively eliminating the majority of contaminating debris. This technique works well for the recovery of protozoan cysts, coccidian oocysts (*Cryptosporidium* and *Isospora*) and some helminth eggs. The technique is unreliable for the recovery of heavier, operculated eggs of some trematodes, unfertilized *Ascaris* eggs, and nematode larvae. Protozoan trophozoites are destroyed by the procedure and the specific gravity of the reagent must be carefully monitored.

The zinc sulfate flotation technique can be used on fresh, formalin-fixed, SAF, and PVA specimens. A suggested step-by-step procedure for the zinc sulfate flotation technique is described in Procedure 2–4.

Sheather's sugar flotation is particularly effective for the recovery of *Cryptosporidium* and *Isospora* oocysts. Unpreserved or formalin-fixed stool specimen is combined with Sheather's sugar solution, centrifuged, and the surface film is extracted for slide preparation. Wet mounts of the concentrate are examined for the

PROCEDURE 2–3
Formalin-Ethyl Acetate Concentration

Purpose

Parasitic elements are concentrated by sedimentation to improve the recovery of fecal specimens.

Principle

Since the number of parasitic forms on a wet count or stained smear may be too low, concentrating the sample should increase the probability of detecting and identifying any diagnostic parasitic stage. The procedure is efficient for the recovery of helminth eggs, larvae, and protozoan cysts that have been preserved with 10% formalin.

Materials

Preserved fecal material
Funnel/filter device
15 ml conical centrifuge tube
Tapwater
Centrifuge
Discard container
9 ml of 10% formalin
4 ml ethyl acetate
Applicator sticks
Cotton tip swabs
Coverglass
Melted vaspar
Iodine
Saline
Compound microscope

Method

1. A large amount of preserved fecal material (4–6 ml) is poured through a funnel/filter device to give a sediment of ½ to ¾ ml in a 15 ml conical centrifuge tube.
2. Add tapwater to the 15 ml mark. Centrifuge at 650 X g (gravity) forces (1,500–1,600 rpm) for one minute.
3. Decant supernatant into a discard container.
4. Add 8–9 ml of 10% formalin to the conical tube and resuspend sediment.
5. Add approximately 3–4 ml of ethyl acetate. Stopper the tube and shake it vigorously for

30 seconds. Hold the tube so the stopper is directed away from your face. After 15–30 seconds, carefully remove the stopper.
6. Centrifuge for one minute at 500 X g.

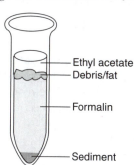

Sedimentation tube after centrifugation.

7. Four layers should result:
   a. the ethyl acetate layer
   b. the debris plug
   c. the formalin layer
   d. the sediment
8. With an applicator stick, free the debris plug from the sides of the tube. Carefully decant the top three layers. Wipe the sides of the tube with a cotton tip swab. Mix the sediment with the small amount of fluid that drains back from the sides of the tube.
9. Add a few drops of 10% formalin to the sediment if necessary.
10. Prepare both a saline and iodine wet mount from the sediment. The suspension should be dense enough to read a newspaper print in each solution.
11. Cover each preparation with a coverglass and seal with melted vaspar to prevent dehydration.
12. Systematically scan the entire saline prep under low-power magnification (10x) and iodine prep under high dry (40x). Examine for helminth eggs, larvae, or protozoan cysts.

Quality Control

1. Check formalin and saline each time they are used. Reagents should appear clear, without any visible contamination.
2. Concentrate known positive specimens and verify organism recovery at least quarterly and after the centrifuge has been recalibrated.

(continues)

PROCEDURE 2–3
Formalin-Ethyl Acetate Concentration *(continued)*

Expected Results

1. Protozoan cysts, helminth eggs, and larvae may be seen and identified. Protozoan trophozoites are less likely to be seen.

2. Results obtrained should be confirmed by a permanent stain (Trichrome) smear. Some protozoa are very small and difficult to be identified by the direct wet smears alone.

---

presence of oocysts using phase-contrast microscopy. Oocysts will appear as rounded, refractile structures containing visible sporozoites. The modified Sheather's sugar flotation technique is described in Procedure 2–5.

Permanent Stains

It is often impossible to determine the exact identification of intestinal protozoa on the basis of observations made by direct wet mount or concentration techniques. Even the most experienced microscopist may have difficulty with the detection and identification of some of the smaller protozoans without the detailed cytologic morphology revealed by the permanent stain. Once stained, a coverslip is affixed to the smear with sealant, such as Permount, and the slide is examined using an oil immersion lens (1000X total magnification). Such slides serve as permanent records of the parasites found and can be kept for years, or sent to a reference laboratory when further investigation is required. Many institutions use parasite positive slides as a teaching resource for laboratory students and medical residents. The permanent stained slide is an essential part of the complete ova and parasite examination.

Fresh or preserved stool specimens can be used for the preparation of the slide. A small amount of sample is rolled over the surface of a clean microscope slide with an applicator stick to form a thin, transparent film. When PVA or SAF samples are used, care should be taken to spread the specimen to the edges of the slide for better adhesion during staining. Slides should be allowed to air dry completely before staining. If fresh stool is received, slides should be prepared in a similar manner and immediately placed into Schaudinn's fixative for a minimum of 30 minutes before staining.

There are three permanent stains that are widely used for routine diagnostic parasitology: iron hematoxylin, Wheatley's trichrome stain, and the modified acid-fast stain. Most laboratories use one of the first two stains for routine testing and the modified acid-fast stain for the identification of coccidia.

The iron hematoxylin stain was developed over a century ago and is noted for creating fine morphologic detail. The classic staining procedure was time consuming and laborious but current modifications have shortened the procedure and made it more applicable to routine diagnostic testing. Iron hematoxylin stains intestinal protozoa (both trophozoites and cysts) with great detail, but helminth eggs and larvae may be obscured by excess stain. A suggested iron hematoxylin staining procedure is described in Procedure 2–6.

Wheatley's trichrome stain (a modification of the Gomori stain) is one of the most commonly used stains for demonstration of intestinal parasites. The procedure is simple and less time consuming than the iron hematoxylin method and produces uniformly well stained smears. Background material appears greenish in color and protozoa have a blue-green to purple cytoplasm with red to purple-red nuclear material and inclusions. The variations in color provide more contrast than the iron hematoxylin procedure. A suggested trichrome staining procedure is described in Procedure 2–7.

The modified acid-fast stain has become a routine part of the ova and parasite examination for the identification of *Cryptosporidium*, *Isospora*, and *Cyclospora*. These organisms are small and yeast-like in appearance and do not stain well with iron hematoxylin or trichrome stain. The modified acid-fast staining procedure differentiates the above organisms, which retain the carbofuchsin and stain bright red to purple against blue staining background material. A suggested modified acid-fast staining procedure is described in Procedure 2–8.

COLLECTION OF SPECIMENS OTHER THAN FECES

In the pages that follow, you will find short descriptions of some of the other types of specimens that may be received in the laboratory for parasite studies. In each case, proper collection and processing techniques

PROCEDURE 2–4
Zinc Sulfate Flotation Technique

Principle

The floatation procedure facilitates the separation of protozoan trophozoites, cysts and certain helminth eggs from background debris through the use of high specific gravity zinc sulfate solution.

Materials

Preserved fecal material
15 ml conical centrifuge tube
Funnel/ gauze filter device
0.85% saline solution
Centrifuge
1.18 or 1.20 specific gravity zinc sulfate solution
Clean glass microscope slide
22 × 22 mm coverslip
Biohazard discard container

Method

1. Transfer a pea size sample of fresh stool (about 4 g) into 10 ml of 5 or 10% formalin. Mix thoroughly and let stand for a minimum of 30 minutes for fixation. If the specimen has already been preserved in formalin, or SAF, resuspend the mixture.

2. Strain a sufficient quantity of the specimen through wet gauze (no more than 2 layers) into a 15 ml conical centrifuge tube. Usually, 8 ml of the formalin-stool suspension from step 1 or 3–4 ml of a previously preserved specimen should be sufficient.

3. Fill the remainder of the tube with 0.85% saline and centrifuge for 10 minutes at 500 X g. The amount of sediment obtained should be approximately 0.5 to 1 ml. Too much or too little sediment will affect the concentration procedure.

4. Decant the supernatant fluid, resuspend the sediment in 0.85% saline, and centrifuge for 10 minutes at 500 X g. This second wash can be eliminated if the supernatant resulting from step 3 is light tan to clear.

5. Decant the supernatant and resuspend the sediment in 1 to 2 ml of zinc sulfate. Fill the tube with additional zinc sulfate to within 2–3 mm of the rim.

6. Centrifuge for 2 minutes at 500 X g. Allow the centrifuge to come to a complete stop without interference. The centrifugation of the sample should result in two layers: a small amount of sediment in the bottom of the tube and a layer of zinc sulfate. The protozoan cysts and some helminth eggs will be in the surface film; heavier eggs will be in the sediment.

7. Without removing the tube from the centrifuge, withdraw 1 or 2 drops of the surface film with a Pasteur pipette or a wire loop.

8. Add a 22 × 22 mm coverslip to the preparation. Iodine may also be added to the preparation to enhance morphologic detail.

9. Using the low power objective (10x), systematically scan the entire area of the coverslip.

10. If something suspicious is observed, a more detailed study can be made with the 40x objective.

Quality Control

1. The specific gravity of the zinc sulfate should be frequently monitored. When fresh stool is received for processing, a specific gravity of 1.18 should be maintained. If formalin preserved sample is used, the specific gravity of the zinc sulfate solution should be adjusted to 1.20.

2. Concentrate known positive specimens and verify organism recovery at least quarterly and after the recalibration of the centrifuge. All QC results must be properly recorded.

Expected Results

Protozoan trophozoites and/or cysts and some helminth eggs and larvae may be recovered. Operculated eggs and heavy helminth eggs will not float in the zinc sulfate. These organisms may be found in the sediment. Oocysts of *C. parvum* may also be seen in the concentrate sediment.

PROCEDURE 2–5
Modified Sheather's Sugar Flotation for *Crytposporidium*

Principle

The Sheather's flotation procedure uses the specific gravity of the sugar solution to separate the rounded oocysts of *Cryptosporidium* from background debris.

Materials

Fecal suspension
Sucrose
Tap water
Phenol
12 ml conical centrifuge tube
Applicator stick
Centrifuge
Wire loop
Clean, dry glass microscope slide
22 × 22 mm coverslip
Phase contrast microscope

Method

Sheather's Sugar Solution:

Sucrose	500 g
Tap water	320 ml
Phenol	6.5 g

Boil sugar solution until clear. Using a fume hood, *carefully* add phenol and stir. Allow to cool to room temperature.

1. In a 12 ml conical centrifuge tube, add 1 to 2 ml fecal suspension.
2. Fill the conical tube 3/4 full with Sheather's sugar flotation solution.
3. Stir the mixture vigorously with an applicator stick.
4. Add sugar solution to within 1 to 2 cm of the rim of the tube.
5. Centrifuge at 500 X g for 10 minutes.
6. Using a wire loop, transfer the surface film to a microscope slide.
7. Cover with a 22 × 22 mm coverslip, and observe with phase-contrast microscopy.

Quality Control

Concentrate known positive specimens and verify organism recovery at least quarterly and after the recalibration of the centrifuge. All QC results must be properly recorded.

Expected Results

Oocysts of *Cryptosporidium* will appear rounded and refractile and the sporozoites within will be well defined.

---

will be considered along with an indication of the more commonly recovered organisms. It should be noted that, in most cases, collection in a sterile container is recommended, pending the request for other diagnostic tests such as bacteriologic culture. Standard precautions should always be maintained. A summary of the information can be found in Table 2–1.

Cellophane Tape Prep

The cellophane tape prep, or Scotch tape test, is one of the most commonly used procedures for the recovery of *Enterobius vermicularis* (pinworm) eggs. During the night, the adult female worm migrates out of the anus and deposits her eggs around the perianal region. Following the procedure describes in Procedure 2–9, specimens should be collected in the morning, before the patient bathes or defecates. A diagnosis of pinworm infection is based on the recovery of typical oval shaped, thick-walled eggs of *Enterobius vermicularis*. Eggs are often fully embryonated when observed. This identical procedure has also proven helpful in the recovery of *Taenia* eggs.

A variety of commercially prepared collection kits are available. Patients are generally children, so parents or caretakers should be given clear instructions regarding the proper collection technique. Patients should not be considered negative until at least four consecutive negative slides have been obtained.

Sigmoidoscopy Material

Sigmoidoscopic procedures may be ordered on patients with suspected amebiasis or may be performed

PROCEDURE 2–6
Iron Hematoxylin Staining Procedure

Principle

The iron hematoxylin staining method is one of a number of procedures available for permanent stains of fecal specimens. This process facilitates the identification of trophozoites and cysts, and the confirmation of species, and can be a permanent record of organisms recovered.

Materials

Freshly prepared fecal slides
70% alcohol
70% alcohol with iodine
Tap water
4% ferric ammonium sulfate solution
Iron hematoxylin staining solution
0.25% ferric ammonium sulfate solution
95% alcohol; 100% alcohol; xylol
Permount
Coverslip

Method

1. Prepare thin layer fecal smears and place in Schaudinn's fixative with acetic acid for 30 minutes.
2. Dehydrate in 70% alcohol for 15 minutes.
3. Wash in 70% alcohol with iodine to remove fixative for 3 minutes.
4. Wash in 70% alcohol for 3 minutes.
5. Rinse in tap water.
6. Place in 4% ferric ammonium sulfate solution for 15 minutes, which acts as a mordant.
7. Rinse in tap water.
8. Stain with iron hematoxylin staining solution for 10 minutes.
9. Rinse with tap water.
10. Decolorize in 0.25% ferric ammonium sulfate for 12 minutes.
11. Rinse in running water for 5 minutes.
12. Dehydrate in 70% alcohol for 5 minutes.
13. Dehydrate in 95% alcohol for 5 minutes.
14. Dehydrate in 100% alcohol for 5 minutes.
15. Dehydrate in 100% alcohol for 5 minutes.
16. Clear in xylol for 5 minutes.
17. Clear in xylol for 5 minutes.
18. Mount in Permount for examination.
19. Examine using an oil immersion lens.

Quality Control

Known positive fecal slides should be processed with each run of stained slides to verify the recovery of organisms and the quality of the staining process (particularly when the reagents have been changed). The results should be properly recorded.

Expected Results

When properly stained, protozoan trophozoites and cysts will appear blue-gray to almost black. The background material stains a pale gray or blue color.

---

to monitor the progress of disease. Material obtained from the procedure may be in the form of an aspirate, tissue biopsy or scraping. The material should be processed immediately. Preferably, one portion of the specimen should be fixed in PVA with Schaudinn's for the preparation of permanent stained smears and an additional portion should be placed in 5 or 10% formalin or SAF. Formalin fixed material is preferred for fluorescent antibody studies. Biopsy material is usually processed through histologic procedures. In addition to *Entamoeba histolytica*, *Cryptosporidium parvum* or *Giardia lamblia* are also commonly recovered in sigmoidoscopic specimens.

Aspirates

Material aspirated from lung or liver abscesses is often helpful for diagnosing infections with *Entamoeba histolytica*. Such material should be examined in direct wet mount and on permanent stained slides. Culture techniques, using bovine serum based medium, such as Diamond's or TYI-S-33 medium, are also routinely used by some labs for the recovery of *Entamoeba*.

Following open surgery for cyst removal, it is not uncommon to receive aspirations from lung or liver cysts for the confirmation of hydatid disease. Cyst material can be examined directly, or mixed with a drop of 10% KOH, for the presence of hydatid sand (scolices) or

PROCEDURE 2–7
Wheatley's Modification of Gomori's Trichrome Stain

Principle

This stain is a rapid, simple procedure that produces uniformly well-stained smears of intestinal protozoa, as well as human cells, yeast cells, and artifact material. It facilitates the identification of trophozoites and cysts, and the confirmation of species, and can be a permanent record of organisms recovered.

Materials

Prepared fecal slides
10 coplin jars
70% ethanol plus iodine
70% ethanol
Trichrome stain
90% glacial acetic acid alcohol
95% ethanol
Absolute alcohol
Carboxylene
Xylene
Permount
Microscope slides
22 × 40 mm coverslips
Compound microscope

Method

1. Place prepared slide(s) into the first coplin jar. Stain smears according to the staining time given:

COPLIN JAR	REAGENT	STAINING TIME
1	70% ethanol plus iodine	10–20 minutes
2	70% ethanol	5 minutes
3	70% ethanol	5 minutes
4	Trichrome stain	8 minutes
5	90% glacial acetic acid alcohol	3–5 seconds (briefly dip in and out)
6	95% ethanol	rinse briefly
7	95% ethanol	rinse briefly
8	absolute alcohol	5 minutes
9	carboxylene	5 minutes
10	xylene	10 minutes

2. Remove slide from coplin jar 10 and add several drops of permount onto smear. Carefully place a 22 × 40 mm coverslip on the smear. Avoid bubble formation.
3. Allow smear to dry overnight or 1 hour at 37°C.
4. Examine smear microscopically with 100x objective. Examine at least 200 to 300 oil immersion fields.

Quality Control

1. Prepare and stain a smear of PVA fixed fecal specimen containing protozoa or PVA-preserved negative stool specimen to which buffy coat cells have been added weekly.
2. Include a QC smear when the decolorizing reagent has been changed, a new lot of reagents have been added, or new reagents have been added to the dish.
3. Cover all staining dishes to prevent evaporation.
4. If xylene becomes cloudy, replace before staining.

Expected Results

1. Protozoan trophozoites and cysts will be readily seen.
2. Cytoplasm of trophozoites or cysts stain blue-green. Chromatin material, chromotoidal bodies, red blood cells (ingested), and bacteria stain red or purplish-red.
3. Background material appears green; larvae or eggs stain red.

PROCEDURE 2–8
Modified Kinyoun Acid-Fast Stain

Principle

Cryptosporidium, *Isospora*, and *Cylospora* species have now been recognized as causes of severe diarrhea in immunodeficient patients and transient diarrhea in immunocompetent individuals. Since the oocysts cannot be detected on a trichrome-stained smear, modified Kinyoun acid-fast stain is recommended. The following procedure may be used on formalin-fixed material or sediments from formalin-ethyl acetate concentrations.

Materials

Prepared fecal smears, including a positive smear of *Cryptosporidium parvum*
Staining set-up
Carbofuchsin stain
Tapwater
3% HCl (acid-alcohol)
Brilliant Green K stain
Permount
Coverglass
Forceps
Compound microscope

Method

1. Flood smear(s) with carbofuchsin stain. You will be given one slide positive for *C. parvum* and a slide without *C. parvum*. Your instructor may also choose to include an unknown smear as well. Let stand at room temperature for 5 minutes. *Do not heat.*

2. Rinse with tapwater and drain.
3. Decolorize with 3% HCl (acid-alcohol) for 2 minutes, or until no more color runs off the slide.
4. Rinse with tap water and drain.
5. Counterstain with Brilliant Green K stain for 2 minutes.
6. Rinse with tap water and drain.
7. Thoroughly air dry smear(s).
8. Place a drop of permount onto the smear and cover with a coverglass.
9. Examine smear microscopically with 40x objective. Examine at least 200–300 high-power fields.

Quality Control

1. A positive control slide of *Cryptosporidium parvum* and a negative control slide without *C. parvum* from 10% formalin preserved specimen will be stained and processed with each staining batch run and with each new reagent prepared.
2. Check preparation of sample (macroscopically) for adherence to the slide.

Expected Results

1. Oocysts of *Cryptosporidium*, *Isospora*, and *Cylospora* species will be readily seen.
2. Cylospora oocysts (8–9 microns in diameter) are twice the size of *Cryptosporidium* oocysts (4–5 microns in diameter) and tend to be acid-fast variable.
3. There is usually a range of color intensity of the oocyst from pink to red to deep purple.

---

characteristic hooklets. Such findings confirm the diagnosis of *Echinococcus* infection. Negative findings do not rule out the possibility of hydatid disease, as some cysts are sterile.

Duodenal aspirates are most often evaluated for *Giardia lamblia*, *Strongyloides stercoralis* or *Cryptosporidium*. This type of fluid specimen may require concentration by centrifugation prior to direct examination for motile organisms and permanent staining. To avoid invasive intubation procedures, a simple method for sampling duodenal contents has been

developed. The technique, called the Entero-test, consists of a weighted length of nylon yarn coiled within a gelatin capsule (Figure 2–8). An extended piece of the yarn is taped to the patient's cheek and the capsule is swallowed. The capsule material dissolves in the patient's stomach, and the yarn is carried into the patients duodenum. After 4–6 hours of incubation, the line is retrieved and the material adhering to the yarn is examined microscopically.

Bronchoscopy procedures yield fluid specimens, such as bronchial washings and bronchoalveolar lavages, that

Table 2-1

Specimen Type		Examination Technique	Possible Parasites
Cellophane Tape Prep		Direct Exam	*Enterobius vermicularis*
Sigmoidoscopy Material		Direct Exam Permanent Stain	*Entamoeba histolytica* Intestinal Protozoa *Cryptosporidium parvum*
Aspirates			
	Duodenal	Direct Exam Permanent Stain	*Giardia lamblia* *Isospora belli* *Strongyloides stercoralis* *Cryptosporidium parvum*
	Liver or Lung Abscess	Direct Exam Permanent Stain Culture	*Entamoeba histolytica* *Entamoeba histolytica* *Entamoeba histolytica*
	Liver or Lung Cyst	Direct Exam with KOH	*Echinococcus* species
	Bronchoscopy Material	Centrifuged, Direct Exam Permanent Stain	*Pneumocystis carinii* *Toxoplasma gondii* *Cryptosporidium parvum*
Sputum		Direct Exam N-acetyl-cysteine concentrate	*Paragonimus westermani* *Strongyloides stercoralis* *Ascaris lumbercoides* Hookworm *Entamoeba histolytica* *Echinococcus* species
Mouth Scrapings		Direct Exam Permanent Stain	*Entamoeba gingivalis* *Trichomonas tenax*
Nasal Discharge		Direct Exam Permanent Stain	*Naegleria fowleri* *Naegleria fowleri*
Corneal Scrapings		Culture Calcofluor White Stain Histologic Processing	*Acanthamoeba* species *Acanthamoeba* species *Acanthamoeba* species
Tissue Biopsy			
	Skin Ulcer	Culture Histologic Processing	*Leishmania* species *Leishmania* species
	Skin Snip	Direct Exam Histologic Processing	*Onchocerca volvulus* *Mansonella streptocerca*
	Lymph Node	Histologic Processing	*Leishmania* species *Trypanosoma* species *Toxoplasma gondii*

(continues)

Table 2–1 *(continued)*			
Tissue Biopsy *(continued)*			
	Bone Marrow	Histologic Processing Permanent Stain	*Leishmania* species *Trypanosoma* species *Toxoplasma gondii*
	Muscle	Histologic Processing	*Trichinella spiralis*
Urine		Centrifuged Direct Exam	*Schistosoma haematobium* Microfilariae *Trichomonas vaginalis*
Urethral Discharge		Direct Exam	*Trichomonas vaginalis*
Vaginal Discharge		Direct Exam	*Trichomonas vaginalis*
Prostatic Secretions		Direct Exam	*Trichomonas vaginalis*
Blood		Direct Exam Permanent Stain	*Plasmodium* species *Babesia* species *Leishmania* species *Trypanosoma* species Microfilariae

PROCEDURE 2–9
Cellophane Tape Prep for Pinworm (and *Taenia*)

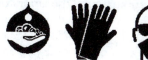

Principle

The adult female *Enterobius vermicularis* migrates out of the anus at night and deposits her eggs over the perianal area. Eggs can be collected for examination using the cellophane tape procedure for the recovery of pinworm.

Materials

8 cm piece of clear (not frosted) cellophane tape
Wooden tongue depressor
Clean, dry microscope slide

Method

1. Cut a piece of *clear* cellophane tape approximately 1 × 8 cm in length. At each end, fold the sticky surfaces together for about 1 cm to create two non-sticky handles.
2. Stretch the tape evenly, sticky side out, over one end of a wooden tongue depressor, holding the non-sticky ends in place firmly with the thumb and forefinger.
3. Apply the tape to the anal region, covering as much of the exposed area as possible.
4. Remove the tape and apply to a clean, dry microscope slide, sticky side down. Press firmly.
5. Examine for eggs under low power (10x).

Expected Results

The characteristic ovoid eggs of *Enterobius vermicularis* adhere to the cellophane tape and can be seen microscopically in positive specimens.

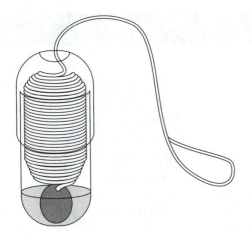

FIG 2–8 Entero test

may be examined for *Pneumocystis carinii*, *Toxoplasma gondii*, or *Cryptosporidium parvum*. This type of fluid specimen should be concentrated by centrifugation prior to the preparation of slides for permanent stain.

Sputum

Expectorated sputum from patients is not one of the more commonly received specimens for parasite studies, but a variety of different parasites may be responsible for symptoms of pneumonia or pneumonitis. Migrating larval forms of *Strongyloides stercoralis*, *Ascaris lumbercoides*, or hookworm may be recovered. Pulmonary amebic abscesses can result in an expectorant that contains blood, epithelial cells, and *Entamoeba histolytica* trophozoites. Patients with pulmonary hydatid disease (*Echinococcus* species) may produce deep sputum specimens that contain scolices from ruptured cysts. Finally, sputum is considered the specimen of choice for the recovery of the eggs of the lung fluke *Paragonimus westermani*. In patients with paragonimiasis, sputum may be thick and tinged with brownish specks called "iron filings," which represent packets of eggs.

Sputum specimens should be collected in the early morning and forwarded to the laboratory in a tight sealing, sterile container. A proper specimen should be from the lower respiratory passages, not saliva. The material can be examined in direct wet mount with saline or iodine or can be concentrated using N-acetyl-L-cysteine and centrifugation. N-acetyl-L-cysteine is a mucolytic agent that is used to digest mucoid specimens to release parasitic elements.

Mouth Scrapings and Nasal Discharge

Entamoeba gingivalis and *Trichomonas tenax* cause parasitic infections of the oral mucosa and gingiva. In most cases, they are associated with poor oral hygiene and can be recovered from mouth scrapings, particularly in material from around the gumline or pyorrheal pockets. Nasal discharge is collected and examined for the presence of *Naegleria fowleri*. In each case, specimens should be obtained in a sterile, airtight container or swab and examined by direct wet mount for the presence of parasites. Permanent stained smears may also have diagnostic value.

Corneal Scrapings

Diagnosis of *Acanthamoeba* keratitis is best achieved by examination of corneal scrapings. Such scrapings, obtained by the physician, should be placed in a sterile airtight container. Scrapings can be directly inoculated onto non-nutrient agar plates (Culbertson's medium) seeded with a suspension of live *E. coli*. Plates are incubated and examined daily for 10 days for *Acanthamoeba* cysts. Scrapings can also be examined directly using calcofluor white stain, or processed as a histologic specimen.

Tissue/Biopsy Material/Skin Snips

Tissue biopsy specimens are often submitted on patients suspected of cutaneous parasitic infections, including *Leishmania braziliensis*. Specimens should be surgically removed and submitted to the laboratory in sterile saline to prevent dehydration. Biopsy material can then be cultured onto Nicolle-Novy-McNeal (NNN) medium and examined weekly for the presence of *Leishmania* promastigotes. Material can also be used to prepare touch prep slides for Giemsa staining or for histologic processing.

Other types of tissue biopsies, skin snips suspected for *Onchocerca volvulus*, and bone marrow and lymph node specimens should be processed by histology and reviewed by the pathologist.

Urine/Genital Specimens

Urine is the specimen of choice for the recovery of *Schistosoma haematobium* eggs and can also be indicated for the detection of microfilariae: *Wuchereria*, *Onchocerca*, *Loa*, and *Brugia*. In addition, *Trichomonas vaginalis* trophozoites are often recovered in the urinary sediment of infected females and males and in vaginal and prostatic secretions. Urine is collected into a wide-mouth, sterile container with a tight fitting lid and forwarded to the laboratory immediately.

The specimen is centrifuged and the sediment is examined microscopically.

Urethral and vaginal discharge specimens and prostatic secretions are examined in direct wet mount for the presence of *Trichomonas vaginalis*. Under low power (10x) and reduced light, *T. vaginalis* demonstrates a jerky motility if present. Multiple specimens may be needed to recover the organism.

Cerebrospinal Fluid

On rare occasion, sterile fluids, such as CSF, may be infected with parasitic organisms. There are certain genera that gravitate to the central nervous system: *Naegleria, Acanthamoeba, Toxoplasma* and *Trypanosoma*. Patients with these infections generally exhibit symptoms of meningitis and a lumbar puncture is performed. Cerebrospinal fluid is collected in a sterile, tight sealing container. The sample should be concentrated by centrifugation, and the sediment examined in wet mount for the presence of motile trophozoites. Permanent stained smears should also be prepared. Additionally, some of the concentrated sediment can be cultured on non-nutrient agar seeded with *Escherichia coli*, incubated and examined for parasite cysts.

PREPARATION OF BLOOD SMEARS FOR PARASITE EXAMINATION

Blood is the specimen of choice for the recovery of parasites such as *Plasmodium* species, *Babesia* species, *Trypanosoma* species, *Leishmania donovani* and the microfilariae (except *Onchocerca volvulus*). Species identification of these organisms is generally based on the examination of permanent stained blood films.

Blood samples may be obtained from the fingertip, earlobe, or venipuncture and may be anticoagulated or non-anticoagulated. Ethylene diamine tetra-acetic acid (EDTA) is the anticoagulant of choice for venipuncture specimens.

The timing of specimen collection can be influenced by the patient's travel history and clinical symptoms. Many of the organisms in question exhibit a natural periodicity in the blood. The intraerythrocytic parasites, like *Plasmodium* species and *Babesia* species, are best recovered from blood samples collected toward the end of a paroxysmal episode. Thick and thin blood smears should be prepared and stained with Giemsa or Wright's stain.

Time of collection is also important for the recovery and identification of the microfilariae of filarial nematodes. *Wuchereria bancrofti* and *Brugia malayi* exhibit a **nocturnal periodicity,** therefore blood samples should be collected after 10 P.M. when the microfilariae are most likely to be present. If *Loa loa* is suspected, blood should be drawn during mid-day (11 A.M. to 1 P.M.). *Loa loa* has a **diurnal periodicity**. Patients with a travel history to the South Pacific may be tested for a strain of *Wuchereria bancrofti* which is **nonperiodic**. Peripheral blood specimens for these patients, as well as those suspect of leishmaniasis and trypanosomiasis, are randomly collected. In each case, thin smears should be prepared and permanently stained.

The success of blood film preparation depends on the use of clean, unscratched, grease-free slides. Even new slides should be alcohol-cleaned and thoroughly dried before using. Two kinds of blood smears may

---

PROCEDURE 2–10
Thin and Thick Blood Smear Preparation

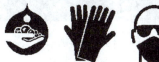

Thin Blood Smear

The thin blood film is made in the same manner as a blood smear used for a differential count in hematology. The suggested "Push Slide Technique"

assures that the thin area of the slide has one layer of evenly distributed cells. For best results, slides should be alcohol-cleaned, grease-free, and thoroughly dry.

1. Place a small drop of blood near one end of an alcohol-cleaned microscope slide.

(Figure A)

(continues)

PROCEDURE 2–10
Thin and Thick Blood Smear Preparation (continued)

2. Using a second clean slide as a "push slide" or spreader, back the spreader into the blood at a 30° angle.

(Figure B)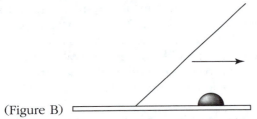

3. In one continuous movement, draw the blood across the slide

(Figure C)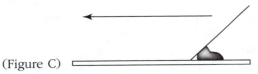

A properly made smear will have a thick end and a thin end that tapers to a feathered edge. Most of the area of the slide will be a thin layer one cell thick.

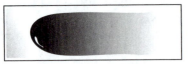

Thick Blood Smear

1. Place 2–3 small drops of whole blood close together at one end of an alcohol-cleaned, dry slide.
2. With one corner of another clean slide, mix the drops together in a circular motion over an area of 2 cm in diameter (about the size of a nickel). **
3. Mixing should continue for at least 30 seconds to prevent formation of fibrin strands. (If anti-coagulated blood is used, this step should be eliminated.)
4. Slides should be allowed to air dry thoroughly at room temperature. Do not heat.
5. Dry slides should be laked to remove hemo-globin. This can be accomplished by placing the slides in buffer solution prior to staining or in the Giemsa solution itself.

If slides are not to be stained immediately, they should be laked in buffer prior to storage. As time passes, the removal of hemoglobin will become more difficult.

** Note: If the slide has not been properly cleaned or the blood is too thick, the blood may flake off the slide during staining.

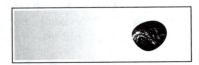

PROCEDURE 2–11
Wright's Staining Procedure of Thick and Thin Blood Smears

Principle

Wright's stain is a permanent stain for blood smears that contains fixative (alcohol) and stain in one solution. Smears do not require fixation before staining.

Materials

Blood sample
Clean, dry glass microscope slide
Wright's stain
Staining rack

(continues)

PROCEDURE 2–11
Wright's Staining Procedure of Thick and Thin Blood Smears (continued)

Phosphate-buffered water
Distilled water

Thin Smears

1. Place slides on a level staining rack and cover the surface with commercially prepared Wright's stain. Let stand for 1 to 3 minutes.
2. Add an equal volume of phosphate-buffered water to the slide. Mix by gently blowing on the surface of the fluid.
3. After 4 to 8 minutes, flood the slide with phosphate buffer, rinsing off the stain.
4. With a paper towel, wipe off the excess stain from the bottom of the slide and stand upright to air dry.

Thick Smears

Before staining, thick blood films should be laked in distilled water to lyse the red cells and then air dried. The staining procedure is the same as for thin smears.

Quality Control

Known positive slides should be stained and examined for quality control purposes.

Interpretation of Thick and Thin Smears

Erythrocytes	Light tan, reddish, or buff
White Blood Cells	
Nuclei	Bright blue
Cytoplasm	Light blue
Eosinophilic granules	Bright red
Intra-erythrocytic Parasite:	
Cytoplasm	Pale blue
Nuclear material	Red
Inclusions/dots	Stain poorly
Microfilariae:	
Sheath	Stains poorly
Nuclei	Pale to dark blue

be made — thick and thin. Thick smears are typically used for screening purposes, particularly in cases where malaria or babesiosis is suspected and the parasitemia may be low. Thin smears are suggested for the observation of morphologic detail and species iden-

tification. A suggested procedure for making both types of smears is described in Procedure 2–10.

Once the slides have been prepared and allowed to air dry at room temperature, permanent staining should follow. Slides should not be stored for

PROCEDURE 2-12
Giemsa Staining Procedure of Thick and Thin Blood Smears

Principle

Giemsa stain is a permanent stain for blood smears that contains separate fixative (methanol) and stain solutions.

Thin Smears

1. Fix blood films in absolute methanol (acetone-free) for 30 seconds.
2. Allow slides to air dry at room temperature.
3. Prepare a solution of 1 part Giemsa stock to 10 to 50 parts buffered (pH 7.0–7.2). Immerse slides in stain 10–60 minutes. **

(continues)

PROCEDURE 2-12
Giemsa Staining Procedure of Thick and Thin Blood Smears (continued)

4. Dip slides briefly in phosphate buffered water or rinse with tap water. With a paper towel, wipe off the excess stain from the bottom of the slide.

5. Drain thoroughly in a vertical position and allow to air dry.

** Fresh working stain should be made daily. For each new batch of working stain, test slides should be stained and examined to determine the best dilution/time ratio. As a general rule, if the stain dilution is 1:20, staining time is 20 minutes; if stain dilution is 1:30, staining time is 30 minutes, and so forth.

Thick Smears

A greater volume of blood can be examined for parasitic forms when using thick smears, but the organisms may lack the morphologic definition needed for species identification.

Perform the same procedure as for thin smears, starting at step 3.

Lack of methanol fixation allows for lysis of red cells in the Giemsa staining solution.

Quality Control

Known positive slides should be stained and examined with each new batch of stain for quality control purposes.

Interpretation of Thick and Thin Smears

Erythrocytes	Pale red
White Blood Cells	
Nuclei	Purple
Cytoplasm	Pale purple
Eosinophilic granules	Deep pink to purple
Intraerythrocytic Parasite:	
Cytoplasm	Blue
Nuclear material	Red to purple-red
Inclusions/dots	Red
Microfilariae:	
Sheath	Stains poorly
Nuclei	Blue to purple

---

prolonged periods or stain retention and morphologic distortion may result. There are two permanent stains that are commonly used in the clinical laboratory to stain parasites — Wright's stain and Giemsa stain. Wright's stain is typically a hematologic stain which combines a fixative and stain in one solution. A suggested procedure for the Wright's stain is described in Procedure 2–11. In the Giemsa staining procedure (Procedure 2–12) the stain and fixative are separate. Giemsa stain, preferred by many parasitologists, provides significant morphologic detail for the species identification of blood parasites.

SUMMARY

The recovery and identification of parasites from clinical samples of all types is highly dependent on proper collection, handling and processing of the specimen. Fecal specimens are the most commonly received specimen for parasite studies. Stools should be examined within the recommended time guidelines,

or they should be preserved. Formalin, PVA and SAF are typical preservatives.

The macroscopic exam, including stool consistency, may give an indication of the form of the parasite that might be present. The types of procedures used to recover parasites include: direct wet mounts, concentration techniques, and permanent stained preparations. Techniques such as sedimentation and flotation remove debris and concentrate the number of organisms in the sample. Permanent smears stained with iron hematoxylin, trichrome or modified acid-fast stain are often required for confirmation of parasite identification. In some instances, cultivation techniques are also used.

The type of specimen to be examined depends on the parasite and the site of infection in the host. Table 2–1 summarizes the types of specimens submitted, processing techniques, and expected parasites. *Plasmodium* species, *Babesia* species, *Trypanosoma* species, *Leishmania* species and the microfilariae (except *Onchocerca volvulus*) are recovered from permanently stained thick and thin blood smears. Giemsa stain is recommended.

REVIEW QUESTIONS

1. *Acanthamoeba* keratitis is best diagnosed using:
   a. urine
   b. corneal scrapings
   c. skin biopsy
   d. feces

2. The specimen of choice for the diagnosis of *Plasmodium* species, *Babesia* species, and filarial nematodes is:
   a. whole blood
   b. stool
   c. sputum
   d. bronchoalveolar lavage

3. The iodine mount is used to demonstrate all the following characteristics *except*:
   a. motility
   b. glycogen mass
   c. cytoplasm
   d. chromatin material

4. If *Cryptosporidium parvum* or *Isospora belli* are suspected, the permanent smear should be stained with:
   a. Gram stain
   b. Gomori's stain
   c. Modified acid-fast stain
   d. Wright's stain

5. The specimen of choice for the recovery of *Schistosoma haematobium* eggs is:
   a. blood
   b. stool
   c. sputum
   d. urine

6. Nocturnal periodicity must be considered in the collection of blood specimens for the diagnosis of:
   a. *Loa loa*
   b. *Wuchereria bancrofti*
   c. *Babesia microti*
   d. *Trypanosoma cruzi*

7. The Cellophane Tape Prep is used for the diagnosis of:
   a. *Trichomonas vaginalis*
   b. *Entamoeba histolytica*
   c. *Enterobius vermicularis*
   d. *Schistosoma haematobium*

8. Sheather's sugar flotation technique is particularly effective for the recovery of:
   a. *Cryptosporidium parvum*
   b. *Trichinella spiralis*
   c. *Fasciolopsis buski*
   d. *Loa loa*

9. Thick and thin blood smears are prepared for the detection of intra-erythrocytic parasites. The thick smear is used to detect light parasitic infections and the thin smear is for:
   a. detection of eosinophilia
   b. enumeration of white blood cells
   c. evaluation of cysts
   d. species identification

10. Consistency of the stool may indicate the form of the parasite that might be present. Formed stools are more likely to contain:
    a. trophozoites only
    b. cysts only
    c. sporozoites
    d. no parasites

CASE STUDY

An unpreserved stool sample arrives in the clinical laboratory of St. Joseph Hospital at 10:30 A.M. The requisition slip and sample are properly labeled with the patient's name, hospital number, physician and time of collection (11:30 P.M.). The request is for an ova and parasite exam. The specimen within the container appears to have a watery consistency.

Questions

1. Should the specimen be processed for ova and parasite exam?

2. What form of the protozoan parasite would you expect to find?

▶ **BIBLIOGRAPHY**

Beal, C. B., Viens, P., Grant, R. G. L., & Hughes, J. M. (1970). A new technique for sampling duodenal contents: Demonstration of upper small-bowel pathogens. *American Journal of Tropical Medicine and Hygiene*, 19, 349–352.

Beaver, P. C., Jung, R. C., & Cupp, E. W. (1984). *Clinical parasitology* (9th ed.). Philadelphia: Lea & Febiger.

Benson, H. J. (1998). *Microbiological applications: Laboratory manual in general microbiology* (7th ed.). Boston: McGraw-Hill.

Brooke, M. M., & Goldman, M. (1949). Polyvinyl alcohol-fixative as a preservation and adhesive for protozoa in dysenteric stools and other liquid material. *Journal of Laboratory Clinical Medicine*, 34, 1554.

Faust, E. C., D'Antoni, J. S., Odom, V., Miller, M. J., Perez, C., Sawitz, W., Thomen, L. F., Tobie, J., & Walker, J. H. (1938). A critical study of clinical laboratory techniques for the diagnosis of protozoan cyst and helminth eggs in feces. *American Journal of Tropical Medicine*, 18, 169–183.

Garcia, L. S., & Bruckner, D. A. (1993). *Diagnostic medical parasitology* (2nd ed.). Washington, DC: American Society of Microbiology.

Garcia, L. S., Shimizu, R. Y., Shum, A. C., & Bruckner, D. A. (1993). Evaluation of intestinal protozoan morphology in polyvinyl alcohol preservative: comparison of zinc-based and mercuric chloride-based compounds for use in Schaudinn's fixative. *Journal of Clinical Microbiology*, 31, 307.

Howard, B. J., Keiser, J. F., Smith, T. F., Weissfeld, A. S., & Tilton, R. C. (1994). *Clinical and pathogenic microbiology* (2nd ed.). St. Louis: Mosby-Year Book.

Ingersoll, F. W., & Marshall, J. R. (1999). *Study guide and laboratory manual to accompany essentials of diagnostic microbiology*. Albany, NY: Delmar Publishers.

Levine, J. A., & Estevez, E. G. (1983). Methods of concentration of parasites from small amounts of feces. *Journal of Clinical Microbiology*, 18, 786–788.

Markell, E. K., John, D. K., & Krotoski, W. A. (1999). *Medical parasitology* (8th ed.). Philadelphia: W. B. Saunders.

Melvin, D. M., & Brooke, M. M. (1982). *Laboratory procedures for the diagnosis of intestinal parasites* (3rd ed.). U. S. Department of Health, Education, and Welfare publication no. (CDC) 82-8282. Washington, DC: Government Printing Office.

Sawitz, W. G., & Faust, E. C. (1942). The probability of detecting intestinal protozoa by successive stool examinations. *American Journal of Tropical Medicine*, 22, 131–136.

Shimeld, L.A. (1999). *Essentials of diagnostic microbiology*. Albany, NY: Delmar Publishers.

Talaro, K. P., & Talaro, A. (1999). *Foundations in microbiology* (3rd ed.). Boston: WBC McGraw-Hill.

Zeibig, E. A. (1997). *Clinical parasitology*. Philadelphia: W. B. Saunders.

CHAPTER THREE
Immunoassays for Human Parasites

LEARNING OBJECTIVES

After reading and studying this chapter, the student should be able to:

- List and explain the various methodologies used for the detection of parasites.
- List the advantages and disadvantages of currently available assays for antibodies and antigens of human parasites.
- Know the sensitivities, specificities and predictive values for available immunoassays for parasites.
- Describe currently available tests for antibody detection of parasites.
- Describe methods for antigen detection of parasites.
- Determine the relative usefulness of immunoassays compared to traditional microscopic analyses for ova and parasites.
- Describe the use of nucleic acid probes (including the polymerase chain reaction, or PCR) in the diagnosis of parasitic infections.
- Know the applicability of various immunoassays and nucleic acid probes for parasites to the clinical microbiology laboratory.

KEY TERMS

Agglutination
(a-GLU-tin-AY-shun)
Bentonite flocculation (BF)
(BEN-toe-nite flok-u-LAY-shun)

Complement fixation (CF)
(KOM-ple-ment fiks-AY-shun)
Counterimmunoelectrophoresis (CIE) (Koun-ter-im-u-no-ee-LEK-tro-for-EE-sis)

Direct fluorescent antibody
(DFA) (di-REKT floor-ES-ent AN-ti-bod-ee)
Enzyme immunoassay (EIA)
(EN-zime IM-u-no-ASS-ay)

(continues)

KEY TERMS (continued)

Enzyme-linked
   immunosorbent assay
   (ELISA) (EN-zime-linkt IM-u-
   no-SOR-bent ASS-ay)
Fluorescent antibody (FA)
   (floor-ES-ent AN-ti-bod-ee)
Immunoassay
   (IM-un-o-ASS-ay)
Immunoblot (IB)
   (IM-u-no-blot)

Immunodiffusion (ID)
   (IM-u-no-di-FU-shun)
Immunoelectrophoresis (IE)
   (IM-u-no-e-LEK-tro-for-EE-
   sis)
Indirect fluorescent antibody
   (IFA) (IN-di-rekt floor-ES-ent
   AN-ti-bod-ee)
Indirect hemagglutination
   (IHA) (IN-di-rekt HEEM-a-
   GLU-tin-AY-shun)

Latex agglutination (LA)
   (LAY-teks a-GLU-tin-AY-shun)
Nucleic acid probe
   (nu-KLEE-ik A-sid PROBE)
Polymerase Chain Reaction
   (PCR) (po-LIM-er-ase CHAYN
   ree-AK-shun)

INTRODUCTION

Traditional methods for the detection of human parasitic infections are usually based on the microscopic detection of diagnostic morphological forms, such as gametocytes, merozoites, cysts, trophozoites, ova, larvae or adult parasites in body specimens, such as feces, urine, blood, or tissue. These methods are laborious and subjective, and costly in terms of labor. Their value is directly proportional to the availability of highly trained and skilled personnel.

Non-microscopic methods for the diagnosis of parasitic diseases include antibody and antigen detection (collectively called immunodiagnostic assays or **immunoassays**) and the use of **nucleic acid probes**, which are small pieces of DNA or RNA complementary to the nucleic acid of the parasite. For convenience, both immunoassays and nucleic acid probes will be discussed in this chapter.

The **polymerase chain reaction (PCR)** involves the use of amplification procedures to greatly increase the quantity of target-specific DNA to enhance the sensitivity of nucleic acid probes in the detection of parasites.

Immunoassays for antibodies and antigens include a variety of methods. The detection of serum antibodies is called serology. The **complement fixation (CF)** technique has been available for many years for antibody detection. It relies on the binding of serum complement which occurs during an antigen-antibody reaction. This "fixation " of complement prevents the complement from reacting with cells sensitized with other antigen-antibody complexes. To indicate the presence of "unfixed" complement, red blood cells are sensitized with specific antibodies. Cell lysis indicates the presence of "unfixed" complement; the absence of hemolysis indicates that the complement has been bound in the test antigen-antibody complex, and is unavailable to react with sensitized blood cells. The test is labor-intensive, and has been largely replaced by newer methods.

The **fluorescent antibody (FA)** method involves the use of a fluorescent dye (fluorescein isocyanate) linked (conjugated) to serum antibody (or antigen) which fluoresces under ultraviolet light. The observation of this fluorescent tag suggests the presence of an antigen-antibody complex. The **direct fluorescent antibody (DFA)** test is generally used to detect antigen, using a fluorescein-labeled monoclonal antibody produced *in vitro* against the parasite. When the labeled antibodies are applied to a slide containing the parasite, the organism fluoresces when viewed by fluorescent microscopy. The **indirect fluorescent antibody (IFA)** test, using a fluorescein-labeled parasite antigen, is mostly used to detect antibody in human serum. Unlabeled parasite antigens may also be used. After applying known antigens to a slide, patient serum is added . After binding between antigen and antibody has occurred, the slides are washed to remove excess serum, then are covered with a fluorescent dye conjugated to anti-human globulin. Binding of the fluorescent dye indicates the presence of the appropriate antibody in the patient's serum.

Agglutination reactions involve the binding of antibodies to particulate antigens. When latex particles are used to suspend the antigen, this method is known as **latex agglutination (LA)**. When these antigens react with specific antibodies, visible agglutination, or clumping of the particles occurs. A variation of this method, known as **indirect hemagglutination (IHA)**, involves the use of protein antigens bound to red blood cells. When particles of bentonite are coated with antigen, the assay is referred to as the **bentonite flocculation (BF)** test.

Immunodiffusion (ID) (or gel diffusion) techniques are used to visualize precipitation reactions between antigens and antibodies in a gel. The double-diffusion assay, known as the Ouchterlony method, uses two wells cut in an agar gel medium, one filled with antibody, and one with antigen. Following diffusion of reactants, lines of precipitation occur when the ratio of antigen and antibody is in optimal proportions. **Counterimmunoelectrophoresis (CIE)**, similar to immunodiffusion, refers to the movement of antigen and antibody toward each other through a gel medium, when an electric current is passed through a buffer solution. This method is more sensitive than passive immunodiffusion.

Immunoelectrophoresis (IE) involves the electrophoretic separation of antigens in a gel, followed by diffusion of antibodies from serum placed in a trough extending parallel to the electrophoretic path. Lines of precipitation form, depending on the antibodies present in the serum. The **immunoblot (IB)** assay (also called the Western Blot assay) involves a technique whereby antigens are separated by electrophoresis and blotted onto a nitrocellulose membrane. After binding to the membrane, antigens are subsequently identified by staining with labeled antibodies.

The **enzyme-linked immunosorbent assay (ELISA)** or **enzyme immunoassay (EIA)** involves the use of enzyme-labeled antigens and antibodies, and is analogous to the fluorescent antibody method with an enzyme used as a label in place of the fluorescein dye. Two enzymes often used are horseradish peroxidase, and alkaline phosphatase. After binding of antigen and antibody takes place, a colorimetric substrate is added. A color change resulting from the enzyme-substrate interaction indicates a positive reaction. The intensity of the color is proportional to the concentration of the antigen-antibody complex. There are many modifications of this technique used to enhance sensitivity.

INTESTINAL PROTOZOA

Immunoassays are available for several members of the intestinal protozoa. Various methods exist for the diagnosis of amebiasis, giardiasis, and cryptosporidiosis.

Entamoeba histolytica

Intestinal amebiasis is usually diagnosed by the detection of characteristic trophozoites and cysts in fecal specimens. Serological methods may be particularly helpful in the diagnosis of extra-intestinal infection with *Entamoeba histolytica*, when the usual diagnostic cysts and trophozoites are often not present in the stool. Amebiasis may be diagnosed using ID, CIE, IHA, CF, IFA, LA, and EIA techniques for serum antibody. CF tests tend to give nonspecific, and variable results. EIA and IHA methods are quite sensitive, however antibody titers persist for years, making interpretation difficult. Titers of IFA and ID tests often decline following successful therapy, providing a useful tool to monitor the patient's therapeutic response. Antibody titers may not correlate with the clinical status of the patient, or the intensity of infection. Tests for antibodies to amebae have approximately 90% sensitivity for amebic liver abscesses, and 70% for amebic colitis. Overall, serum antibody is present in 85–95 % of cases of invasive disease. Serologic assays have proven useful as an epidemiologic tool to determine the prevalence of disease in a certain population.

Commercial kits using EIA and IFA methods are available to detect antigen in stool specimens. Two morphologically identical species of *Entamoeba*, *E. histolytica* and *E. dispar*, may infect humans. *E. histolytica* is the pathogenic form, able to invade tissue, causing systemic disease. *E. dispar* is considered to be nonpathogenic. Certain antigen detection methods are specific for the pathogenic *E. histolytica*. Others do not distinguish between the two species. These forms may also be distinguished using nucleic acid probes. PCR methods, although not commercially available, have been developed to detect specific gene sequences found in pathogenic *E. histolytica*.

Giardia lamblia

Giardiasis is usually diagnosed by the detection of characteristic trophozoites and cysts in fecal specimens. However, the intermittent passage, or low numbers, of *Giardia lamblia* cysts and trophozoites in stool often makes a diagnosis of giardiasis difficult. Serological assays for antibody to *G. lamblia* lack sensitivity. This may be because of variations in the immune response to *Giardia* among individuals in different populations. The humoral antibody response may also vary with the isolate.

Antigen detection methods have been more successful in the diagnosis of giardiasis. The presence of small amounts of *Giardia* antigen in feces is a better indication of active giardial infection than the detection of antibodies in serum, and represents a more significant clinical finding. DFA, IFA and EIA techniques have been developed for the detection of *G. lamblia* antigen in stool specimens. FA techniques have the advantages of allowing microscopic examination under low power magnification, and detection of low numbers of parasites. Certain EIA assays have shown sensitivities and specificities comparable to or better than those of microscopic examination for cysts or trophozoites. Sensitivity and specificity of 98% and 100%, respectively, have been reported. Kits are commercialy available. PCR methods have also been used on stool specimens, with limited success.

Cryptosporidium parvum

The modified acid-fast smear is the most common method of detecting the oocysts of *Cryptosporidium parvum* in stool specimens. Serological assays for antibody lack sensitivity. DFA, IFA, and EIA methods for antigen detection are commercially available, and are considered to be more sensitive and specific than available microscopic methods. These methods have reported sensitivities of 94% or greater, and can provide rapid screening of large numbers of stool specimens. They would be extremely helpful in an outbreak of cryptosporidiosis. Several commercial kits combine antibodies to both *Giardia lamblia* and *Cryptosporidium parvum*, to allow detection of both parasites, using a single assay. Sensitive PCR methods have been developed, but are not available for routine use.

BLOOD/BODY FLUID/TISSUE PROTOZOA

Immunodiagnostic assays exist for certain blood/body fluid/tissue protozoa. Methods are available for the diagnosis of leismaniasis, Chagas' disease, African trypanosomiasis, malaria, babesiosis, toxoplasmosis, and pneumocystosis.

Leishmania

The diagnosis of leishmaniasis is traditionally based on the demonstration of amastigotes in clinical specimens, such as tissues or aspirates. Serological methods available for the diagnosis of leishmaniasis include CF, CIE, IFA, and EIA. The IFA and CF tests are used by the Centers for Disease Control; cross-reactions may occur with trypanosome antibodies. Antibody detection may be useful to diagnose visceral leishmaniasis, but is much less reliable for cutaneous leishmaniasis. Most serological methods lack sensitivity and specificity, but are sometimes used for epidemiological studies. Monoclonal antibodies and DNA probes may enhance the diagnosis of leishmaniasis. PCR has also been shown to be effective, particularly in immunocompromised patients.

Trypanosomes

Examination of blood smears for *Trypanosoma cruzi* is the most commonly used method for the diagnosis of Chagas' disease. This test is most useful during the early acute phase of disease, or during relapse. Serological assays are preferable to diagnose chronic infection. Available methods include CF, IHA, IFA, EIA, and agglutination. EIA and IFA methods are most sensitive; however the CF test is more specific. PCR methods are more sensitive and specific than traditional tests, and are useful to diagnose acute and chronic infections of Chagas' disease, as well as to monitor therapy.

African trypanosomiasis (sleeping sickness) may be diagnosed by detecting the trypomastigotes of *Trypanosoma brucei gambiense*, or *T. brucei rhodesiense* in peripheral blood, lymph node aspirates, bone marrow, or cerebrospinal fluid specimens, stained by the Giemsa method. Serological assays available include LA and IFA. A commercially available agglutination assay is called the Card Agglutination Trypanosomiasis Test (CATT). PCR has also been used.

Malaria and Babesiosis

The diagnosis of malaria and babesiosis is usually made by the observation of typical developmental stages in thick and thin blood smears, stained by the Giemsa method. Limitations of microscopic methods include the difficulty for detection of malarial parasites, or infected red blood cells sequestered in the deep tissues. Skill is required for preparation and interpretation of slides. Babesiosis may be difficult to diagnose because of the low numbers of infected red blood cells, or the confusion of the parasite with those causing malaria.

Rapid diagnostic methods are designed to be as sensitive and specific as microscopy. IFA methods have been used to detect antibody to both *Babesia* and, with limited success, *Plasmodium* species. Cross-reactions between the two parasites may occur. PCR methods have been used in the diagnosis of both babesiosis and malaria.

Toxoplasma and Pneumocystis

Toxoplasmosis may be congenitally acquired, and may have devastating consequences for the fetus. The diagnosis of toxoplasmosis may be made by demonstration of tachyzoites in blood, body fluids, or tissue sections, or by detection of cysts in tissue. Serological methods for antibody detection are more suitable for most laboratories, and have been widely used to diagnose active infections. Although in most cases of *Tox-*

oplasma infection the detection of IgG and IgM antibodies is diagnostic, recent studies have shown that detection of IgA antibodies is helpful in the diagnosis of acute and congenital infections. In these cases, IgM and IgA antibodies are the earliest sign of infection. Since these antibodies are unable to cross the placenta, the presence of either antibody in the neonate is diagnostic for *Toxoplasma* infection. The titers of these antibodies increase during the first few weeks of infection, and often remain high for at least one year. Immunocompromised patients, especially those having AIDS, or patients with ocular infections, may show no evidence of an antibody response. Serological methods available for the diagnosis of toxoplasmosis include IFA, EIA, CF, IHA, and agglutination. IFA and EIA are most commonly used. Molecular amplification techniques, especially PCR, have proven to be very sensitive for the diagnosis of toxoplasmosis, especially in the immunocompromised patient, but may be available only in research settings.

Pneumocystosis refers to pneumonia caused by *Pneumocystis carinii* (*Pneumocystis carinii* pneumonia or PCP). Traditional methods for the diagnosis of this infection include mainly invasive procedures, such as open-lung biopsy, bronchial biopsy, and bronchoalveolar lavage (BAL). Observation of characteristic cysts is diagnostic for infection. Serologic procedures for specific antibody, including CF, IFA, LA, and EIA have been evaluated, but most assays appear to lack acceptable sensitivity and specificity. Also, many normal individuals possess antibody to this common parasite. It may be necessary to collect acute and convalescent serum specimens to demonstrate a fourfold or greater rise in antibody titer in order to confirm a diagnosis.

Antigen detection, using FA techniques, is currently an acceptable method for the diagnosis of this infection. The availability of monoclonal antibodies has enhanced the sensitivity and specificity of these assays. Kits utilizing monoclonal antibodies are commercially available. PCR methods offer the possibility of rapidly and accurately making a diagnosis of pneumocystis infections.

HELMINTHS

Immunodiagnostic assays are available for the detection of the nematodes, *Strongyloides stercoralis*, *Toxocara* species, *Trichinella spiralis*, and filarial worms and the trematodes, *Fasciola hepatica*, *Paragonimunmus westermani*, and the schistosomes. Methods have also been developed to diagnose the cestode infections, cysticercosis and hydatid disease.

Strongyloides stercoralis

The diagnosis of strongyloidiasis is usually made by the detection of rhabditiform larvae in human feces, during the routine examination of stool specimens for ova and parasites. The presence of this parasite in immunocompromised patients may lead to the hyperinfection syndrome, which is often fatal. Serological methods for diagnosis include EIA, IFA, and IHA. EIA appears to have greater sensitivity than IFA or IHA. Antibody detection assays should use antigens derived from the infective filariform larvae of *S. stercoralis*, for the greatest sensitivity and specificity. Cross-reactions with other nematodes may occur.

Toxocara species

The dog and cat ascarids in the genus *Toxocara* cause visceral larva migrans and ocular larva migrans in humans, mostly in children. The diagnosis of infection may be made by the histologic demonstration of larvae in tissue, since typical diagnostic stages are not found in human feces. Serologic methods are preferred, and may be the only confirmatory assays available. The EIA performed with larval antigens appears to be the most sensitive serodiagnostic assay available.

Trichinella spiralis

The diagnosis of trichinosis is usually made by demonstration of larvae in muscle tissue. Recommended serological methods include the EIA used as a screening test, and the BF test used for confirmation, since the EIA is more sensitive and remains positive longer, and the BF is more specific. CIE is also available for the diagnosis of trichinosis. The development of antibody to *T. spiralis* is directly proportional to the infective dose of larvae. Serial specimens should be collected, to demonstrate seroconversion. Detectable antibody usually first appears about one month after infection, and peaks in the second or third month following infection.

Filarial Nematodes

The diagnosis of infection with filarial nematodes is usually made by the observation of microfilariae in blood, urine, or skin. Concentration procedures may be necessary to visualize the parasites. The microfilariae of various filarial nematodes may be distinguished by the presence or absence of a sheath, and the morphology of nuclei in the tails of the parasites. Histological examination of tissue biopsies may also be used to make a diagnosis of filariasis. Although several serologic assays are available for the diagnosis of this disease, including EIA, IHA and IFA, they lack sensitivity and specificity. However, immunoassays may be helpful when low numbers of parasites are present. The presence of circulating antigens has been used diagnostically, and to monitor therapy, with limited success. PCR shows promise in this role.

Fasciola hepatica

In cases of fascioliasis, stool examination usually reveals the characteristic eggs of the liver fluke, *F. hepatica*. Serological assays used in the diagnosis of fascioliasis include EIA and IB. Although cross-reactions may occur with schistosome antibodies, immunoassays are useful to diagnose acute and chronic disease, in the absence of a positive examination of feces for ova and parasites. Serologic tests are also helpful for early diagnosis of fascioliasis (antibodies may be detectable within three weeks, as opposed to the appearance of eggs in the stool at about six weeks), and as a test of cure following therapy.

Paragonimus westermani

The diagnosis of infection with the lung fluke, *P. westermani*, is usually made by finding characteristic eggs in human feces, as well as sputum. Immunoassays for antibodies in serum or pleural effusions may also be used to detect pulmonary and extra-pulmonary infections, and may be useful in monitoring therapy. These tests may only be available in endemic areas, and specialized reference laboratories. EIA, IB, and CF assays have been used to detect paragonimiasis. The use of monoclonal antibodies has improved the sensitivity and specificity of immunoassays for parasite antigens in the detection of active infection.

Schistosomes

The diagnosis of schistosomiasis is usually made by the detection of characteristic eggs in stool specimens (*S. mansoni* and *S. japonicum*), or urine specimens (*S. haematobium*). Detection of antibodies to schistosomes may be helpful when eggs are not detected in feces or urine. Although many serologic assays, (including EIA, IHA and IFA) have been developed for the diagnosis of schistosomiasis, cross-reactions have been noted with other helminthic infections. EIA assays have been used as screening tests to detect serum antibodies in endemic areas. EIA methods have also been used to detect antigen in serum and urine of infected patients.

Cysticercosis

Cysticercosis refers to the presence of the larval stage of the pork tapeworm, *Taenia solium*, in human tissue. Serological tests used for the diagnosis of this disease include IB, CF, IFA, IHA, ID, IE, and EIA. The Centers for Disease Control IB assay using purified *T. solium* antigens appears to be the test of choice for the diagnosis of cysticercosis, having a specificity of 100%, and a high sensitivity. The numbers and stages of development of cysticerci are the most important factors in determining IB results. EIA methods are less sensitive than IB, and less specific, cross-reacting with other helminthic antigens. PCR assays have been developed to distinguish between *T. saginata* and *T. solium*. These tests are useful to identify carriers of *T. solium*, and to interrupt the transmission of human cysticercosis. An IB kit is also commercially available.

Hydatid Disease

Serological assays available for the diagnosis of echinococcosis (hydatid disease) caused by *Echinococcus granulosis* or *E. multilocularis* include IB, ID, IFA, IHA, CF, LA, IE, and EIA. Test results are variable, since antibody response depends on the cyst viability and location in the body. Some individuals harboring cysts lack antibodies. A very sensitive and specific EIA has been developed for the diagnosis of hydatid disease. IB may be used to monitor therapy, but the IHA and EIA may remain positive for many years following infection. A combination of assays has been suggested to diagnose echinococcosis. EIA or IHA may be used as a screening test, followed by IB or ID tests to confirm positive results. False positive reactions may occur with other helminthic infections and immune disorders. Antibody assays have had variable success in monitoring therapy outcome.

Antigen assays might be useful as additional tests in antibody-negative individuals, but are not currently available in the United States. PCR assays have been developed to detect mRNA from fine-needle biopsy specimens in cases of infection with *E. multilocularis*.

SUMMARY

Human parasitic infections are traditionally diagnosed by the microscopic or macroscopic observation of characteristic stages of development of the parsite. Trophozoites and cysts of intestinal protozoans, or eggs and larvae of intestinal helminths, may be present during active infections. Blood smears for malaria and trypanosomiasis are commonly used methods of diagnosis.

A variety of immunoassays exist to detect antibodies and antigens of human parasites. These assays are often more sensitive and specific than routine microscopic methods. Intestinal protozoan infections, such as amebiasis, giardiasis, and cryptosporidiosis may be diagnosed by antibody or antigen detection. Immunoassays are often tests of choice for several blood/body fluid/tissue parasites, especially for toxoplasmosis. Helminthic infections, such as cysticercosis are usually confirmed using immunodiagnostic methods. The use of monoclonal antibodies, DNA probes and PCR technology has vastly improved methods to detect parasitic infections.

Available immunoassays and molecular diagnostic methods used in the diagnosis of parasitic infections are summarized in Table 3–1.

Table 3–1 ▶ Immunoassays and Nucleic Acid Probes Used in the Diagnosis of Parasitic Diseases

Parasite	Antibody Detection	Antigen Detection	Nucleic Acid Probes
Entamoeba histolytica	EIA, IFA, ID, CIE, IHA, LA	EIA, IFA	PCR
Giardia lamblia		DFA, IFA, EIA	PCR
Cryptosporidium parvum		DFA, IFA, EIA	
Leishmania species	CF, CIE, IFA, EIA		PCR
Trypanosoma species	CF, IHA, IFA, EIA, A		
Toxoplasma gondii	IFA, EIA, CF, IHA, A		PCR
Pneumosystisis carinii	CF, IFA, LA, EIA	FA	PCR
Strongyloides stercoralis	EIA, IFA, IHA		
Toxocara species	EIA		
Trichinella spiralis	EIA, BF, CIE		
Filarial nematodes	EIA, IHA, IFA		PCR
Fasciola hepatica	EIA, IB		
Paragonimus westermani	EIA, IB, CF		
Schistosomes	EIA, IHA, IFA		
T. solium (cysticercosis)	IB, CF, IFA, IHA, ID, IE, EIA		
Echinococcus species	IB, ID, IFA, IHA, CF, LA, IE, EIA		PCR
Plasmodium species	IFA		PCR
Babesia species	IFA		PCR

A-agglutination; BF-bentonite flocculation; CF-complement fixation; CIE-counterimmunoelectrophoresis; DFA-direct fluorescent antibody; EIA-enzyme immunoassay; IB-immunoblot; ID-immunodiffusion,; IE-immunoelectrophoresis; IFA-indirect fluorescent antibody; IHA-indirect hemagglutination; LA-latex agglutination; PCR-polymerase chain reaction

REVIEW QUESTIONS

1. A technique used to amplify the amount of DNA to increase the sensitivity of nucleic acid probes is :

   a. latex agglutination (LA)

   b. complement fixation (CF)

   c. polymerase chain reaction (PCR)

   d. immunodiffusion (ID)

2. Serological methods are particularly useful to detect extra-intestinal infections with:

   a. *Entamoeba dispar*

   b. *Entamoeba histolytica*

   c. *Entamoeba coli*

   d. *Giardia lamblia*

3. An antigen detection method has partially replaced a modified acid-fast technique for the detection of:

   a. *Cryptosporidium parvum*

   b. *Entamoeba histolytica*

   c. *Entamoeba coli*

   d. *Giardia lamblia*

4. Because of confusion from morphological features, immunological methods have been useful to distinguish between parasites causing the following diseases:

   a. malaria and babesiosis

   b. toxoplasmosis and pneumocystosis

   c. cysticercosis and hydatid disease

   d. fascioliasis and strongyloidiasis

5. Immunoassays may be used to diagnose _____ in place of histological demonstration of larvae in tissues.

   a. malaria and babesiosis

   b. toxoplasmosis and pneumocystosis

   c. cysticercosis and hydatid disease

   d. trichinosis and toxocaral infection

6. Which cestode infections may be confirmed using serological methods?

   a. malaria and babesiosis

   b. toxoplasmosis and pneumocystosis

   c. cysticercosis and hydatid disease

   d. fascioliasis and strongyloidiasis

7. The detection of antibodies to _____ is important, to prevent the hyperinfection syndrome often associated with this parasite.

   a. *E. histolytica*

   b. *G. lamblia*

   c. *T. solium*

   d. *S. stercoralis*

8. The Centers for Disease Control recommend the immunoblot assay, using purified parasite antigens, to detect which of the following parasites?

   a. *E. histolytica*

   b. *C. parvum*

   c. *S. stercoralis*

   d. *T. solium*

9. For which parasitic disease are immunoassays not currently available?

   a. malaria

   b. microsporidiosis

   c. cysticercosis

   d. visceral larva migrans

10. Combination diagnostic kits are commercially available to detect which two parasitic diseases?

    a. giardiasis and amebiasis

    b. cryptosporiosis and malaria

    c. cryptosporidiosis and giardiasis

    d. fascioliasis and schistosomiasis

CASE STUDY

The patient was a 24-year old female graduate student who had attended a university in Mexico for the past few years. She had been in good health until the day of her visit to the emergency department of a California hospital, after suffering from a severe headache and having a seizure at home. Although the neurological examination was unremarkable, a computed tomagram (CT) scan of the brain showed multiple intracranial lesions. A serological test for HIV was negative. Serum and CSF specimens were taken for serological tests, which confirmed the diagnosis.

Questions

1. What diagnoses must be considered in this case?

2. What parasite causes this disease?

3. How do people acquire this infection?

4. What risk factor exists in the patient's history?

5. How would you confirm the clinical diagnosis of this parasitic infection?

► BIBLIOGRAPHY

Faubert, G. (2000). Immune response to Giardia duodenalis. *Clinical Microbiology Review*, 13, 35–54.

Garcia, L. S. & Bruckner, D. A. (1997). *Diagnostic medical parasitology* (3rd ed.). Washington, DC: ASM Press.

Gonzalez, L. M., Montero, E., Harrison, L. J. S., Parkhouse, R. M. E., & Garate, T. (2000). Differential diagnosis of *Taenia saginata* and *Taenia solium* infection by PCR. *Journal of Clinical Microbiology*, 38, 737–744.

Gradus, M. S. (2000). Cryptosporidium and public health: From watershed to water glass. *Clinical Microbiology Newsletter*, 22 (4)4, 25–32.

Koneman, E. W., Allen, S. D., Janda, W. M., Schreckenberger, P. C., & Winn, Jr, W. C. (1997). *Color atlas and textbook of diagnostic microbiology* (5th ed.). Philadelphia: Lippincott.

Markell, E. K., Voge, M. A., & John, D. T. (1992). *Medical parasitology* (7th ed.). Philadelphia: W. B. Saunders.

Petrie, W. A., & Singh U. (1999). Diagnosis and management of amebiasis. *Clinical Infectious Disease*, 29, 1117–1125.

Tizard, I. R. (1984). *Immunology: An introduction*. Philadelphia: W. B. Saunders.

Walls, K. W., & Smith, J. W. (1979). Serology of parasitic infections. *Laboratory Medicine*, 10, 329–336.

Wilson, M., Schantz, P., & Pieniazek, N. (1995). Diagnosis of parasitic infections: Immunologic and molecular methods. In Murray, P. R., Baron, S. J., Pfaller, M. A., Tenover, F. C., & Yolken, R. H.(Eds.) *Manual of clinical microbiology* (6th ed.). (pp. 1159–1170). Washington, DC: ASM Press.

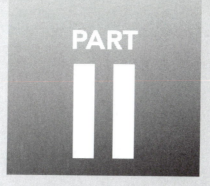

PART

II

Protozoa

CHAPTER FOUR

Intestinal Amebae

LEARNING OBJECTIVES

After reading and studying this chapter, the student should be able to:

- List the clinically significant intestinal amebae found in humans.
- List and describe characteristics used to identify intestinal amebae.
- Describe the typical life cycle of intestinal amebae and note the species that may also exhibit extra-intestinal development.
- Compare the morphological characteristics of intestinal amebic trophozoites, including size, descriptions of cytoplasm, karyosomes, inclusions, and numbers and characteristics of nuclei.

- Compare the morphological characteristics of intestinal amebic cysts, including size, descriptions of cytoplasm, karyosomes, inclusions, and numbers and characteristics of nuclei.
- Describe the pathogenesis of intestinal amebiasis in humans.
- Describe the treatment of infection with pathogenic amebae.
- Describe the prevention of infection with pathogenic amebae.

KEY TERMS

Binary fission
   (BI-na-ree FI-shun)
Central body
   (SEN-trul BOD-ee)
Chromatin (KRO-ma-tin)

Chromatoidal bar
   (KRO-ma-TOY-dal bar)
Commensals (ko-MEN-sals)
Cyst (SIST)
Dysentery (DIS-in-te-ree)
Excystation (EGG-sis-TA-shun)

Glycogen mass
   (GLI-ko-jen mass)
Karyosome (KAR-ee-o-som)
Pathogen (PATH-o-jen)
Pseudopod (SOO-do-pod)
Trophozoite (TRO-fo-ZO-ite)

INTRODUCTION

Human infection with amebae is known as amebiasis. The amebae are classified in the subphylum Sarcodina, in the phylum Sarcomastigophora. These parasites are characterized by the presence of **pseudopods** (extentions of the cytoplasm, which act as organelles of locomotion). All amebae, except one, exist in two forms. These forms are the **trophozoite** (the motile, actively feeding, multiplying form, susceptible to destruction outside the host), and the **cyst** (the dormant, non-feeding resistant stage, which is significant in the transmission of amebae from host to host). Amebae multiply by **binary fission** (splitting of the parent cell, after duplication of cytoplasm and genetic material, into two equal cells).

The diagnosis of amebiasis is made in the laboratory by the examination of stool specimens for the presence of trophozoites and cysts. Trophozoites are more likely to be found in liquid stool specimens, while cysts are generally more numerous in formed stools. Important characteristics used to identify amebae include the number and structure of nuclei, especially the presence and location of **chromatin** (genetic material found in the nucleus), particularly along the inner nuclear membrane, (peripheral nuclear chromatin). Most amebic trophozoites have a single nucleus, while the cysts are usually multinucleate. The number of nuclei is characteristic for each species of amebae. All intestinal amebae have **karyosomes** (clumps of chromatin material found within the nuclei) . The size, configuration and location of the karyosomes are distinctive for each ameba and are helpful in identification.

The trophozoite cytoplasm may be finely or coarsely granular. It may be vacuolated, and may have a variety of inclusions., such as red blood cells, bacteria, or yeasts. The cyst cytoplasm is usually finely granular. Inclusions may be found in the cytoplasm. **Glycogen masses** (masses of food stored as glycogen) may be present in the cysts of certain species of amebae. **Chromatoidal bars** (rod-shaped masses of RNA) are also characteristically found. These bodies may be rodlike, with rounded, or splinter-like ends.

The characteristic features of the trophozoites and cysts of intestinal amebae are demonstrated in Figure 4–1.

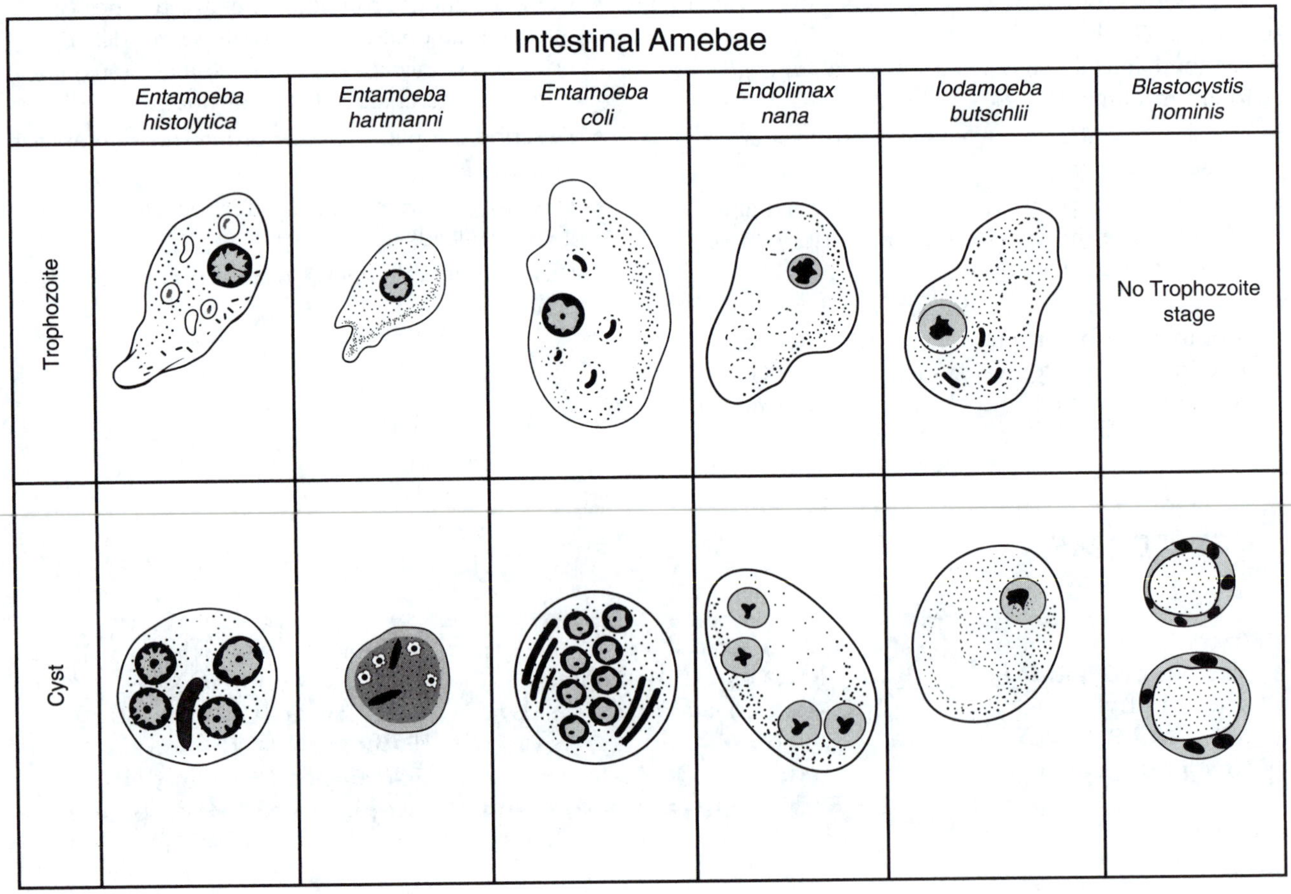

FIG 4–1 Characteristic Features of Trophoziotes and Cysts of Intestinal Amebae

INTESTINAL AMEBAE

The intestinal amebae may be recognized and identified by observation of the appearance of trophozoites and cysts in stained and unstained preparations. The only truly significant **pathogen** (disease-causing microbe) among the amebae is *Entamoeba histolytica*. This pathogen causes amebic **dysentery** (a gastrointestinal illness characterized by diarrhea, with blood and mucus in the stools). With the exception of *Blastocystis hominis*, the remaining amebae discussed in this chapter are considered to be **commensals**, which are not known to cause human illness. Their importance lies in the need to distinguish them from *E. histolytica*, as well as to provide evidence of exposure to fecally-contaminated food or water.

Entamoeba histolytica/ Entamoeba dispar

Morphology

Trophozoite: *Entamoeba histolytica* is the most pathogenic of the intestinal amebae found in humans, although morphologically indistinguishable nonpathogenic strains of *E.dispar* exist. The trophozoites of *E. histolytica* measure 10–60 micrometers (μm) (Figure 4–2). Trophozoite cytoplasm is finely granular, and may contain inclusions. Ingested bacteria and yeast are usually absent, although nonpathogenic strains, which tend to be somewhat smaller, may contain bacteria. The presence of red blood cells is diagnostic for *E. histolytica*. The single nucleus has peripheral nuclear chromatin, which is usually evenly distributed in a beadlike arrangement, with a small, central, compact karyosome. Movement is progressive and purposeful, and is characterized by protrusion of a clear pseudopod.

Cyst: The spherical cyst of *E. histolytica* measures 10–20 μm (Figure 4–3). The mature cyst contains 4 nuclei, while the immature cyst may contain fewer than 4. It is imperative to carefully focus up and down using the microscope, to accurately count the nuclei at different planes. The presence of evenly distributed peripheral nuclear chromatin is important in the identification of *E. histolytica*. All species of the genus *Entamoeba*, but no other genus of amebae, possess peripheral nuclear chromatin in different arrangements.

The karyosome is tiny and usually centrally located with evenly distributed peripheral nuclear chromatin. The elongated chromatoidal bars have blunt, smooth, rounded ends. Glycogen vacuoles may be present in immature cysts, but usually disappear as cysts mature.

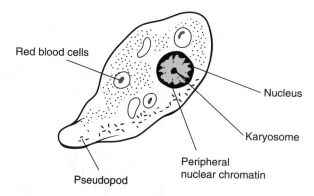

FIG 4–2 *E. histolytica* trophozoite

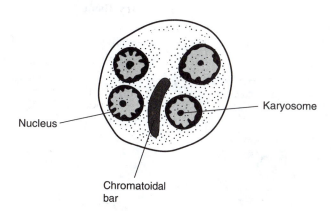

FIG 4–3 *E. histolytica* cyst

Life Cycle

The life cycle of all amebae is similar, and is shown in Figure 4–4. The invasive stage, however, involving extra-intestinal infection, is seen only with *E. histolytica*. Following ingestion, the mature cyst passes through the stomach and into the small intestine. **Excystation** occurs in the lower ileum, when the cyst develops into the trophozoite form. Binary fission follows, and trophozoites continue to multiply in the lumen of the colon. Trophozoites often become encysted. These immature cysts are passed in the feces, or develop to maturity before being excreted. Both stages of cysts plus trophozoites may be found in the feces, although trophozoites are usually only found in liquid feces. Occasionally trophozoites invade the wall of the colon, multiply, and pass into the circulation.

Transmission and Pathogenesis

E. histolytica has a wide geographic distribution and is considered one of the most important human protozoan parasites. It is now recognized that clinical isolates of *E histolytica* may be divided into pathogenic and nonpathogenic strains (zymodemes), called *E. histolytica* and *E. dispar*, respectively. For the purposes

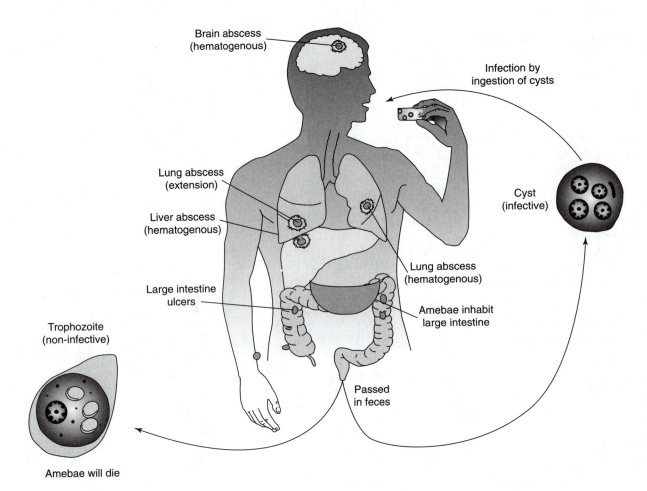

FIG 4–4 Life cycle of *Entamoeba histolytica*.

of this text, we will confine our discussion to *E. histolytica*.

Amebiasis is usually acquired by ingestion of contaminated water or food containing amebic cysts, although transmission as a sexually transmitted disease by male homosexuals has occured. Asymptomatic carriers may also transmit disease. Incubation is variable, from several days to months. Symptomatic patients may have abdominal pain and diarrhea. When dysentery develops, bloody diarrhea may ensue. Ulcers may form in the appendix, cecum, and other parts of the colon. The characteristic flask-shaped ulcer appears to be raised, with a small mucosal opening, and an eroded area beneath the surface. Symptoms may resemble ulcerative colitis or diverticulitis. *E. histolytica* trophozoites may invade the wall of the colon, enter the circulation, and spread hematogenously, causing the development of extra-intestinal abscesses. Multiple amebic abscesses may develop, especially in the liver, but also in the brain or lung.

Laboratory Diagnosis

Differentiation among intestinal amebae is based on morphologic examination of fecal preparations for the presence of parasites. Actively motile amebic trophozoites are commonly seen in direct wet mount preparations made from liquid or soft fecal specimens from infected patients. However the preferred method involves concentration techniques, and particularly, permanent smears stained by the trichrome method. This procedure and others are described in Chapter 2. Other specimens suitable for examination include sigmoidoscopic aspirates and aspirates obtained from liver abscesses. Although trophozoites in fresh specimens seen on wet mount are usually ameboid in shape, fixation frequently causes these structures to round up or become elongated.

Serological procedures, including the indirect hemagglutination assay (IHA), the enzyme-linked immunosorbent assay (ELISA), and the indirect immunofluorescent (IFA) assay are available. These tests are particularly useful in the diagnosis of extra-intestinal infection with *E. histolytica*. Certain methods are also helpful in monitoring the patient's therapeutic response. In addition to antibody detection, commercial kits may be used to detect parasite antigens in stool specimens. Special techniques, such as enzyme electrophoresis or DNA probes may be used to distinguish the pathogenic *E. histolytica* from the non-pathogenic *E. dispar*.

Treatment and Prevention

The presence of *E. histolytica* requires treatment of the patient regardless of symptoms. Amebicidal agents available for the treatment of amebiasis are divided into two classes, luminal amebicides, such as iodoquinol or diloxanide furoate, and tissue amebicides, including metronidazole, chloroquine and dehydroemetine. No resistance to these agents has been reported.

The human acts as the reservoir for infection with *E. histolytica*. The cysts of this parasite are hardy and often transmitted in infected water. They are resistant to environmental effects, including chlorination. A combination of filtration and chemical treatment is required to ensure a parasite-free water supply. Close attention to maintaining sanitary conditions is essential to avoid transmission of this parasite.

Entamoeba hartmanni

Morphology

Trophozoite: *E. hartmanni* looks similar to *E. histolytica*, but is much smaller (Figure 4–5). For this reason, it was previously known as "small-race histolytica." The trophozoite measures 5–12 µm, with a small, discrete karyosome, which may be centrally located, or which may be eccentric. When seen on a wet mount, the parasite demonstrates non-progressive motility. Although bacteria may be present, no red blood cells are ingested.

Cyst: The cyst of *E. hartmanni* measures 5–10 µm. Although the mature cyst, like *E. histolytica*, contains 4 nuclei, only 2 nuclei are frequently seen. Chromatoidal bars will usually look like those found in *E. histolytica*.

Life Cycle

The life cycle of *E. hartmanni* is similar to *E. histolytica*, but lacking the extra-intestinal phase. Following excystation in the lower ileum, binary fission occurs, and trophozoites continue to multiply in the

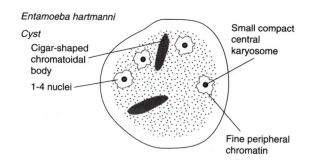

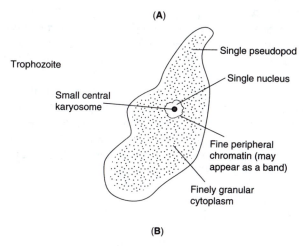

FIG 4–5 *Entamoeba hartmanni*. **A.** cyst and **B.** trophozoite.

lumen of the colon. Immature and mature cysts, as well as trophozoites, may be found in the feces.

Transmission and Pathogenesis

Amebiasis caused by *E. hartmanni* is acquired by ingestion of water or food containing mature cysts. This ameba is considered to be a nonpathogenic commensal. Infections are asymptomatic

Laboratory Diagnosis

The standard examination for ova and parasites is the most commonly used procedure to detect infection with *E. hartmanni*. Care must be taken to accurately measure the trophozoites and cysts, using a calibrated ocular micrometer, to distinguish them from the pathogenic *E. histolytica*.

Treatment and Prevention

E. hartmanni is considered nonpathogenic, therefore, no treatment is warranted. Since ingestion of contaminated water containing cysts is the usual means of transmission, good sanitation practices should be employed to prevent infection.

Entamoeba coli

Morphology

Trophozoite: The trophozoite of *E. coli* measures 15–50 μm (Figure 4–6). The coarsely granulated cytoplasm is usually described as "dirty," containing many vacuoles, as well as bacteria, yeast and debris. In the single nucleus, peripheral nuclear chromatin is unevenly distributed in clumps, with a large, discrete eccentric karyosome. The characteristic motility of *E. coli* is sluggish and non-progressive, with blunt pseudopods.

Cyst: The usually spherical, sometimes oval, cyst (Figure 4–7) measures 10–35 μm, and contains 8 nuclei, and as many as 16 nuclei, when mature. Immature cysts contain 8 nuclei or fewer. Peripheral chromatin is granular and unevenly distributed. Chromatoidal bars, if present, tend to have sharp, pointed, splinterlike ends.

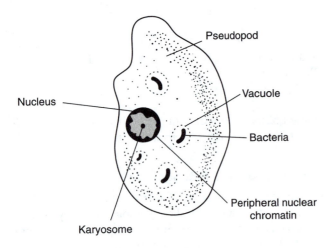

FIG 4–6 *E. coli* trophoziote

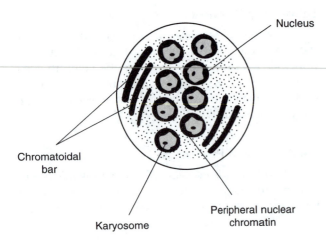

FIG 4–7 *E. coli* cyst

Life Cycle

The life cycle of *E. coli* is similar to other amebae, except for the extra-intestinal stage found in *E. histolytica*.

Transmission and Pathogenesis

Infection with *E .coli* is asymptomatic. Transmission of infection is caused by ingestion of food or water contaminated with amebic cysts. Transmission by flies and cockroaches has been reported.

Laboratory Diagnosis

Diagnosis of *E. coli* infection is made using the standard examination of fecal specimens for ova and parasites. The permanent stained smear is recommended for the detection of this parasite.

Treatment and Prevention

No treatment is recommended for the nonpathogen *E. coli*. Prevention of infection is accomplished by avoidance of contaminated food or water. Protection of food and drink from flies and cockroaches is required to stop transmission.

Endolimax nana

Morphology

Trophozoite: Trophozoites of *Endolimax nana* measure 6–12 micrometers (Figure 4–8); the granular cytoplasm is usually described as "clean"or finely vacuolated, with some nuclear variation. Bacteria may be present. No peripheral chromatin is present in the single nucleus. Normally, only karyosomes are visible, and are large and blotlike. Wet mounts reveal amebae with blunt pseudopods; motility is sluggish and non-progressive.

Cyst: The round to oval cyst (Figure 4–9) contains 4 nuclei, with blotlike karyosomes visible when mature; cysts measure 5–10 μm and have no visible chromatoidal bars.

Life Cycle

The life cycle of *E. nana* is similar to that described for *E. histolytica*, without an extra-intestinal phase.

Transmission and Pathogenesis

Infection with *E. nana* occurs after ingestion of cysts in contaminated food or water, and results in asymptomatic infection.

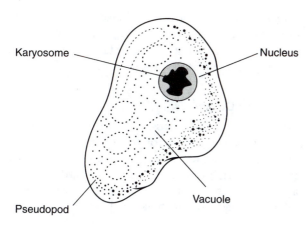

FIG 4–8 *Endolimax nana* trophoziote

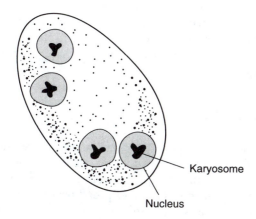

FIG 4–9 *Endolimax nana* cyst

Laboratory Diagnosis

Diagnosis of infection is made by examination of fecal specimens for parasites.

Treatment and Prevention

No treatment is necessary; prevention involves avoidance of comtaminated food and water.

Iodamoeba butschlii

Morphology

Trophozoite: The *Iodamoeba butschlii* trophozoite (Figure 4–10) measures 8–20 μm, with coarsely vacuolated cytoplasm containing debris, including bacteria and yeast. A large karyosome usually fills much of the intranuclear space. Chromatin granules radiating from the karyosome may result in the "basket nucleus" appearance of this parasite. No peripheral chromatin is seen. Motility is sluggish and non-progressive.

Cyst: The cyst measures 5–20 μm, with no visible chromatoidal bars (Figure 4–11). It frequently contains

a large glycogen vacuole, which, when fresh, stains reddish brown with iodine. In permanent stains, the glycogen vacuole appears as a clear unstained space. The cyst contains a single nucleus, which is seldom seen in iodine stained preparations. If seen in permanent stained smears, a large karyosome may be present in an eccentric position.

Life Cycle

The life cycle of *I. butschlii* resembles that of other nonpathogenic amebae, although no nuclear multiplication occurs in the cyst form. Therefore the mature cyst contains only a single nucleus.

Transmission and Pathogenesis

The infection is asymptomatic and is transmitted by the fecal-oral route.

Laboratory Diagnosis

Diagnosis is by the examination of fecal specimens for the parasite.

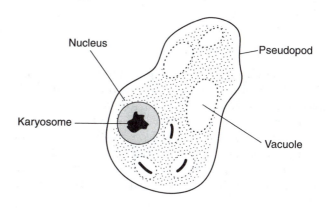

FIG 4–10 *Iodamoeba butschlii* trophozoite

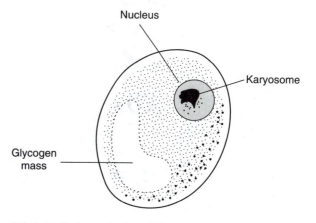

FIG 4–11 *Iodamoeba butschlii* cyst

Treatment and Prevention

No treatment is necessary; infection is prevented by avoiding contaminated food and water.

Blastocystis hominis

Morphology

The **central body** (a clear, transparent area resembling a vacuole) form is usually observed in stool specimens. The spherical to oval vacuolated form measures 6–15 μm, and appears refractile in wet mounts. A clear central area, resembling a large vacuole, is surrounded by 3 to 7 granules around the periphery (Figure 4–12). The iodine stain emphasizes the peripheral granules.

Life Cycle

Although the life cycle of *B. hominis* has not been fully described, stages appear to include the amebic form, the cyst form, and the central body or vacuolated form. The latter stage is the one usually found in human feces, although the amebic form may occasionally be seen in diarrheal stool specimens. The parasite reproduces by binary fission or sporulation; the central body is also involved in sexual and asexual reproduction. *B. hominis* feeds on bacteria and debris in the intestine.

Transmission and Pathogenesis

Although commonly found as a normal resident of the intestinal tract, *Blastocystis hominis* is considered to be a potential pathogen, if present in large numbers. In patients with no other obvious reason for their diarrhea, nausea, abdominal pain or vomiting, moderate numbers of this parasite are believed to be responsible for their symptoms. It has been suggested, however, that these patients may have an additional undetected pathogen that is responsible for their symptoms. The mode of transmission is not known; however, it is assumed that the infection is acquired by ingesting contaminated food or water.

Laboratory Diagnosis

Infection with *B. hominis* is detected by examination of stool specimens for the presence of characteristic vacuolated forms. A permanent stained smear, such as the trichrome stain, is the preferred method for detection of this parasite, although iodine stained smears are also used to make a diagnosis.

Treatment and Prevention

When *B. hominis* is present in moderate to high numbers in symptomatic patients, the treatment of choice is metronidazole. This agent is also effective against other protozoa. An alternate choice is iodoquinol.

SUMMARY

Although six species of amebae may cause intestinal infection in humans, *E. histolytica* is the only true pathogen in this group. As well as causing amebic dysentery, this parasite may spread beyond the intestine, causing abscesses in the liver and other organs. Infection with nonpathogenic amebae may represent ingestion of fecally-contaminated water or food, since amebiasis is spread by the fecal-oral route. Only *E. histolytica* infection requires treatment. Therefore it is imperative to differentiate this parasite from the other commensals in this group. Key characteristics of the trophozoites and cysts of intestinal amebae are summarized in Table 4–1.

Although the pathogenicity of *Blastocystis hominis* has been controversial, it is currently believed that, in the absence of other pathogens, large numbers of this parasite may be responsible for symptoms of gastroenteritis.

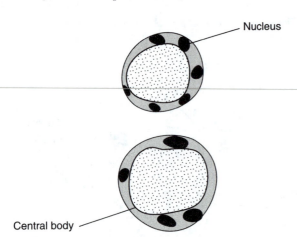

Nucleus

Central body

FIG 4–12 *Blastocystis hominis*

Table 4–1 ▶ Key Characteristics of Intestinal Amebae

AMEBAE	TROPHOZOITE	CYST
Entamoeba histolytica	10–60 µm Finely granular cytoplasm Evenly distributed peripheral nuclear chromatin Small, central, compact karyosome Inclusions: ingestion of RBC is diagnostic Progressive motility	10–20 µm Mature cyst contains 4 nuclei Elongated chromatoidal bars with blunt, smooth ends Small, central, compact karyosome
Entamoeba hartmanni	5–12 µm Finely granular cytoplasm Evenly distributed peripheral nuclear chromatin Central, compact karyosome Inclusions: bacteria, no RBC Non-progressive motility	5–10 µm Mature cyst contains 4 nuclei Elongated chromatoidal bars with blunt, smooth ends Central, compact karyosome
Entamoeba coli	15–50 µm Coarsely granular cytoplasm Unevenly distributed peripheral nuclear chromatin Large, discrete, eccentric karyosome Inclusions: bacteria, yeast, debris Sluggish, non-progressive motility	10–35 µm Mature cyst contains 8 nuclei Splinter shaped chromatoidal bars with sharp, pointed ends Large, eccentric karyosome
Endolimax nana	6–12 µm Granular cytoplasm No peripheral chromatin Karyosomes are large and blotlike Inclusions: bacteria Sluggish, non-progressive motility	5–10 µm Mature cyst contains 4 nuclei No peripheral chromatin Large karyosomes, but smaller than trophozoite No visible chromatoidal bars
Iodamoeba butschlii	8–20 µm Granular, vacuolated cytoplasm No peripheral chromatin Large karyosomes Inclusions: bacteria, yeast Sluggish, non-progressive motility	5–20 µm Mature cyst contains 1 nucleus No peripheral chromatin Large karyosome, with granules on 1 side No visible chromatoidal bars Prominent glycogen vacuole

REVIEW QUESTIONS

1. The most significant pathogen among the amebae is:
   a. *Entamoeba coli*
   b. *Endolimax nana*
   c. *Entamoeba histolytica*
   d. *Entamoeba hartmanni*

2. Ingestion of red blood cells is characteristic of:
   a. *E. histolytica*
   b. *E. hartmanni*
   c. *Blastocystis hominis*
   d. *Iodamoeba butschlii*

3. A _____ is a clump of genetic material found in the nucleus of amebae.
   a. pseudopod
   b. karyosome
   c. chromatoid body
   d. cyst

4. Peripheral nuclear chromatin is *absent* in:
   a. *E. nana*
   b. *E. histolytica*
   c. *E. hartmanni*
   d. *E. coli*

5. A total of 16 nuclei may be found in the ameba:
   a. *E. histolytica*
   b. *E. nana*
   c. *E. coli*
   d. *E. hartmanni*

6. Nonpathogenic strains of _____ are mophologically indistinguisable from *E. histolytica*.
   a. *Entamoeba dispar*
   b. *E. coli*
   c. *E. hartmanni*
   d. *E. nana*

7. Large, blotlike karyosomes are found in:
   a. *E. dispar*
   b. *E. coli*
   c. *E. hartmanni*
   d. *E. nana*

8. A large glycogen vacuole, usually appearing as a clear space in permanent stains, is characteristic of:
   a. *Endolimax nana*
   b. *Iodamoeba butschlii*
   c. *Blastocystis hominis*
   d. *Entamoeba hartmanni*

9. Amebiasis may be transmitted by:
   a. food
   b. water
   c. sexual activity
   d. all of the above

10. Extra-intestinal infection may occur with infections caused by:
    a. *E. coli*
    b. *E. hartmanni*
    c. *E. nana*
    d. *E. histolytica*

CASE STUDY

A previously healthy 28-year old man, who had recently returned from a trip to Mexico, was seen by his family physician for crampy abdominal pain, malaise, slight fever and bloody, mucoid diarrhea. Liquid stool specimens were collected and submitted for culture for enteric bacterial pathogens, as well as parasites.

Stool cultures were negative for bacterial pathogens, examination for ova and parasites was positive for motile trophozoites in the saline wet mount, and ameboid trophozoites with finely granular cytoplasm and ingested red blood cells in the permanent trichrome stain.

Questions

1. What intestinal parasite would you consider in making a diagnosis?

2. How can you differentiate pathogenic from nonpathogenic species of this parasite?

3. Is this parasite capable of causing extra-intestinal infection? What organ is most commonly involved?

4. How is this parasite transmitted?

5. Should this patient be treated? How?

▶ BIBLIOGRAPHY

Garcia, L. S. & Bruckner, D. A. (1997). *Diagnostic medical parasitology* (3rd ed.). (pp. 6–33). Washington, DC: ASM Press.

Shimeld, L. & Rodgers, A. T. (1999). Intestinal and atrial protozoans. In Shimeld, L. (Ed.) *Essentials of diagnostic microbiology*. (pp. 572-589). Albany, NY: Delmar Publishers.

Leber, A. L. & Novak, S. M. (1999). Intestinal and urogenital amebae, flagellates and ciliates. In Murray, P. R., Baron, S. J., Pfaller, M. A., Tenover, F. C., & Yolken, R. H. (Eds.) *Manual of clinical microbiology* (7th ed.). (pp. 1391-1404). Washington, DC: ASM Press.

CHAPTER FIVE
Free-living Amebae

LEARNING OBJECTIVES

After reading and studying this chapter, the student should be able to:

- Define the key terms.
- List and describe the characteristics of *Naegleria fowleri* and *Acanthamoeba* species.
- Describe the life cycles of the clinically significant free-living protozoans.

- Discuss the transmission and pathogenesis of *Naegleria fowleri* and *Acanthamoeba* species.
- Identify methods of treatment and prevention for primary amebic meningoencephalitis.
- Identify methods of treatment and prevention for granulomatous amebic encephalitis and amebic keratitis.

KEY TERMS

Acanthopodia (ah - kan - thoh - poh - dee - ah)
Amebic keratitis (a - mee - bik/ ker - ah - tie - tis)
Ameboflagellate (a - mee -bow - flaj - e - late)
Cribriform plate (krib - ri - form/ plate)

Free-living (free/ living)
Granulomatous amebic encephalitis (gran - u - low - ma -tus/ a- mee - bik/ en - sef -ah -lie -tis)
Intrathecal (in -trah - thee - kal)

Nuchal rigidity (new - kul/ ri - jid - i - tee)
Primary amebic meningoencephalitis (pri- mar-ee/ a - mee - bik/ men- in- go-en - sef -ah -lie-tis)

INTRODUCTION

The **free-living** amebae are a large and diverse group of protozoan organisms that inhabit fresh and salt water, decaying organic matter and damp soil. Only two genera of these ubiquitous amebae have been implicated in occasional infection of human tissue. The most notable potential pathogens are *Naegleria fowleri* and less commonly *Acanthamoeba* species (Figure 5–1). The organisms are numerous in the environment and a chance encounter usually does not result in disease. On rare occasions, however, the consequence is quite severe. *Naegleria fowleri* is the etiologic agent of **primary amebic meningoencephalitis (PAM)**, a rapidly progressive, fatal infection of the central nervous system. *Acanthamoeba* spp. have been associated with a subacute, more chronic condition of the central nervous system, ***granulomatous amebic encephalitis***, **amebic keratitis** (a chronic infection of the cornea) and skin ulcerations. A comparison of the two amebic CNS infections is highlighted in Table 5–1.

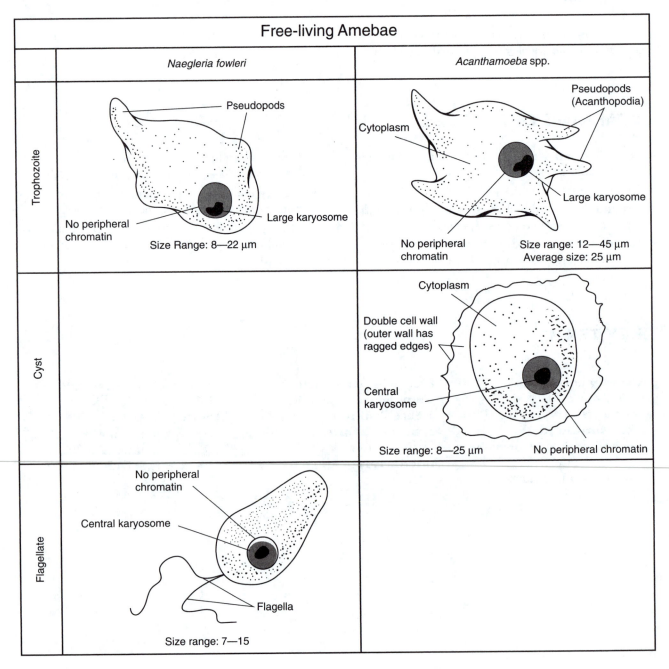

FIG 5–1 Free-living amebae

Table 5–1 ▶ CNS Infections Caused by Free-living Amebae		
	Granulomatous Amebic Encephalitis	**Primary Amebic Meningoencephalitis**
Causative organism:	*Acanthamoeba* species	*Naegleria fowleri*
Risk group:	Immunocompromised, chronically ill	Generally healthy children and young adults with a history of swimming or diving
Transmission:	Respiratory or skin with hematogenous spread to CNS	Nasal instillation, follows olfactory nerve to CNS
Clinical course:	Slow, chronic progression	Rapid, fulminant (death within 7 days untreated)
Diagnostic stages in: CSF	Trophozoite	Trophozoite
Biopsy tissue	Trophozoite and cyst	Trophozoite
Characteristics:	Trophozoite: 10–45 μm Spiny acanthopodia Single nucleus, large central karyosome Cyst: 10–20 μm, rounded, double walled, single nucleus	Trophozoite: 7–20 μm Large, broad pseudopods Single nucleus, large central karyosome

NAEGLERIA FOWLERI

Morphology

Naegleria belongs to the family Vahlkampfiidae. Members of this family are characterized as **ameboflagellates**, having both an ameboid and flagellate stage in their life cycle. *Naegleria fowleri* is the agent of primary amebic meningoencephalitis (PAM) also known as Naegleriasis.

Primary amebic meningoencephalitis is a fulminant, purulent infection of the brain and meninges. Since first being identified in 1965, more than 140 cases of PAM caused by *N. fowleri* have been reported worldwide. Only a few of those cases have been reported in the United States each year.

A similar pattern links the cases both clinically and epidemiologically. PAM tends to be a disease of the warm summer months. The majority of the victims are otherwise healthy children or young adults who have a recent history of swimming or diving in fresh or brackish water. Contaminated swimming pools, stagnant ponds, freshwater lakes and streams, thermal springs and spas, have all been implicated as sources of infection. During periods of drought and elevated temperatures, concentrations of *Naegleria fowleri* increase as they feed on large populations of bacteria in these warmed water sources. More recent cases indicate that the organism may also be transmitted via inhalation of contaminated dust.

Life cycle

The life cycle of *Naegleria fowleri* consists of three stages: an amebic trophozoite, a biflagellate form, and a more resistant cyst form. The amebic trophozoite is the only stage that exists in humans. See Figure 5–2 for the complete life cycle.

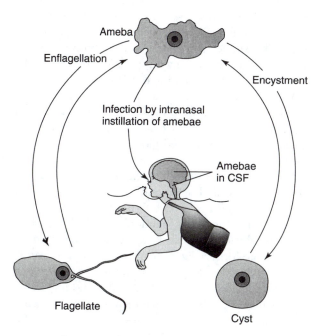

FIG 5–2 Life cycle of *Naegleria fowleri*

The organism enters the host's nasal cavity and infects the mucous membranes and the paranasal sinuses. Amebic trophozoites penetrate the **cribriform plate** (perforated portion of the ethmoid bone) and follow the olfactory nerve to the brain. The organisms then multiply in the tissues of the central nervous system and may be isolated from cerebral spinal fluid.

The ameba transforms into its biflagellate form when in water, a characteristic which may be induced in the laboratory to aid in diagnosis. The cyst form is found in the environment but not in host tissues.

Transmission and Pathogenesis

Naegleria fowleri enters the brain via the nasal mucosa and olfactory nerve to cause primary amebic meningoencephalitis (PAM). The disease progresses rapidly with dramatic symptoms and is usually fatal.

PAM has a nonspecific clinical presentation resembling other types of meningoencephalitis. The incubation period is generally 3–7 days accompanied by the prodromal symptoms of headache and fever. These early symptoms rapidly progress to frank meningitis with the onset of nausea and vomiting, **nuchal rigidity** (stiff neck), confusion and coma. Death usually occurs in 3–6 days following the onset of these serious symptoms.

Laboratory Diagnosis

Laboratory diagnosis can be made by finding motile trophozoites of *Naegleria fowleri* (Figure 5–3) in saline and wet preps of fresh spinal fluid, nasal discharge or tissue biopsy. The organism moves in a directional manner by extension of large, broad pseudopods. The trophozoite measures 7–20 micrometers (μm) and has a finely granular cytoplasm which may contain vacuoles. The single nucleus contains a prominent central karyosome which may appear to be surrounded by a halo. Peripheral chromatin is absent.

A hematologic examination of the spinal fluid reveals many white blood cells (predominantly neutrophils) and red blood cells. Biochemical analysis notes markedly decreased glucose and elevated protein values.

Although infection with *Naegleria fowleri* is rare, the rapid progress of disease leads to a very high mortality rate. Diagnosis is usually made at autopsy. Prepared brain biopsy specimens of lesions show *Naegleria fowleri* trophozoites, but not cyst forms.

Flagellate forms (Figure 5–4) of this parasite can be induced within 2–20 hours by transferring the ameboid form from tissue or CSF to water and incubating at 37 degrees C. This characteristic helps to differen-

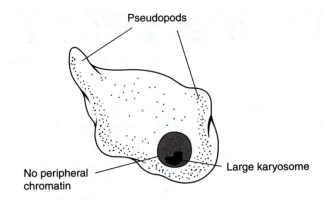

Size Range: 7–20 μm

FIG 5–3 *Naegleria fowleri* trophozoite.

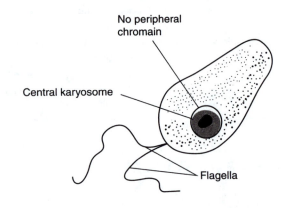

Size Range: 7–15 μm

FIG 5–4 *Naegleria fowleri* flagellate form.

tiate trophozoites of *Naegleria fowleri* from those of *Acanthamoeba* spp. which have no such flagellate form.

The organism may also be recovered using a cultivation technique which involves overlaying non-nutrient agar plates with living *Escherichia coli* bacteria, prior to inoculation with the suspected specimen. The plates are incubated at 37 degrees C and examined daily. The amebae feed on the available bacteria in an aerobic environment as they would do in their natural habitat. This produces cleared tracks visible within the areas of bacterial growth.

Although not routinely performed in most laboratories, laboratory techniques such as PCR and indirect fluorescent antibody procedures may be used to identify these organisms at the species level. These tests are offered by reference laboratories, such as the Centers for Disease Control and Prevention.

Treatment and Prevention

The progress of meningoencephalitis caused by *Naegleria* is so rapid that, unfortunately, the patient often dies before a definitive diagnosis can be made. The possibility of a cure for PAM depends on the early and aggressive treatment with intravenous and **intrathecal** (into the spinal canal) Amphotericin B. Combination treatment with Amphotericin B and miconazole or rifampin has also been shown to be effective in rare cases.

There is no easy solution for controlling *Naegleria* because of its extensive distribution and its ability to withstand adverse environmental conditions. However, public and private swimming pools, hot tubs and baths should be properly maintained and adequately chlorinated to prevent growth of the organism.

ACANTHAMOEBA SPECIES

Morphology

Acanthamoeba belong to the family of Ancanthamoebidae and, unlike *Naegleria*, they never produce flagella. *Acanthamoeba* are known to produce a chronic infection of the central nervous system, called granulomatous amebic encephalitis (GAE). They can also produce an ocular manifestation in the form of a keratitis and skin ulcers.

Life cycle

The life cycle of *Acanthamoeba* spp. consists of a slow moving amebic trophozoite and a resistant cyst form that is found in the environment and may also be recovered from host tissues. The complete life cycle of *Acanthamoeba* spp. can be seen in Figure 5–5.

The trophozoite form is characterized by spiny cytoplasmic projections termed **acanthopodia** (Figure 5–6). Trophozoite size may vary from 10–45 micrometers. The karyosome is large and centrally placed within the nucleus. Peripheral chromatin is absent.

Acanthamoeba spp. cysts are rounded and smaller, ranging in size from 10–20 micrometers. Cysts have a single nucleus and are double walled, with the outer wall having a wrinkled appearance (Figure 5–7). The cyst of *Acanthamoeba*, like those of *Naegleria*, are resistant to dessication and mild chlorination, and can be carried by water and through the air.

Transmission and Pathogenesis

Granulomatous amebic encephalitis has an insidious onset and, unlike PAM caused by *Naegleria* spp.,

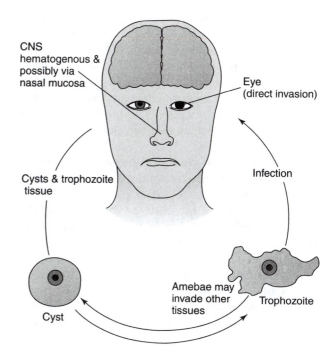

FIG 5–5 Life cycle *Acanthamoeba* species.

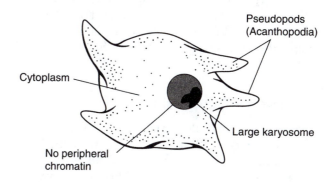

Size Range: 12–45 µm
Average Size: 25 µm

FIG 5–6 *Acanthamoeba* species trophozoite.

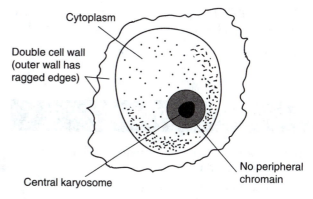

FIG 5–7 *Acanthamoeba* species cyst.

a much longer course. Those affected are generally immunocompromised or chronically ill. GAE is not associated with swimming pools as is PAM. CNS infection is acquired hematogenously by the inhalation/aspiration of trophozoites and cysts, resulting in pneumonitis, or through skin and mucosal ulceration with direct vascular invasion. The incubation period is questionable and may take weeks to months to progress.

The relatively slow process of tissue invasion tends to stimulate granuloma formation. Single or multiple focal lesions develop over a prolonged period marking the chronic nature of the disease. Symptoms of GAE gradually develop and may include headache, fever, fatigue, stiff neck, and altered mental status.

Acantamoebic keratitis is a chronic infection of the cornea that has been well documented since the 1980s. The population at risk are those contact lens wearers using homemade non-sterile saline cleansing solutions. The amebae may also be introduced through corneal trauma.

Infection of the eye with *Acanthamoeba* spp. leads to the development of painful refractory corneal ulcers. Patients experience a gradual loss of vision and tissue damage that clinically resembles infection with viral agents, such as herpes simplex. This confusion can hamper the early detection and treatment of suspected cases.

Laboratory Diagnosis

Patients with GAE deteriorate slowly over a period of weeks to months. Diagnosis can be made by finding characteristic trophozoites in spinal fluid specimens, or both cyst and trophozoite forms in brain biopsy tissue. Scrapings from cutaneous or corneal lesions may also yield cysts and trophozoites indicative of *Acanthamoeba* spp. Indirect immunofluorescent staining techniques may be used for diagnostic testing.

Like *Naegleria fowleri*, *Acanthamoeba* spp. can be cultured on non-nutrient agar which has been overlaid with viable *E. coli* bacteria. The amebae utilize the bacteria as a food source and leave visible "tracks"

on the agar. Permanent smears stained with Geimsa or calcofluor white can aid in the identification of cysts and trophozoites found in clinical specimens or cultures.

Treatment and Prevention

Because of the chronic nature of GAE, symptoms develop gradually over a prolonged period of time and the disease may be overlooked. Treatment with sulfamethazine has been suggested; however, most cases are only diagnosed at autopsy.

Therapies that have been used to treat amebic keratitis include ketoconazole, miconazole, propamidine, pentamidine isothianate, and rifampin. The sooner treatment is begun, the better the prognosis. In many cases the patient loses sight in the affected eye and corneal replacement may be required.

SUMMARY

Naegleria fowleri and *Acanthamoeba* spp. are both free-living amebae that have been linked to rare, but serious, opportunistic infections in humans. *Naegleria fowleri* is found in stagnant water and may be acquired by nasal instillation during swimming. It causes a rapidly progressive fatal infection of the brain and meninges, termed primary amebic meningoencephalitis. Diagnosis of PAM is made by finding the trophozoite form in CSF or brain biopsy tissue.

Acanthamoeba spp. have been associated with a more chronic type of brain infection identified primarily in immunocompromised individuals. The disease is known as granulomatous amebic encephalitis. CNS infection is subsequent to vascular dissemination from the lungs or cutaneous lesions.

Acanthamoeba spp. may also cause keratitis or corneal ulceration in contact lens wearers who use non-commercially prepared, homemade lens solutions. Diagnosis is made by the identification of characteristic cyst and trophozoite forms in corneal or skin scrapings or biopsies of affected skin or brain tissue.

REVIEW QUESTIONS

1. The etiologic agent of primary amebic meningoencephalitis is:

   a. *Acanthamoeba* species

   b. *Naegleria fowleri*

   c. *Giardia lamblia*

   d. *Plasmodium vivax*

Choose the best response for each of the following questions.

2. Amebic keratitis is a condition caused by:

   a. *Trypanosoma cruzi*

   b. *Naegleria fowleri*

   c. *Leishmania donovani*

   d. *Acanthamoeba* species

3. The cyst of *Acanthamoeba* species is characterized by:

a. broad pseudopods

b. multiple nuclei

c. spiny cytoplasmic projections

d. a double walled structure with wrinkled appearance

4. All of the following are true with regard to *Acanthamoeba* infection, *EXCEPT*:

a. may cause corneal ulceration

b. may cause a chronic infection of the CNS

c. only trophozoites are found in biopsy tissue

d. trophozoites are characterized by spiny cytoplasmic projections

5. The term keratitis refers to:

a. a chronic infection of the cornea

b. amebic dysentery

c. an acute infection of the CNS

d. ulceration of the skin

6. The trophozoite of *Acanthamoeba* species is characterized by:

a. broad pseudopods

b. multiple nuclei

c. spiny cytoplasmic projections

d. a double walled structure with wrinkled appearance

7. Primary amebic meningoencephalitis is usually acquired by children while:

a. eating seafood

b. swimming or diving

c. playing in the park

d. shopping at the mall

CASE STUDY

A 25-year old Caucasian male medical resident is seen in the emergency room with complaints of headache, ocular pain, and blurred vision. The patient's medical record notes that he wears contact lenses but has had no previous history of eye infections. Further questioning revealed that the resident had just finished a 36 hour on-call rotation and has a history of rinsing his contact lenses in homemade cleaning solution. The emergency physician ordered an eye culture for bacterial identification and sensitivity and a calcofluor white stain of the corneal scraping. The culture was reported as negative after 48 hours. The calcofluor white stain revealed rounded, double walled cysts measuring 17 μm in diameter. Each cyst had a single nucleus.

Questions

1. What protozoan parasite is suggested by these findings?

2. What diagnosis correlates with the patient history and the laboratory findings?

3. How is the parasite acquired?

▶ BIBLIOGRAPHY

Beaver, P. C., Jung R. C., & Cupp E. W. (1984). *Clinical parasitology* (9th ed.). (pp. 136–145). Philadelphia: Lea & Febiger.

Berger, S. T., Mondino B. J., (1990). Successful medical management of *Acanthamoeba* keratitis. *American Journal of Opthalmology, 110*, 395.

Butt, C. G. (1966). Primary amebic meningoencephalitis. *New England Journal of Medicine, 274*, 1473–1476.

Hawley, H. B., Czachor, J. S., Malhotra, V., Funkhouser, J. W., & Visvesvara, G. S. (1997). *Acanthamoeba* encephalitis in patients with AIDS. *The AIDS Reader,* 7(4), 131–134.

Kilvington, S., Larkin, D. F. P., (1990). Laboratory investigation of *Acanthamoeba* keratitis. *Journal of Clinical Microbiology, 28,* 2722.

Ma, P., Visvesvara, G. S., Martinez, A. J., Theodore, F. H., Daggett, P. M., & Sawyer, T.K. (1990). *Naegleria* and *Acanthamoeba* infections: Review. *Review of Infectious Diseases, 12,* 490.

Mahon, C. & Manuselis, G. (1995). *Textbook of diagnostic microbiology.* (pp. 741–742, 1030–31). Philadelphia: WB Saunders.

Shimeld, L.A. (1999). *Essentials of diagnostic microbiology.* (pp. 591–592). Albany, NY: Delmar Publishers.

Taylor, J.P., Hendricks, K.A., & Dingley, D.D. (1996). Amebic meningoencephalitis. *Infectious Medicine, 13*(12), 1017, 1021–1024, 1052.

U.S. Food and Drug Administration, Center for Food Safety & Applied Nutrition, *Foodborne pathogenic microorganisms and natural toxins handbook, bad bug book:* Acanthamoeba *spp.,* Naegleria fowleri *and other amoebae.* Washington, DC: Author.

Visvesvara G.S., & Balamuth W. (1975). Comparative studies on related free-living and pathogenic amebae with special reference to *Acanthamoeba. Journal of Protozoology, 22,* 245–256.

Yeoh, R., Warhurst, D.C., & Falcon, M.G. (1987). *Acanthamoeba* keratitis. *British Journal of Opthalmology, 71,* 500.

CHAPTER SIX

Intestinal and Atrial Flagellates and Ciliates

OUTLINE

INTESTINAL FLAGELLATES

Giardia lamblia (gee-ARE-dee-a LAM-blee-a)

Chilomastix mesnili
(KILE-o-MAS-tiks mes-NIL-ee)

Enteromonas hominis
(EN-ter-o-mon-as HOM-in-is)

Retortamonas intestinalis
(re-TOR-ta-MO-nis in-TEST-tin-AL-is)

Trichomonas hominis
(TRIK-o-MO-nas HOM-in-is)

Dientamoeba fragilis (di-EN-ta-MEE-ba FRA-jil-is)

ATRIAL FLAGELLATES

Trichomonas vaginalis
(TRIK-o-MO-nas va-gin-AL-is)

Trichomonas tenax (TRIK-o-MO-nas TEE-naks)

INTESTINAL CILIATES

Balantidium coli (BAL-an-TID-ee-um KO-li)

LEARNING OBJECTIVES

After reading and studying this chapter, the student should be able to:

- List the clinically significant intestinal flagellates and ciliates found in humans.
- List and describe characteristics used to identify intestinal flagellates and ciliates.
- Describe the typical life cycle of intestinal flagellates and ciliates.
- Compare the morphological characteristics of intestinal flagellates, and ciliate trophozoites and cysts.

- Describe structures unique to flagellates, which allow for their identification in the laboratory
- Describe the pathogenesis of giardiasis.
- Describe the pathogenesis of balantidiasis
- Describe the treatment and prevention of infections with pathogenic flagellates and ciliates.

KEY TERMS

Axoneme (AKS-o-neem)
Axostyle (AKS-o-stil)
Cilia (SIL-ee-a)
Costa (KOSS-ta)
Cytopyge (SI-toe-pige)

Cytostome (SI-to-stom)
Flagella (fluh-JEL-a)
Hyaline knob (HI-a-lin nob)
Median bodies
(MEE-dee-in bod-ees)

Sucking disc (SUHK-ing disk)
Undulating membrane
(UN-du-la-ting MEM-brain)

INTRODUCTION

The presence of whiplike structures known as **flagella** is characteristic for the members of the phylum Sarcomastigophora, subphylum Mastigophora. Flagellates show a great deal of diversity. Most flagellates are free-living, and most intestinal flagellates are non-pathogenic for man. Although flagella are characteristic for members of this group, they are not always visible in microscopic preparations. Certain morphologic characteristics of flagellate trophozoites and cysts are similar to amebae, although specific structures are unique to this group of protozoans. An **axoneme** refers to the portion of a flagellum located intracellularly. The wavy membranous structure attached to the outer portion of some flagellates is called an **undulating membrane**. An **axostyle**, consisting of a pair of axonemes, is a rodlike structure that provides rigidity to certain flagellate cells. The ciliates, found in the phylum Ciliophora, are characterized by the presence of short, numerous organelles of locomotion called **cilia**. *Balantidium coli* is the only pathogen among the ciliates. It is the largest intestinal protozoan to infect man and, unlike intestinal flagellates, which reside mainly in the small intestine, cecum and colon, resides solely in the large intestine.

INTESTINAL FLAGELLATES

Although most of the intestinal flagellates are non-pathogenic, their presence in human feces suggests the ingestion of contaminated food or water. The life cycles of intestinal flagellates, as well as their processes of encystation and excystation, are similar to those of amebae. However, these parasites reside mostly in the small intestine, cecum, and colon. The intestinal flagellates can be recognized by observation of characteristic trophozoites and cysts in stained and unstained preparations of fecal specimens. Characteristic trophozoites and cysts of intestinal flagellates are illustrated in Figure 6–1. Procedures are similar to those described for detection of intestinal amebae.

Giardia lamblia

Morphology

Trophozoite: *Giardia lamblia* is the most common of all intestinal flagellates, and is responsible for most cases of human infection. The trophozoite of *G. lamblia* measures 9 to 20 micrometers in length (Figure 6–2), 5 to 15 micrometers in width, and is oval to pear-shaped. The broad anterior end, containing a **sucking disc**, a concave area which covers half the ventral surface, tapers to a narrow posterior end. The structure of this parasite has often been described as a "smiling face." The two nuclei ("eyes"), lacking peripheral chromatin, but containing large, central karyosomes, are laterally located in the bilaterally symmetrical trophozoite. An axostyle, consisting of two axonemes, divides the flagellate into two halves. Two curved **median bodies** (parabasal bodies), thought to be involved in metabolism, cross the axonemes at an oblique angle, giving the appearance of a "mouth." Four lateral, two ventral, and two caudal flagella are present, although they may be difficult to see. The trophozoite exhibits "falling leaf" motility.

Cyst: The cyst of *G. lamblia* is oval (Figure 6–3) and measures 8 to 18 micrometers in length, and 7 to 10 micrometers in width. The karyosomes tend to be more eccentric than in the trophozoites. In the mature cyst, four median bodies are present, and longitudinal fibers may be observed. There are four nuclei in the mature cyst. The cytoplasm is often retracted away from the cyst wall, creating a clear zone.

Life Cycle

The life cycle of *G. lamblia* is shown in Figure 6–4. The cyst is the infective stage, and is acquired by ingestion. After passage through the stomach, the cyst passes into the small intestine. Excystation occurs in the duodenum; multiplication occurs by longitudinal binary fission, at approximately 8-hour intervals. Trophozoites attach by means of their sucking discs to the mucosa of the duodenum. This attachment prevents dislocation of the parasite by intestinal peristalsis. Encystation occurs as the trophozoites pass into the large intestine. Trophozoites and cysts may be found in the feces, and are diagnostic for this infection. The predominant form is the cyst, as the trophozoites are highly susceptible to environmental conditions outside of the body.

Transmission and Pathogenesis

The most pathogenic intestinal flagellate is *Giardia lamblia*, which causes giardiasis. This parasite, found worldwide, is probably the most common intestinal parasite in the United States. It is found in the gastrointestinal tracts of a variety of mammals, including man. Many water sources, such as ponds, lakes, streams, and so forth, harbor *G. lamblia* cysts, as a result of fecal contamination by animals or man. Since this parasite is generally resistant to chlorine, filtration is necessary to eliminate contamination. Outbreaks have occurred when filtration is not part of the water purification process. Although foods are less frequently implicated as vehicles for infection, contaminated fruits and raw vegetables may transmit disease. Person-to-

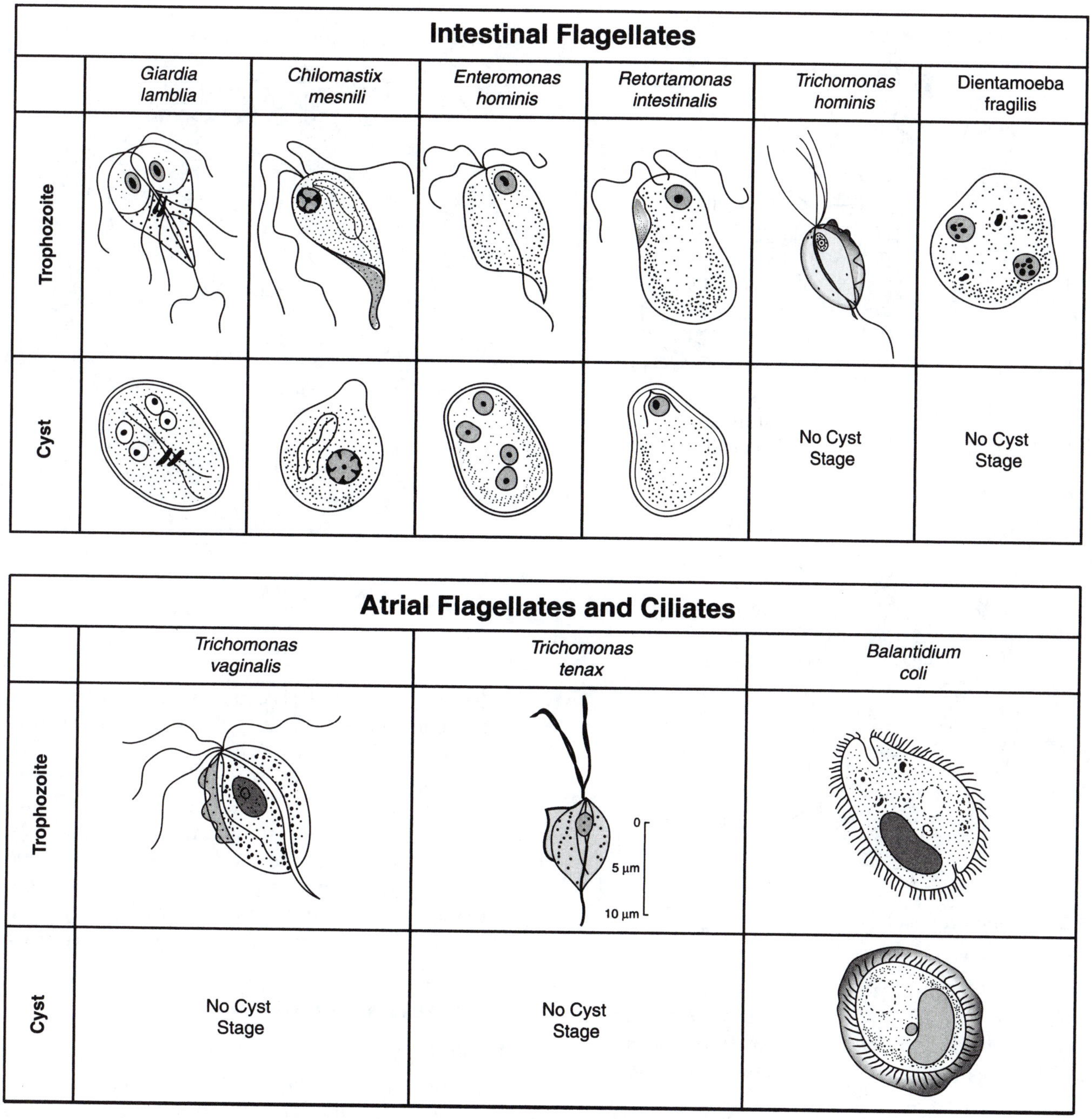

Intestinal Flagellates

	Giardia lamblia	*Chilomastix mesnili*	*Enteromonas hominis*	*Retortamonas intestinalis*	*Trichomonas hominis*	*Dientamoeba fragilis*
Trophozoite						
Cyst					No Cyst Stage	No Cyst Stage

Atrial Flagellates and Ciliates

	Trichomonas vaginalis	*Trichomonas tenax*	*Balantidium coli*
Trophozoite			
Cyst	No Cyst Stage	No Cyst Stage	

FIG 6–1 Characteristic features of trophozoites and cysts of intestinal and atrial flagellates and ciliates

person contact through oral-anal sexual practices may also transmit *G. lamblia*.

After an incubation period of 2 to 3 weeks, symptoms, including watery foul-smelling diarrhea, abdominal cramps, flatulence, anorexia, and nausea may develop. Fat-soluble vitamin deficiencies, folic acid deficiencies, hypoproteinemia with hypogammaglobulinemia and structural changes in intestinal villi may develop. In severe cases, malabsorption syndrome and steatorrhea may result. Weight loss may occur. Patients are often, however, asymptomatic. The parasite attaches to the intestinal mucosa by means of the sucking disc located on the ventral side of the cell.

Laboratory Diagnosis

Differentiation among intestinal flagellates is based on morphological examination of fecal preparations. As with the amebae, liquid or soft fecal specimens from infected patients are more likely to show actively motile trophozoites, while cysts are more likely to be found in formed stools. The presence of either form is

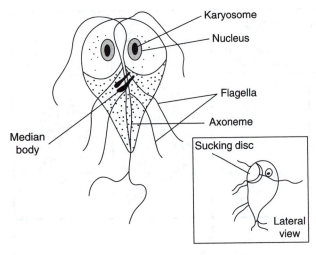

FIG 6–2 *Giardia lamblia* trophozoite

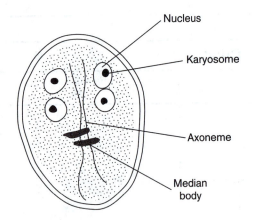

FIG 6–3 *Giardia lamblia* cyst

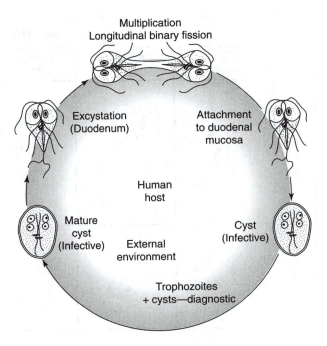

FIG 6–4 Life cycle *Giardia lamblia*

diagnostic for infection. In addition to the wet mount and permanently stained smear of stool specimens, duodenal aspirates may also be examined for the presence of the parasite.

Although serological assays for antibody to *G. lamblia* lack sensitivity, antigen detection methods have been more successful in diagnosing giardiasis. Immunofluorescence methods and enzyme immunoassays have been developed for the detection of *G. lamblia* antigen in stool specimens. Certain tests have shown sensitivities and specificities comparable to or better than those of microscopic examination for cysts or trophozoites.

Treatment and Prevention

The treatment of choice for giardiasis is metronidazole. Alternate choices include quinacrine, tinidazole, furazolidone and paromomycin.

Most cases of giardiasis can be prevented by avoidance of contaminated water. Filtration of water is necessary to avoid transmission of infective cysts of *G. lamblia*, since this parasite is usually resistant to chemicals, such as chlorine. Other preventive measures include protecting water supplies from reservoir hosts, such as beavers, muskrats and voles, exercising good personal hygiene, and proper preparation and cooking of food. Person-to-person transmission through sexual contact can be prevented by safe sexual practices.

Chilomastix mesnili

Morphology

Trophozoite: The trophozoite of *Chilomastix mesnili*, shown in Figure 6–5, is teardrop-shaped, having a rounded anterior end tapering to a narrow posterior end, and measures 5 to 24 micrometers long by 5 to 8 micrometers wide. The single large nucleus, with a small central or eccentric karyosome in the form of chromatin granules, is located anteriorly at the rounded end of the trophozoite. Peripheral nuclear chromatin is absent. A prominent **cytostome**, or oral groove, runs alongside the nucleus, extending one-third to one-half the length of the trophozoite. Four flagella, three extending anteriorly and one extending posteriorly from the cytostome, are present. The trophozoite exhibits stiff, rotary motility. A spiral groove may be seen extending across the ventral surface, resulting in a curve at the posterior end.

Cyst: The cyst of *C. mesnili*, measuring 5 to 10 micrometers by 4 to 6 micrometers (Figure 6–6), is lemon shaped with a distinctive **hyaline knob**, resembling a nipple, at the anterior end. One nucleus, with a large, central karyosome, with no peripheral chromatin, is present, as well as a curved cytostome at one side of the nucleus.

Life Cycle

The life cycle of this flagellate resembles that of *G. lamblia*, except for the stage in the duodenum. The processes of encystation and excystation occur in the small intestine, cecum and colon. The cysts withstand environmental conditions, and are considered to be the infective forms.

Transmission and Pathogenesis.

C. mesnili causes asymptomatic infection. The parasite tends to be prevalent in tropical climates. Transmission occurs by ingestion of infective cysts, and is prevalent when poor sanitary conditions prevail.

Laboratory Diagnosis

Diagnosis of infection with *C. mesnili* is made by the traditional examination of fecal specimens for ova and parasites. Both stained and unstained smears should be examined.

Treatment and Prevention

No treatment is recommended for infection with *C. mesnili*, since the parasite is considered to be nonpathogenic. Prevention of infection is accomplished by good hygiene and careful sanitary practices.

Enteromonas hominis
Morphology

Trophozoite: The oval trophozoite, sometimes flattened on one side, of *Enteromonas hominis*, as shown in Figure 6–7, measures 4 to 10 micrometers in length, and 3 to 6 micrometers in width. The posterior end resembles a tiny tail. The nucleus, having a large central karyosome, is located anteriorly. Peripheral chromatin is absent. Four flagella, three extending anteriorly and one extending posteriorly, are present. A jerky motility is characteristic for this parasite. No cytostome, axostyle, or undulating membrane is present.

Cyst: The cyst is oval (Figure 6–8) and measures 4 to 10 micrometers by 4 to 6 micrometers. One to four nuclei with central karyosomes may be present. These are often paired up at opposite ends of the cyst.

Life Cycle

The life cycle of *E. hominis* is similar to that of other intestinal flagellates, having both a trophozoite and a

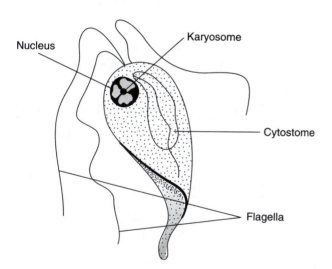

FIG 6–5 *Chilomastix mesnili* trophozoite

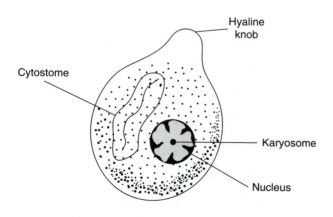

FIG 6–6 *Chilomastix mesnili* cyst

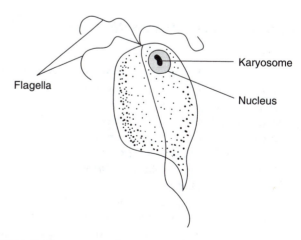

FIG 6–7 *Enteromonas hominis* trophozoite

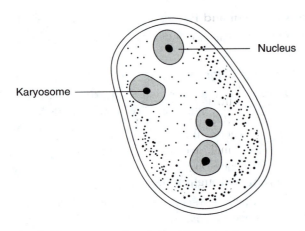

FIG 6–8 *Enteromonas hominis* cyst

cyst stage. The cyst is resistant to environmental conditions and is the infective form.

Transmission and Pathogenesis

E. hominis is found worldwide in both tropical and temperate climates. The ingestion of infective cysts is the mode of transmission of the parasite. Infections are asymptomatic.

Laboratory Diagnosis

The standard examination of stool specimens for trophozoite and cyst forms of this parasite is used to make a diagnosis of infection. The small size of *E. hominis* trophozoites and cysts makes identification difficult.

Treatment and Prevention

This parasite is a nonpathogen, and does not require therapy. Close attention to personal hygiene and avoidance of contaminated water should prevent infection.

Retortamonas intestinalis

Morphology

Trophozoite: The oval trophozoite of *Retortamonas intestinalis* measures 4 to 8 micrometers in length, and 5 to 6 micrometers in width (Figure 6–9). A single nucleus, having a small, central karyosome, is located anteriorly. A cytostome extends opposite the nucleus to about half the length of the trophozoite. Two anterior flagella are present. Like *E. hominis*, this parasite exhibits a jerky motility.

Cyst: The pear-shaped cyst of *R. intestinalis* (Figure 6–10) measures 4 to 8 micrometers in length and 4 to 5 micrometers in width. One nucleus, having a central karyosome, is located anteriorly or centrally.

Two fibrils originating anterior to the nucleus separate around the nucleus, giving the appearance of a bird's beak.

Life Cycle

The life cycle of *R. intestinalis* resembles that of other intestinal flagellates, with a trophozoite and a cyst stage.

Transmission and Pathogenesis

Although rarely reported, this parasite causes asymptomatic infection in humans. It is transmitted by ingestion of infective cysts.

Laboratory Diagnosis

Examination of fecal specimens for trophozoites and cysts is the standard procedure for diagnosis of this infection. However, because of the small size of the

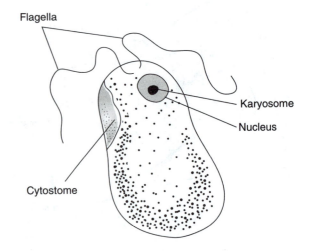

FIG 6–9 *Retortamonas intestinalis* trophozoite

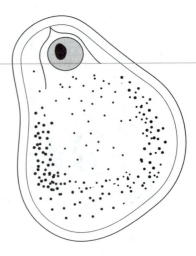

FIG 6–10 *Retortamonas intestinalis* cyst

parasite, a permanent stain is essential. The difficulties encountered in identifying this parasite probably account for the small number of reports.

Treatment and Prevention

No therapy is recommended for infection with this nonpathogen. Good personal hygiene is essential for prevention of infection.

Trichomonas hominis

Morphology

Trophozoite: The trophozoite of *Trichomonas hominis* measures 7 to 18 micrometers by 5 to 8 micrometers, is pear-shaped, and is characterized by the presence of an undulating membrane, extending the length of the cell (Figure 6–11). A rodlike structure called the **costa** connects the undulating membrane to the trophozoite. A central, longitudinal axostyle provides rigidity to the cell. The axostyle curves around the nucleus and extends posteriorly beyond the body of the organism. A cone-shaped cytostome is located opposite the undulating membrane. The single nucleus is located anteriorly, and has a small, central karyosome. Peripheral chromatin is absent. Three to five flagella are present. The parasite exhibits a rapid, jerky motility.

Cyst: There is no known cyst form of *T. hominis*.

Life Cycle

The trophozoites of *T. hominis* reside in the cecum, where they feed on bacteria.

Cell division occurs in the large intestine, but encystation does not occur.

Transmission and Pathogenesis

T. hominis infection occurs worldwide, but especially in warm climates. It is thought that the trophozoite form is probably transmitted in some protective material, such as milk, which would serve to protect the vegetative cells from destruction. Although frequently detected in patients having diarrhea, the parasite is considered to be nonpathogenic. It is suspected that in patients with achlorhydria, milk acts as a shield for the entry of *T. hominis* into the stomach, allowing the organism to survive passage through the stomach and to settle in the small intestine.

Laboratory Diagnosis

Detection of *T. hominis* is difficult because of its small size and poor staining qualities. Flagellar movement from the undulating membrane seen in fresh preparations of fecal material is often helpful in identification of this parasite.

Treatment and Prevention

No treatment is indicated for this nonpathogen. Prevention of infection is accomplished by an emphasis on good hygiene and sanitary conditions.

Dientamoeba fragilis

Morphology

Trophozoite: *Dientamoeba fragilis* does not have external flagella, although it retains certain flagellar characteristics (Figure 6–12). *D. fragilis* was originally classified as an ameba, since it moves in ameboid fashion by means of pseudopods with serrated edges. Although no external flagella are visible, active motility may be exhibited. The trophozoite measures 5 to 16 micrometers, and is roundish, although some variation occurs. One, or more commonly two, nuclei may be present; the delicate nuclear membrane is frequently indistinct. The karyosome of each nucleus consists of

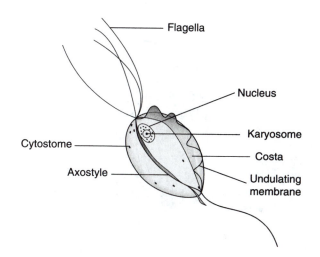

FIG 6–11 *Trichomonas hominis* trophozoite

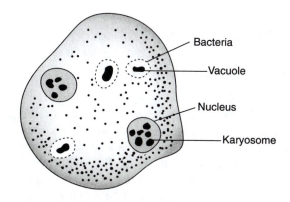

FIG 6–12 *Dientamoeba fragilis* trophozoite

four to eight chromatin granules usually symmetrically located. Peripheral chromatin is absent. Vacuoles containing bacteria may also be present in the cytoplasm.

Cyst: There is no known cyst form of *D. fragilis*.

Life Cycle

Trophozoites of *D. fragilis* reside and multiply in the large intestine. No cysts of this parasite have been identified. The complete life cycle of this parasite is not well understood.

Transmission and Pathogenesis

The pathogenicity of *D. fragilis* remains controversial. Infections are often accompanied by intermittent diarrhea, fatigue, nausea, abdominal pain, vomiting, and flatulence, with low-grade eosinophilia. However, the majority of persons with *D. fragilis* infections remain asymptomatic. Although the mechanism of transmission of *D. fragilis* is unclear, there appears to be an association with, and perhaps transmission within, the eggs of the pinworm, *Enterobius vermicularis*, as well as *Ascaris lumbricoides*.

Laboratory Diagnosis

The standard examination of fecal specimens for trophozoites of *D. fragilis* is recommended. Several specimens should be tested, since intermittent passage of parasites has been noted. Careful examination of a permanent stain is essential for diagnosis, since the parasite tends to stain weakly, often blending into the background.

Treatment and Prevention

Symptomatic patients with *Dientamoeba fragilis* may be treated with tetracycline or iodoquinol. In children, metronidazole is often used. Although fecal-oral transmission has not been proven, careful attention to good hygiene and sanitary practices is recommended, to prevent ingestion of helminth eggs.

ATRIAL FLAGELLATES

Trichomonas vaginalis

Morphology

Trophozoite: The trophozoite of *Trichomonas vaginalis* is very similar to those of other trichomonads, such as *T. hominis*. It measures 8 to 23 micrometers in length, and 5 to 12 micrometers in width (see Figure 6–13). The anterior end is rounded, while the posterior end is tapered. Four to six flagella originate from the anterior end. The undulating membrane is shorter

than that of *T. hominis*, extending only halfway down the side, and the axostyle is usually visible. Granules may be visible near the axostyles. Chromatin is evenly distributed. A single nucleus is present. In wet preps, the parasite exhibits a rapid, jerky motion.

Cyst: There is no known cyst form of *T. vaginalis*.

Life Cycle

The trophozoites of *T. vaginalis* reside on the mucous membranes of the vagina, and feed on bacteria and white blood cells. In infected males, trichomonads commonly reside in the prostate gland or the urethral epithelium. Multiplication occurs by longitudinal binary fission.

Transmission and Pathogenesis

Transmission of *T. vaginalis* is usually by sexual contact. Infected women may be asymptomatic, or they may suffer from burning, itching, and irritation, and produce a profuse foul-smelling, yellowish discharge. Red lesions may be present on the vaginal mucosa. Infected men may be asymptomatic, or suffer from urethritis. In severe cases, involving the prostate gland and upper urogenital system, prostate tenderness and swelling may occur. A thin discharge may reveal *T. vaginalis* trophozoites.

Laboratory Diagnosis

The diagnosis of trichomoniasis is usually made by the observation of motile trophozoites in wet preps of vaginal or urethral secretions. Methods are also available to culture the trichomonads from these secretions. Although permanent stained smears may be examined for *T. vaginalis* trophozoites, false positive and false negative results are common. Specimens should not be refrigerated. The indirect hemagglutination assay

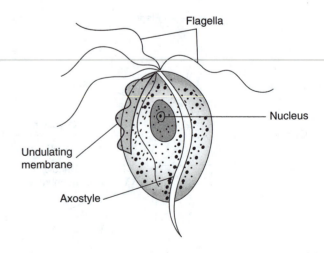

FIG 6–13 *T. vaginalis* trophozoite

has been used for the retrospective diagnosis of this infection, although serologic methods are not routinely available.

Treatment and Prevention

The treatment of choice is metronidazole. Sexual partners should also be treated. Prevention of trichomoniasis is accomplished by the avoidance of unprotected sex, as well as prompt treatment and diagnosis of asymptomatic men.

Trichomonas tenax

Morphology

Trophozoite: The trophozoite of *Trichomonas tenax* has a pyriform shape (see Figure 6–14); it is similar to other trichomonads, but is smaller and more slender than *T. hominis*. It measures 5 to 12 micrometers in length by 7 to 9 micrometers in width. Five flagella originate from the anterior end; four extend anteriorly and one extends posteriorly. The undulating membrane runs almost the full length of the trophozoite, like that of *T. hominis*. The axostyle is characteristic of trichomonads, running along the full body length and beyond. There is a single oval nucleus.

Cyst: There is no known cyst form of *T. tenax*.

Life Cycle

T. tenax is a commensal, and resides in the mouth, especially in cases of pyorrhea, and in patients with poor oral hygiene. The parasites are located primarily in tartar, and around gingival crevices. Like *T. vaginalis*, *T. tenax* trophozoites multiply by longitudinal binary fission.

Transmission and Pathogenesis

Although the means of transmission is not known for certain, exchange of oral secretions by kissing has been suggested as a possible route of infection. Contaminated dishes may also be involved.

Infections are usually asymptomatic.

Laboratory Diagnosis

Diagnosis of infection is accomplished by the observation of characteristic trophozoites in wet preps of gum scrapings. Specimens may be cultured in a manner similar to *T. vaginalis*, but this method is not often used in the clinical setting.

Treatment and Prevention

Since this parasite is considered to be nonpathogenic, treatment is usually not recommended. Infection with *T. tenax* is prevented by the practice of good oral hygiene.

INTESTINAL CILIATES

Balantidium coli is a member of the phylum Ciliophora, and the class Kinetofragminophorea. It is the only pathogenic intestinal ciliate, and the largest intestinal protozoan parasite causing gastroenteritis in man.

Balantidium coli

Morphology

Trophozoite: The oval trophozoite of *B. coli* measures 30 to 100 micrometers in length, and 30 to 80 micrometers in width (Figure 6–15). It tapers at the anterior end, where a cytostome is located. Two nuclei are present in the trophozoite, a large, kidney-shaped macronucleus, and a small, round micronucleus, located adjacent to the macronucleus. Cilia, which tend

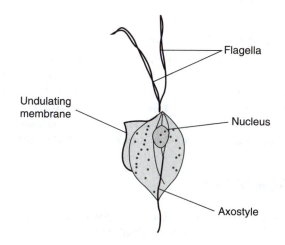

FIG 6–14 *T. tenax* trophozoite

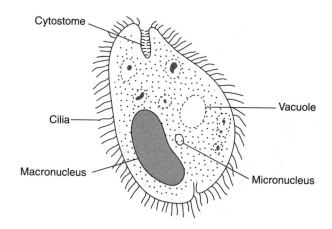

FIG 6–15 *Balantidium coli* trophozoite

to be longer at the anterior end, are present along the periphery of the trophozoite. Contractile vacuoles are usually present in the cytoplasm. The **cytopyge** is the excretory pore, and is located opposite the cytostome. Ingested bacteria may also be found in the cytoplasm.

Cyst: The round to elliptical cyst of *B. coli* measures 45 to 65 micrometers (Figure 6–16). A kidney-shaped macronucleus is present, as well as a small, round, often indistinct micronucleus, lying adjacent to the macronucleus. Cilia are located within the two layers of the cyst wall, but may be absent in mature cysts.

Life Cycle

The life cycle of *B. coli* (Figure 6–17) is similar to that of *E. histolytica*. Ingestion of infective cysts through food and water initiates the infection. Excystation occurs in the small intestine. Trophozoites multiply by transverse binary fission, mainly in the cecum and ileum, and also in the lumen of the colon. Encystation also occurs in the lumen of the colon. Multiplication of *B. coli* nuclei does not occur in the cyst stage.

Transmission and Pathogenesis

B. coli may cause a form of gastroenteritis called balantidiasis, which is characterized by abdominal pains, and bloody diarrhea, often resembling infection with *E. histolytica*. The incidence of infection with *B. coli* is low, although the parasite is distributed worldwide. Pigs are a known reservoir for the parasite. The infection is transmitted by the fecal-oral route, and, occasionally, from person-to-person. Infected food handlers may be implicated in the spread of this disease. In the severe form of balantidiasis, abscesses and ulcers may form in the mucosa and submucosa of the large intestine, and may resemble amebic dysentery. Chronic infection may occur, and some patients are asymptomatic. Extraintestinal infections in the liver, lungs, and other organs may occur, but this is rare.

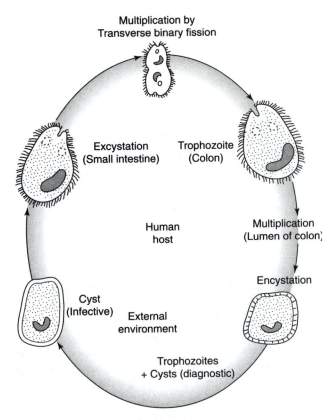

FIG 6–17 Life cycle *Balantidium coli*

Laboratory Diagnosis

Diagnosis of infection with the only pathogenic ciliate, *Balantidium coli*, is accomplished by examining stool specimens by wet prep and permanently stained smears. The parasite may also be revealed in sigmoidoscopy material. The parasite is recognized by its large size, as well as by the presence of a layer of cilia surrounding the trophozoite stage. The cilia located between the two cyst wall layers are often not recognizable.

Treatment and Prevention

Good personal hygiene and proper sanitary conditions are effective measures of preventing infection with *B. coli*. Also caution should be taken in dealing with pigs, which may also transmit the organism.

Suggested antimicrobial agents used for balantidiasis include tetracycline, metronidazole, and iodoquinol

SUMMARY

Intestinal and atrial flagellates and ciliates may cause serious illness in humans. Pathogenic parasites must be distinguished from commensal forms. The number and structure of nuclei, karyosomes, flagella or cilia

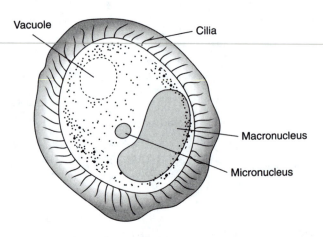

FIG 6–16 *Balantidium coli* cyst

may be useful in characterizing different species. Other characteristics, such as the presence or structure of an undulating membrane, cytostome, axoneme, and axostyle may also be useful. The pathogenic ciliate, *B. coli,* is usually recognized by its large size, large macronucleus and small micronucleus, and the presence of cilia on the trophozoite form. Although non-pathogenic intestinal flagellates need not be treated, they may signify ingestion of contaminated water or food. Key characteristics of the trophozoites and cysts of intestinal and atrial flagellates and ciliates are summarized in Table 6–1.

Table 6–1 ▶ Key Characteristics of Intestinal and Atrial Flagellates and Ciliates

FLAGELLATES/CILIATES	TROPHOZOITE	CYST
Giardia lamblia	9–20 µm by 5–15 µm Pear-shaped or teardrop shaped with 2 nuclei, linear axonemes, curved median bodies, and 8 flagella; sucking disc Falling leaf motility	8–18 µm by 7–10 µm Round to oval with 4 nuclei, axonemes and median bodies
Chilomastix mesnili	5–24 µm by 5–8 µm Teardrop shaped Prominent cytostome 1 nucleus 4 flagella Stiff, rotary motility	5–10 µm by 4–6 µm Lemon shaped with 1 nucleus, and anterior knob or "nipple" cytostome
Enteromonas hominis	4–10 µm by 3–6 µm Oval shape 1 nucleus 4 flagella Jerky motility	4–10 µm by 4–6 µm Oval shape 1–4 nuclei
Retortamonas intestinalis	4–8 µm by 5–6 µm Oval or pear-shaped 1 nucleus 2 flagella Jerky motility	4–8 µm by 4–5 µm Pear shaped 1 nucleus
Trichomonas hominis	7–18 µm by 5–8 µm Pear-shaped 4–6 flagella 1 nucleus Undulating membrane extends the full length of the organism Axostyle present Rapid, jerky motility	No cyst form
Dientamoeba fragilis	5–16 µm Ameba-like shape 1 or 2 nuclei No visible flagella Debris in cytoplasm; pale staining Active motility Pseudopod present	No cyst form

(continues)

Table 6–1 *(continued)*

FLAGELLATES/CILIATES	TROPHOZOITE	CYST
Trichomonas vaginalis	8–23 μm by 5–12 μm Pear-shaped 1 nucleus 4–6 flagella Prominent axostyle Undulating membrane extends halfway down the length of the organism Rapid, jerky motility	No cyst form
Trichomonas tenax	5–12 μm by 7–9 μm Pear-shaped 1 nucleus 5 flagella Undulating membrane extends the full length of the organism Axostyle protrudes beyond posterior end Rapid, jerky motility	No cyst form
Balantidium coli	30–100 μm by 30–80 μm Very large ovoid shape Large bean-shaped macronucleus Small spherical micronucleus Numerous cilia Cytostome/cytopyge	45–65 μm Oval or spherical shape Large macronucleus

REVIEW QUESTIONS:

1. The most common intestinal parasitic protozoan causing gastroenteritis in the United States is
   a. *Giardia lamblia*
   b. *Chilomastix mesnili*
   c. *Dientamoeba fragilis*
   d. *Balantidium coli*

2. The largest human intestinal parasitic protozoan is
   a. *Giardia lamblia*
   b. *Chilomastix mesnili*
   c. *Dientamoeba fragilis*
   d. *Balantidium coli*

3. Excystation of the cysts of *G. lamblia* occurs in the
   a. ileum
   b. colon
   c. duodenum
   d. stomach

4. A sucking disc covers half the ventral surface of
   a. *Giardia lamblia*
   b. *Chilomastix mesnili*
   c. *Dientamoeba fragilis*
   d. *Balantidium coli*

5. A parasite considered to be a flagellate, but which lacks external flagella, is
   a. *Giardia lamblia*
   b. *Chilomastix mesnili*
   c. *Dientamoeba fragilis*
   d. *Balantidium coli*

6. The flagellate _____ is recognized by the presence of a prominent cytostome, which runs approximately one-third the length of the trophozoite.

   a. *Enteromonas hominis*

   b. *Chilomastix mesnili*

   c. *Retortamonas intestinalis*

   d. *Trichomonas hominis*

7. An undulating membrane is present along the length of the trophozoite of

   a. *Retortamonas intestinalis*

   b. *Chilomastix mesnili*

   c. *Enteromonas hominis*

   d. *Trichomonas hominis*

8. A large kidney-shaped nucleus is characteristic of the parasite

   a. *Giardia lamblia*

   b. *Chilomastix mesnili*

   c. *Dientamoeba fragilis*

   d. *Balantidium coli*

9. The parasite _____ does not form cysts, existing only in the trophozoite form.

   a. *Giardia lamblia*

   b. *Chilomastix mesnili*

   c. *Dientamoeba fragilis*

   d. *Balantidium coli*

10. A hyaline knob gives the cyst form of _____ the appearance of a lemon.

   a. *Giardia lamblia*

   b. *Chilomastix mesnili*

   c. *Dientamoeba fragilis*

   d. *Balantidium coli*

CASE STUDY

A 24-year old hiker had recently returned from a camping trip to Colorado. While camping, she had obtained drinking water from an untreated stream. Several weeks after returning home, she presented to her family physician with profuse, watery diarrhea, crampy abdominal pain, and foul-smelling flatulence.

Stool specimens were negative for enteric bacterial pathogens, but wet mounts demonstrated binucleate pear-shaped trophozoites showing a "falling leaf" type of motility. A permanent trichrome stain confirmed the diagnosis.

Questions

1. What is the name of the parasite causing the patient's illness? What is the infectious stage of this parasite?

2. How does this parasite avoid being dislodged by intestinal peristalsis?

3. How does this parasite sometimes result in malabsorption?

4. How is this parasite transmitted? How can transmission be prevented?

5. How is this illness treated?

▶ **BIBLIOGRAPHY**

Garcia, L. S. & Bruckner, D. A. (1997). *Diagnostic medical parasitology* (3rd ed.). (pp. 34–53). Washington, DC: ASM Press.

Zeibig, E. A. (1997). *Clinical parasitology*. (pp. 37–60). Philadelphia: W. B. Saunders.

Leber, A. L. & Novak, S. M. (1999). Intestinal and urogenital amebae, flagellates and ciliates. In Murray, P. R., Baron, S. J., Pfaller, S. J., Tenover, F. C. & Yolken, R. H. (Eds.) *Manual of clinical microbiology* (7th ed.). (pp. 1391–1404). Washington, DC: ASM Press.

Koneman, E. W., Allen, S. D., Janda, W. M., Schreckenberger, P. C., & Winn, W. C. Jr. (1997). *Color atlas and textbook of diagnostic microbiology* (5th ed.). (pp. 1071–1176). Philadelphia: Lippincott.

CHAPTER SEVEN

Blood and Tissue Flagellates:
Leishmania species

OUTLINE

**LEISHMANIA TROPICA COMPLEX — OLD
WORLD CUTANEOUS LEISHMANIASIS**

(leesh - may - nee - uh / trop - i - kuh)

**LEISHMANIA MEXICANA COMPLEX — NEW
WORLD CUTANEOUS LEISHMANIASIS**

(leesh - may - nee - uh / mex - i - can - a)

**LEISHMANIA BRAZILIENSIS COMPLEX —
MUCOCUTANEOUS LEISHMANIASIS**

(leesh - may - nee - uh / bra - zil - ee - en - sis)

**LEISHMANIA DONOVANI COMPLEX —
VISCERAL LEISHMANIASIS**

(leesh - may - nee - uh / don - o - va - nee)

LEARNING OBJECTIVES

After reading and studying this chapter, the student
should be able to:

- Define the key terms.
- For each hemoflagellate cited, state the geo-graphic distribution.
- Describe the morphologic characteristics of the protozoans in this chapter.
- Briefly describe the life cycle of each hemoflagel-late cited.
- Identify the hosts and vector for each organism.

- List the infective stage and diagnostic state of each organism.
- Describe the mechanism of pathogenesis for each organism.
- Discuss the clinical presentation of each disease.
- Name the specimen of choice for the diagnosis and/or recovery of each hemoflagellate.
- Identify means of treatment and prevention for each parasite.

KEY TERMS

Amastigote (a-mast-i-goat)
Anergic (an-erj-ik)
Chiclero ulcer
  (chik-ler-oh/ ul-sir)
Cutaneous (ku-tay-nee-us)
Espundia (esp-un-dee-ah)
Hemoflagellate
  (hemo-flaj-el-ate)
Kala azar (ka-lah/ ah-zar)

Kinetoplast (kin-et-oh-plast)
Leishmaniasis
  (leesh-man-eye-ah-sis)
Montenegro skin test
  (mon-ten-e-grow)
Mucocutaneous
  (mu-ko-ku-tay-nee-us)
Oriental sore
  (or-ee-en-tal/ sore)

Pain bois (pan/ bwah)
Promastigote (pro-mast-i-goat)
Sandfly (sand-fly)
Uta (oo-tah)
Visceral (vis-sir-al)
Zoonosis (zoo-no-sis)

INTRODUCTION

The family Trypanosomatidae contains the flagellated protozoa that parasitize the blood and tissues of the human host: genus *Leishmania* and genus *Trypanosoma* (Chapter 8). Collectively, these organisms are called the **hemoflagellates**. They are transmitted by insect vectors, in which they undergo a portion of their life cycle and, depending on the species, may exist in two or more of the four morphologic forms illustrated in Figure 7–1. The characteristics of each of the forms are listed in Table 7–1.

Leishmaniasis is a significant public health problem. World Health Organization statistics suggest that there are 12 million people currently infected with the disease in 88 countries around the world. Another 350 million individuals in those areas are at risk of becoming infected. It is estimated that the number of new cases grows by 2 million each year and only about 600,000 of those cases are reported.

The increased incidence of leishmaniasis is related to man's encroachment into the sandfly habitat. Economic development in the form of mining, harvesting lumber, and expanding cultivation in the primary forests, as well as rapid urbanization worldwide, have elevated the number of reported cases.

The *Leishmania* species that infect humans are studied as group complexes based on the clinical presentation of the disease they cause: **cutaneous**, **mucocutaneous**, and **visceral** leishmaniasis. Cutaneous leishmaniasis is generally a localized infection

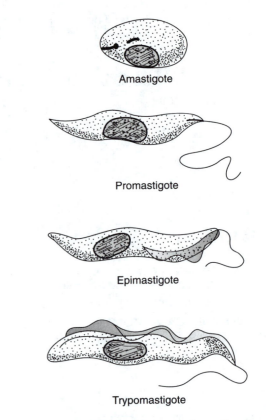

FIG 7–1 Morphologic forms seen in hemoflagellates

of the capillaries of the skin. The mucocutaneous type of disease tends to cause lesions of the skin and mucous membranes, specifically, of the oral and nasal

TABLE 7–1 ▶ Morphologic Characteristics of Hemoflagellate Forms

Characteristic	Amastigote	Promastigote	Epimastigote	Trypomastigote
Size	5 by 3 μm	9–15 μm	9–15 μm	12–35 μm
Shape	Oval to round	Long and slender	Long and slightly wider	"Spindle shaped" U or C shape in blood films
Nucleus	One, eccentric	One, central	One, in posterior end	One, anterior to kinetoplast
Kinetoplast	Present, consisting of dot-like blepharoplast with small axoneme and parabasal body	Anterior end of the organism, no undulating membrane	Anterior to the nucleus, with half-body undulating membrane	Posterior, gives rise to full-body length undulating membrane
Flagellum	Absent	Single, anterior free flagellum	Single, anterior free flagellum	Single, anterior free flagellum

mucosa. Systemic or visceral leishmaniasis presents with more generalized symptoms leading to enlargement of the internal organs, especially the liver, lymph nodes and spleen. The organisms are indistinguishable in appearance but may be differentiated based on geographic distribution, pathogenesis, kinetoplast DNA (kDNA) analysis, DNA hybridization and serologic testing.

Members of the genus *Leishmania* have an **amastigote** (nonflagellate, intracellular morphologic stage) and **promastigote** (a long, slender morphologic form containing a free flagellum that extends anteriorly from the axoneme) stage in their life cycle and a vertebrate and invertebrate host. Typically, the vector is the female of one of a variety of species of tiny phlebotomine **sandflies** (*Phlebotomus, Lutzomyia*). The *Leishmania* are intracellular parasites inhabiting human macrophages and other cells of the reticuloendothelial system in the amastigote form. The protozoa are drawn into the insect as it takes a blood meal, and within the insect's gut, they multiply and transform into promastigotes. The flagellated promastigotes migrate to the proboscis of the fly from which they may be introduced to a new host as the insect takes its next meal. The generalized life cycle of *Leishmania* species can be seen in Figure 7–2.

LEISHMANIA TROPICA COMPLEX — OLD WORLD CUTANEOUS LEISHMANIASIS

Morphology

Old World cutaneous leishmaniasis, also know as **Oriental sore**, Delhi boil and dry or urban cutaneous leishmaniasis, is caused by the organisms of the *Leishmania tropica* complex. The complex encompasses three clinically significant and serologically distinct species: *Leishmania tropica, Leishmania aethiopica,* and *Leishmania major.* All these organisms are vectored by tiny sandflies (*Phlebotomus*) measuring two to three mm in length. The geographic distribution of each *Leishmania* species varies; these are listed in Table 7–2.

Cutaneous leishmaniasis is a chronic disease that is characterized by the production of dry, raised, ulcerated lesions at bite sites. Lesions usually occur on areas of skin not typically covered by traditional clothing.

Life cycle

Phlebotomus sandflies serve as the vector for all three members of the *Leishmania tropica* complex. Only the female sandfly transmits the parasites, becoming infected herself as she draws a blood meal from an infected human or mammalian host.

Within the gut of the insect, the amastigote forms transform into promastigotes and multiply. Fully developed promastigotes then migrate in large numbers to the pharynx of the now infectious sandfly. When the fly feeds again, the organisms are transmitted to a new host.

Within the mammalian host, the parasite is engulfed by reticuloendothelial cells within which amastigotes multiply repeatedly by binary fission. When the host cell can no longer accommodate the parasite load, the cell ruptures and the newly released amastigotes invade new macrophages and perpetuate the cycle.

The life cycle of the various medically significant *Leishmania* species is similar and is diagrammed in Figure 7–2. Differentiation of the various species of *Leishmania* that cause human disease is based on the geographic distribution, clinical presentation, and diagnostic testing. In the case of *Leishmania tropica* complex, the affected tissue is restricted to the reticuloendothelial (RE) cells and lymphoid tissue of the skin, giving a cutaneous presentation.

Transmission and Pathogenesis

Introduced into the skin by the bite of an infected sandfly, promastigotes of the *Leishmania tropica* subspecies are phagocytized by local macrophages. Within these cells, they round up into amastigote forms and multiply. As the host cell ruptures, amastigotes are released to invade new macrophage cells. The repeated cycle of invasion, reproduction and cell rupture leads to tissue destruction.

The incubation period of the disease can vary from several weeks to as long as three years, depending on the species involved, with *Leishmania major* having a more rapid onset and *Leishmania tropica* and *L. aethiopica* being more prolonged. The first sign of cutaneous leishmaniasis is the development of a small red papule at the initial site of the insect bite. There

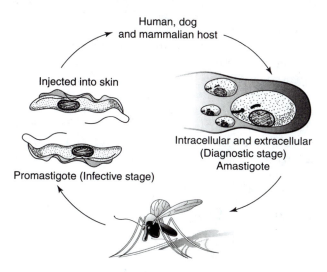

FIG 7–2 Life cycle of *Leishmania* spp.

Human, dog and mammalian host

Injected into skin

Promastigote (Infective stage)

Intracellular and extracellular (Diagnostic stage) Amastigote

Table 7–2 ▶ Geographic Distribution of *Leishmania* species

Leishmania species	Geographic Distribution
Leishmania tropica complex	**Old World Cutaneous Leishmaniasis**
L. tropica	Mediterranean region, Middle East, Armenia, Caspian region, Afghanistan, India and Kenya (particularly in urban areas)
L. aethiopica	Highlands of Ethiopia, Kenya, and Southern Yemen
L. major	Desert regions of Turkmenistan, Uzbekistan and Kazakhstan, Northern Africa and the Sahara, Iran, Syria, Israel and Jordan
Leishmania mexicana complex	**New World Cutaneous Leishmaniasis**
L. mexicana	Belize, Guatemala, and the Yucatan peninsula
L. pifanoi	Amazon river basin and parts of Brazil and Venezuela
L. amazonensis	Amazon basin of Brazil
L. venezuelensis	Forest areas of Venezuela
L. garnhami	Venezuelan Andes
Leishmania braziliensis complex	**Mucocutaneous Leishmaniasis**
L. braziliensis	Mexico to Argentina
L. panamensis	Panama and Columbia
L. peruviana	Peruvian Andes
L. guyanensis	Guiana and parts of Brazil and Venezuela
Leishmania donovani complex	**Visceral Leishmaniasis**
L. donovani	India, Pakistan, Thailand, parts of Africa and the Peoples Republic of China
L. infantum	Mediterranean area, Europe, Africa, the Near East, and parts of the former Soviet Union
L. chagasi	Central and South America

a local granulomatous response leads to the formation of a crateriform lesion. This primary lesion may enlarge to 2 cm or more in diameter (Figure 7–3), be intensely itchy (pruritic) and become subjected to secondary bacterial infections. *L. tropica* and *L. aethiopica* produce dry lesions while the lesions of *L. major* infection are moist and covered with a serous exudate. These cutaneous lesions generally heal spontaneously but may leave serious scars. It should be noted that contact spread of infection is also possible. Patients may produce multiple sores by scratching and auto-inoculating normal skin. Although very rare, transfusion associated leishmaniasis has been documented.

Recovery depends on the development of a cell mediated immune response. In patients with an impaired immunity or the **anergic** patient who is unable to mount an adequate immune response, diffuse cutaneous leishmaniasis (DCL) may occur. DCL is characterized by the presence of multiple nodular lesions, particularly on the face and limbs. These lesions are loaded with parasites and do not heal spontaneously.

Laboratory Diagnosis

Definitive diagnosis of cutaneous leishmaniasis is made by demonstrating the presence of amastigotes in clinical specimens or the presence of promastigotes from material cultured on NNN media. The specimen

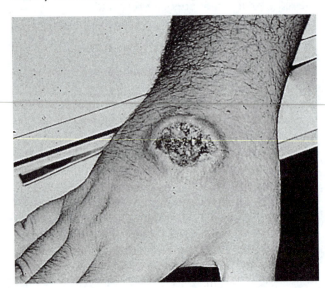

FIG 7–3 Cutaneous leishmaniasis

of choice is an aspiration or biopsy of material taken from an active lesion bed. Giemsa or Wright's stained smears of clinical specimens are examined microscopically for evidence of oval amastigote forms within tissue macrophages (Figure 7–4). When using the Giemsa stain, the cytoplasm of the parasite will stain pale blue and the **kinetoplast** and nucleus will appear red to purple. Species analysis requires more complex testing procedures, such as isoenzyme studies or molecular diagnostic techniques, including polymerase chain reaction (PCR).

The **Montenegro (leishmanin) skin test** is often used for the screening of large populations at risk for infection. Like the tuberculin skin test for tuberculosis, the Montenegro test is a delayed hypersensitivity reaction provoked by a suspension of killed leishmanial promastigotes administered intradermally. A local inflammatory reaction appears at the site of injection usually within 48–72 hours in positive patients.

Serologic tests, including an indirect fluorescent antibody assay, are available through the Centers for Disease Control and Prevention (CDC).

Treatment and Prevention

The drug of choice for the treatment of cutaneous leishmaniasis is sodium stibogluconate (antimony sodium gluconate: Pentostam), which is administered intramuscularly for ten days and may require multiple courses of treatment to induce a clinical response. An alternate drug choice is meglumine antimonate or Glucantime. Amphotericin B and the less toxic antifungal agent ketoconazole have been proven effective in treating patients who are unresponsive to the antimonial compounds or in patients with longstanding infections.

As with other vector transmitted infections, prevention lies in vector and reservoir control. The use of bed netting, insect repellent and residential spraying are effective personal control measures. Rodent control in endemic areas is also effective in reducing transmission. Individuals with active lesions should be promptly treated and their wounds covered to prevent autoinfection and further insect transmission to other individuals.

LEISHMANIA MEXICANA COMPLEX — NEW WORLD CUTANEOUS LEISHMANIASIS

Morphology

The distribution of cutaneous leishmaniasis to the New World extends from southern Texas in the United states, through Mexico, Central and South America. The species most commonly encountered are: *Leishmania mexicana, Leishmania pifanoi, Leishmania amazonensis, Leishmania venezuelensis* and *Leishmania garnhami.*

Leishmania mexicana causes **chiclero ulcer** or Bay sore and is found in Belize, Guatemala and the Yucatan peninsula. *Leishmania pifanoi* is often associated with a more diffuse cutaneous form of the disease and is found in patients from the Amazon river basin, and isolated parts of Brazil and Venezuela. *Leishmania amazonensis* is concentrated in the Amazon basin of Brazil and produces cases of cutaneous and diffuse cutaneous leishmaniasis (DCL). *Leishmania venezuelensis* has been identified as the cause of cutaneous leishmaniasis in more remote forested areas of Venezuela. Venezuelan Andean cutaneous leishmaniasis is caused by *Leishmania garnhami*. The organisms within the *Leishmania mexicana* complex are morphologically indistinguishable, but may be individually identified by monoclonal antibody testing.

The reservoir hosts for these organisms are a diverse group, ranging from forest rodents and opossums to the domestic dog and cat. The primary vector in all cases is a *Lutzomyia* sandfly.

Life cycle

The life cycle of the members of the *Leishmania mexicana* complex is similar to that of other leishmanial organisms (Figure 7–2). Their morphology is indistinguishable. These organisms are transmitted by sandflies of the genus *Lutzomyia*.

Transmission and Pathogenesis

The clinical manifestations of New World cutaneous leishmaniasis are similar to those caused by the Old World species. Promastigote forms are transmitted to the human host by the infected *Lutzomyia* sandfly. The organisms are engulfed by macrophages and multiply intracellularly as amastigotes. The incubation period varies with the species involved.

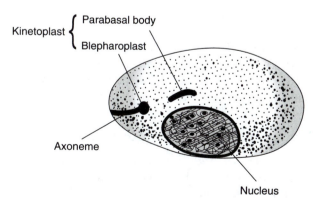

FIG 7–4 Amastigote of *Leishmania* spp.

Leishmania mexicana infection produces a lesion known as chiclero ulcer or Bay sore, which is common among workers who collect chicle gum from the Chicazapote trees in the rainforest in Nicaragua, Guatemala, Belize and the Yucatan peninsula of Mexico.

The clinical manifestation of this form of disease is usually a single cutaneous papule, nodule or ulcer located on the ear or face. Lesions generally heal spontaneously but may cause cartilage destruction and gross disfigurement.

Leishmania pifanoi and *Leishmania amazonensis* may also present with a single lesion, but are more likely to progress to the diffuse cutaneous form of the disease. The majority of patients infected with these species are clustered in the Amazon river basin of Brazil and Venezuela. The clinical presentation of diffuse cutaneous leishmaniasis may be confused with lepromatous leprosy.

Leishmania garnhami and *Leishmania venezuelensis* are both associated with cutaneous leishmaniasis in rural parts of Venezuela. Infection with either organism presents with a solitary lesion that is usually self-limiting.

Laboratory Diagnosis

The diagnosis of cutaneous leishmaniasis must be differentiated from many other infections with similar presentation, including fungal infections, such as sporotrichosis, and bacterial infections, such as impetigo, leprosy and cutaneous tuberculosis. A definitive diagnosis can be made by demonstrating *Leishmania* forms in Giemsa stained smears or cultures of clinical material. Amastigotes will be seen in direct stained smears while promastigotes forms can be obtained from culture on NNN medium. As with the *Leishmania tropica* complex, immunological testing methods are available.

Treatment and Prevention

In most cases, the infections of *Leishmania mexicana* complex are self-limiting and require no specific treatment. If the lesion should endure or threaten cartilaginous structures (ear, nose), then treatment is paramount.

Therapeutic agents used for New World cutaneous leishmaniasis are the same as those discussed previously for the treatment of Oriental sore and Old World leishmaniasis. Antimony compounds are the mainstay, with Pentamidine 2 mg/kg every other day for 7 doses as an useful alternative. Therapeutic success should be monitored with follow-up smears and cultures. Prognosis for most patients is usually favorable.

The same types of preventive measures that are effective in the control of Old World disease are applicable to the New World organisms namely, protective clothing, insect repellents and residential insecticides. Individuals at greatest risk of infection are those who venture into the forested areas to collect chicle gum. Insect repellents applied to the skin and garments along with aerial spraying offer some protection. Treatment of infected individuals will interrupt the spread of disease.

LEISHMANIA BRAZILIENSIS COMPLEX — MUCOCUTANEOUS LEISHMANIASIS

Morphology

There are four members of the *Leishmania braziliensis* complex that have clinical significance: *L. braziliensis*, *L. panamensis*, *L. peruviana*, *L. guyanensis*. These organisms are morphologically indistinguishable upon light microscopy and cause infections throughout the Americas from Mexico to Argentina. As a group, they are responsible for the majority of cases of mucocutaneous leishmaniasis in the New World. The distinguishing feature of these infections is the development of ulcers on or about the oral and nasal mucosa.

L. braziliensis infection, known in Brazil as **espundia**, is the principal cause of mucocutaneous disease in Central and South America. In endemic areas, human infections are **zoonoses** (diseases communicable from animals), acquired as man ventures into the rainforest and becomes part of the transmission cycle between rodents and the sandflies.

L. guyanensis causes disease called **pain bois** (forest yaws) in the Guianas and parts of Brazil and Venezuela. In Panama and Columbia the etiologic agent of mucocutaneous leishmaniasis is *L. panamensis*. In the Peruvian Andes the disease known as **uta** is caused by *L. peruviana*. All species are transmitted by sandflies and all cause considerable morbidity and mortality in the endemic areas.

Life Cycle

The life cycle and morphology of the parasites of *Leishmania braziliensis* complex is similar to those of other *Leishmania* species. The general life cycle is again seen in Figure 7–2.

Transmission and Pathogenesis

Sandflies of the genera *Lutzomyia* and *Psychodopygus* serve as the vector for the organisms of the *Leishmania braziliensis* complex. The primary lesion resulting from the bite of an infected insect tends to develop in the same manner as the Oriental sore. Macrophages ingest the parasites and become heavily laden with replicating amastigotes. Tissue damage ensues as the result of the inflammatory process.

These species of *Leishmania*, however, tend to invade the mucous membranes of the mouth and nasopharynx. The spread is either a direct extension of the primary lesion or metastasis via the bloodstream or lymphatics. The progression of disease may take years, but the resulting disease may produce ulcers that erode soft tissues of the face and palate or form polyp-like appendages in the nasal cavity. Patients commonly present with enlargement of the regional lymph nodes and secondary bacterial infections. Untreated, patients generally succumb to these secondary infections or to starvation if destruction of the oral cavity is extensive.

Diagnosis

As with other cutaneous leishmaniasis, *Leishmania braziliensis* complex infections must be distinguished from other dermal infections. A definitive diagnosis can be made by demonstrating amastigotes of *Leishmania* in Giemsa stained smears of biopsy material from the edge of an active ulcer. Culture methods will produce the promastigote stage. Serologic testing (complement fixation, direct agglutination) and the intradermal reaction (Montenegro skin test) also have diagnostic usefulness.

Treatment and Prevention

Pentavalent sodium antimony (Pentostam) is the treatment of choice for all *Leishmania braziliensis* complex infections. Drugs are administered in the same manner as previously described for Oriental sore. Mucocutaneous infections may be persistent and require a prolonged therapeutic regimen. Cycloguanil pamoate (Camolar) and Amphotericin B (Fungizone) have also been reported effective when administered appropriately. In fact, the approximate cure rate when antimony is used is about 60%, and when Amphotericin B given as 1 mg/kg body weight, intravenously, every other day for 20–30 doses yields a greater than 75% cure rate.

As with New World cutaneous leishmaniasis, those individuals at greatest risk for *Leishmania braziliensis* complex infections are those individuals who frequent the forested habitant of the sandfly. Personal protective measures (protective clothing, insect repellents), vector control, control of reservoir host, and public health educational programs are all effective methods of disease prevention. Prompt treatment of infected individuals also helps to break the cycle of disease transmission.

LEISHMANIA DONOVANI COMPLEX — VISCERAL LEISHMANIASIS

Morphology

Visceral leishmaniasis, also know as **kala azar** or dum-dum fever, is the most severe of the *Leishmania* infections. The causative organisms belong to the *Leishmania donovani* complex, which incorporates *L. donovani*, *L. infantum*, and *L. chagasi*. Again each of the organisms has a distinct geographic distribution. Like the *Leishmania* species previously mentioned in this chapter, *Leishmania donovani* complex organisms parasitize the reticuloendothelial cells. Unlike the previously discussed species, these parasites are viscerotropic. Rather than remaining fixed, infected macrophages disseminate throughout the body.

L. donovani is found widely distributed throughout India, Pakistan, Thailand, parts of Africa, and the People's Republic of China. It is transmitted by *Phlebotomus* sandflies and is generally a disease of juveniles and young adults. In India, man appears to be the only mammalian reservoir, but in other areas, rodents and dogs serve as natural reservoirs.

In the Mediterranean area, Europe, Africa and the near East, as well as parts of the former Soviet Union, *L. infantum* is the predominant species. As its name might imply, infections with this organism occur primarily in young children. Domesticated dogs, other canines and porcupines serve as the natural reservoirs, and the *Phlebotomus* sandfly remains the vector.

Visceral leishmaniasis in the New World (Central and South America) is caused by *L. chagasi*. Foxes and domestic dogs and cats serve as the natural reservoir. Sandflies of the genus *Lutzomyia*, serve as the vector and children are the most susceptible group.

Life cycle

The *Leishmania donovani* complex life cycle is again similar to the *Leishmania* species already discussed. However, there is one noteworthy exception. the infected mononuclear phagocytes do not remain confined to the skin or mucous membranes. Parasitized macrophages are carried by the bloodstream to lymphoid tissue throughout the body, especially to the spleen, liver and bone marrow. Amastigotes multiply in great numbers in these tissues.

Transmission and Pathogenesis

Visceral leishmaniasis is transmitted by sandflies of the genera *Phlebotomus* and *Lutzomyia*. Promastigotes are inoculated into the victim by the insect bite and are subsequently engulfed by tissue macrophages. The onset of disease is generally insidious after a variable incubation period of 3 weeks to 2 years. Rather than remaining fixed, the infected macrophages migrate by lymphatic and hematogenous spread to distant lymphoid tissues throughout the body. For this reason, transmission via blood transfusion is also possible.

Clinically, the patient first presents with a prodrome of headache, malaise, fever, and possible weight loss. Occasionally, abdominal pain may occur. Sometimes the fever may occur in periodic intervals mimicking tertian or quartan malaria. Patients may also experience bouts of diarrhea, consistent with typhoid fever. Physical examination of the affected patient reveals enlargement of the liver and spleen (hepatosplenomegaly) and lymph nodes (lymphadenopathy). In response to the infection, there may be a marked increase in serum globulin levels.

Microscopically, parasitized macrophages may be found in the tissues of the spleen, liver heart, kidneys, lymph nodes, intestines and bone marrow. Rapid proliferation of reticuloendothelial cells within the involved organs leads to organ hypertrophy. Parasitized macrophages may crowd out other hematopoietic cells leading to various degrees of anemia and leukopenia. The infiltration of the intestinal mucosa may result in ulceration and yield malabsorption, and wasting. As the patient becomes more emaciated, the abdominal distention from the hepatosplenomegaly becomes more pronounced. A characteristic hyperpigmentation of the forehead and hands, known in India as kala azar, may also be observed.

The prognosis for untreated cases is poor. The mortality rate can be as high as 95%. Even in chronic cases, death usually occurs from medical complications or bacterial infections within two years of diagnosis. With treatment, the prognosis is usually much better, especially for Indian kala azar. Recovery leads to a lasting immunity. In some patients, a condition called post-kala azar dermal leishmaniasis, or dermal leishmoid, may develop following the treatment with antimony compounds. The clinical presentation of this condition is marked by the appearance of either erythematous or hypopigmented lesions anywhere on the body. A butterfly rash, characteristic of systemic lupus erythematosus, may develop on the malar portion of the face. The dermal lesions, whether a papule or patch, may progress to nodules and resemble lepromatous leprosy. These lesions do contain viable parasites and can serve as a reservoir of infection.

Laboratory Diagnosis

Even when the clinical picture is highly suggestive of kala azar, a definitive diagnosis can only be made by demonstrating the organism. Giemsa stained slides of tissue biopsies from the spleen and liver are often used to demonstrate the diagnostic nonflagellated amastigote stage. The procedure employed to obtain the specimen puts the patient at considerable risk, so bone marrow and lymph node aspirations are often advised. In all incidences, direct examination of stained smears and culture procedures are recommended. Cultured samples will yield promastigote forms. A Giemsa stained buffy coat prep may also reveal intracellular amastigotes.

Patients with visceral leishmaniasis have greatly elevated serum globulin levels. Serologic testing procedures are available for diagnostic purposes. Both the direct agglutination test (DAT) and complement fixation test (CF) are simple and reliable, and available in the endemic areas. Indirect fluorescence and molecular diagnostic techniques are available in more advanced diagnostic laboratories.

The Montenegro (leishmanin) skin test is not reactive in people with active disease, as *Leishmania donovani* complex infection results in a suppression of cell mediated immune responses. The delayed hypersensitivity response becomes reactive following successful treatment.

Treatment and Prevention

The drugs of choice for treating the infections of *Leishmania donovani* complex are pentavalent antimony sodium gluconate (Pentostam) and pentamidine isothionate (Lomidine). The length of therapy is species dependent. Patients with Indian kala azar tend to respond more rapidly to treatment and have the best prognosis. If the disease does not respond to either therapeutic agent, Amphotericin B is used. The highest incidence of treatment failure occurs in African disease. Combination drug regimens exist using either allopurinol or gamma interferon along with Pentostam. These have been shown to be very effective in treating otherwise resistant cases.

Control of *Leishmania donovani* complex infections is best accomplished through the prompt diagnosis and treatment of infected individuals and through reduction of the vector and reservoir populations. The spraying of residential insecticide in homes and sandfly breeding areas effectively interrupts the spread of disease. The personal measures of avoidance of outdoor activities when the sandflies are most active (dusk to dawn), the use of mechanical barriers such as protective clothing, screens and bed netting impregnated with permethrin, and the use of insect repellants liberally applied to the skin continue to be extremely effective measures that are well advised.

SUMMARY

The hemoflagellates are flagellated protozoa that are transmitted by blood-sucking arthropod vectors and infect the tissues and blood of man as well as other mammalian hosts.

The genus *Leishmania* contains several geographically separate species that are responsible for the human disease called leishmaniasis. The organisms are intracellular parasites of the reticuloendothelial cells which are characterized into group complexes based on the migration of infected macrophages. Clinical infections are classified as cutaneous, mucocutaneous or visceral.

Leishmaniasis is a zoonosis transmitted by phlebotomine sandflies with wild rodents and dogs serving as reservoir hosts. Two stages exist in the life cycle. The promastigote can be found in the insect gut and serves as the infective stage. The amastigote is the diagnostic stage found within human cells. The four clinically important group complexes are: the *Leishmania tropica* complex which causes Old World cutaneous leishmaniasis or Oriental sore, the *Leishmania mexicana* complex which causes New World cutaneous leishmaniasis, the *Leishmania braziliensis* complex which causes mucocutaneous leishmaniasis and the *Leishmania donovani* complex which is responsible for visceral leishmaniasis or kala azar. Treatment is generally with antimonial compounds and prevention involves vector and reservoir controls.

REVIEW QUESTIONS

1. The etiologic agent of Oriental sore is:

a. *Leishmania donovani*

b. *Leishmania tropica*

c. *Leishmania braziliensis*

d. *Phlebotomus* and *Lutzomyia*

2. All the clinically significant *Leishmania* species are transmitted by:

a. *Glossina* tsetse fly

b. *Culex* mosquitoes

c. Phlebotomine sandflies

d. Reduviid beetle

3. *Leishmania braziliensis* causes a form of mucocutaneous leishmaniasis in Brazil commonly known as:

a. chiclero ulcer

b. pain bois

c. uta

d. espundia

4. The definitive diagnosis for any of the leishmanial infections is made by finding the parasite in clinical material. The diagnostic stage of the organism is the:

a. amastigote

b. epimastigote

c. promastigote

d. trypomastigote

5. The common name for *Leishmania donovani* infection in India is:

a. Oriental sore

b. espundia

c. kala azar

d. uta

6. In the human host, *Leishmania* spp. tend to proliferate within:

a. reticuloendothelial cells

b. retinal cells

c. renal cells

d. red blood cells

7. All of the following are true regarding hemoflagellates, *except*:

a. they are vectored by blood-sucking insects.

b. they are blood and tissue parasites of human hosts.

c. they include species of the genera *Leishmania* and *Trypanosoma*.

d. they have an amastigote, promastigote and cyst stage in their life cycle.

8. A patient who is anergic is:

a. capable of complete recovery

b. slow and listless

c. unable to mount an immune response

d. capable of having lasting immunity

9. *Leishmania peruviana* is the etiologic agent of:

   a. espundia

   b. uta

   c. pain bois

   d. chiclero ulcer

10. The treatment of choice for *Leishmania mexicana* infection is:

    a. amphotericin B

    b. antimony sodium gluconate

    c. pentamidine isothionate

    d. no treatment, lesions are self-limiting

CASE STUDY

A 24-year old white female presents in a Boston emergency room with complaints of intermittent bouts of fever, anorexia, and abdominal pain. The patient's history revealed that the young woman had recently returned from Africa where she had just completed a two year commitment with the Peace Corps. Her symptoms had become progressively worse over the last four weeks. Upon physical examination, the physician noted marked enlargement of the liver, splenomegaly and generalized lymphadenopathy. A complete blood count (CBC) revealed pancytopenia.

After studying the original laboratory data the physician ordered a bone marrow aspiration/biopsy and serum protein electrophoresis. When the specimens were received in the laboratory, the clinical laboratory scientist made slides from the bone marrow aspirate and prepared the serum specimen for processing. The Giemsa stained slides contained numerous macrophages filled with oval shaped parasitic forms about 2–3 micrometers in length. The organisms appeared to have one nucleus, a parabasal body and an axoneme. The patients serum globulins were markedly elevated.

Questions

1. What disease does the physician suspect?

2. What parasite might be suggested from the patients travel history?

3. What form of the organism was seen in the Giemsa stained bone marrow smears?

4. What vector is responsible for the disease transmission?

5. What is the infective stage of the parasite?

6. What is the recommended treatment?

▶ BIBLIOGRAPHY

Addy, M., & Nandy, A. (1992). Ten years of kala-azar in west Bengal, Part 1. Did post kala azar dermal leishmaniasis initiate the outbreak in 24 Parganas. *W.H.O. Bulletin, 70,* 341–346.

Beaver, P. C., Jung, R. C., & Cupp, E. W. (1984). *Clinical parasitology* (9th ed.). Philadelphia: Lea & Febiger.

Chance, M. L. (1981). The six diseases of WHO: Leishmaniasis. *British Medical Journal, 2,*1245–1247.

Falcoff, E. (1994). Clinical healing of antimony-resistant cutaneous and mucocutaneous leishmaniasis following the combined administration of interferon-γ and pentavalent antimonial compounds. *Transactions of the Royal Society of Tropical Medicine and Hygiene, 88,* 95–97.

Garcia, L. S. & Bruckner, D. A. (1993). *Diagnostic medical parasitology* (2nd ed.). Washington, DC: American Society of Microbiology.

Gustafson, T. L., Reed, C. M., McGreevy, P. B. Pappas, M. C., Fox, J. C., & Lawyer, P. G. (1985). Human cutaneous leishmaniasis acquired in Texas. *American Journal of Tropical Medicine and Hygiene, 34,* 58–63.

Lainson, R. & Shaw, J. J. (1978). Epidemiology and ecology of leishmaniasis in Latin America. *Nature, 273,* 595–600.

Lightner, L. K., Chulay, J. D., & Bryceson, A. D. M. (1983). Comparison of microscopy and culture in the detection of *Leishmania donovani* from splenic aspirates. *Ameri-*

can Journal of Tropical Medicine and Hygiene, 32, 296–299.

Markell, E. K., John, D. K. & Krotoski, W. A. (1999). *Medical parasitology* (8th ed.). Philadelphia: W. B. Saunders.

Sadick, M. (1984). Development of cellular immunity in cutaneous leishmaniasis due to *Leishmania tropica*. *Journal of Infectious Diseases, 150,* 135–138.

Shimeld, L.A. (1999). *Essentials of diagnostic microbiology.* Albany, NY: Delmar Publishers.

World Health Organization. (1990). *Control of the leishmaniases.* W.H.O. Technical Report (Ser. No. 793). Geneva: World Health Organization.

Zeibig, E. A. (1997). *Clinical parasitology.* Philadelphia: W. B. Saunders.

CHAPTER EIGHT

Blood and Tissue Flagellates: *Trypanosoma* species

LEARNING OBJECTIVES

After reading and studying this chapter, the student should be able to:

- Define the key terms.
- For each hemoflagellate cited, state the geographic distribution.
- Briefly describe the life cycle of each hemoflagellate cited.
- Identify the hosts and vector for each organism.
- List the infective stage and diagnostic stage of each organism.
- Describe the mechanism of pathogenesis for each organism.
- Discuss the clinical presentation of each disease.
- Identify means of treatment and prevention for each parasite.

KEY TERMS

Aphasia (ay-FAY-zee-ah)
Cardiomegaly (KAR-dee-oh-MEG-ah-lee)
Chagoma (shag-OH-ma)
Chancre (SHANG-ker)
Congenital transmission (kon-JEN-i-tal)
Dyspnea (DISp-nee-ah)
Edema (e-DEE-ma)
Erythema (ER-i-THEE-ma)
Febrile (FEE-brile)

Glomerulonephritis (glo-MER-u-lo-ne-FRI-tis)
Histiocyte (HIST-ee-oh-CYTE)
Lymphadenopathy (lymph-AD-en-OH-pa-thee)
Kerandel's sign (ker-AN-del-s/sign)
Kissing bug (KISS-ing/bug)
Myalgia (mi-al-jee-ah)
Myocarditis (MY-o-kar-DI-tis)
Parasitemia (para-sit-ee-mia)

Pruritus (pru-RI-tis)
Reduviid bug (re-DO-vid/bug)
Romana's sign (roh-MA-na-s/sign)
Somnolence (SOM-no-lens)
Tsetse fly (*Glossina*) (TSET-see)
Triatomid bug (TRI-ah-TO-mid/bug)
Winterbottom's sign (WIN-ter-BOT-tom-s/sign)

INTRODUCTION

The genus *Trypanosoma* has an abundance of species that have been found to parasitize the blood and tissues of vertebrate hosts and are called hemoflagellates. Although very few species are a threat to humans, all share the characteristic of a complex life cycle which includes a blood sucking invertebrate as an intermediate host and a variety of life cycle stages that are profoundly different from those of the intestinal flagellates (Figure 8–1). At some point in their life cycle, all flagellates of the genus *Trypanosoma* assume the characteristic trypomastigote structure. The body of the parasite elongates into a spindle shape that tapers at both ends. The nucleus is generally centrally located. A kinetoplast at the posterior end gives rise to an undulating membrane, which runs the length of the trypanosome. A single free flagellum is present at the anterior end.

The species of the genus *Trypanosoma* that are medically significant to humans are represented, on the one hand, by *Trypanosoma brucei* variants *gambiense* and *rhodesiense*, which are associated with African sleeping sickness, and on the other hand, by *Trypanosoma cruzi* which causes Chagas' disease or American trypanosomiasis. These two distinctly different forms of trypanosomes vary considerably in their mode of transmission, geographic distribution and clinical presentations (Table 8–1).

TRYPANOSOMA BRUCEI GAMBIENSE

Morphology

African sleeping sickness occurs in two geographically different parts of Africa and has two clinically distinct presentations. However, the causative organisms are morphologically indistinguishable and share a common life cycle (see Figure 8–2).

The two species of trypanosomes which are pathogenic for humans in Africa, namely *Trypanosoma gambiense* and *Trypanosoma rhodesiense,* are part of the group complex *brucei-gambiense-rhodesiense. Trypanosoma brucei* is thought to be the wild type or ancestral form which infects primarily wild game animals. Over time, the parasite has adapted to the human host giving rise to the two variants: *T. gambiense* and *T. rhodesiense.*

Cases of African sleeping sickness can be found throughout a large area of Africa known as the "tsetse fly belt." The **Glossina (tsetse) fly** (Figure 8–3) serves as the intermediate host and vector for both forms of the disease. The threat of trypanosomiasis has virtually excluded habitation by men and domestic animals from almost one-fourth of the African continent.

Gambian trypanosomiasis, caused by *T. b. gambiense,* can be found in the wet lowlands and rainforest of West and Central Africa where the tsetses breed in the moist areas around riverbanks. The infection has a chronic course which ends with central nervous involvement and death after several years of durations.

Life Cycle

Transmission of *Trypanosoma brucei gambiense* from host to host occurs through the bite of an infected tsetse fly. The two species of fly that serve as intermediate host and vector for the Gambian disease are *Glossina palpalis* and *Glossina tachinoides.* Both male and female flies bite man and may serve as a vector.

Parasites are ingested by the fly when it takes a blood meal on an infected mammal, typically human or ungulate (hoofed animals). Within the fly, the parasite begins to multiply. It undergoes several developmental stages within the gut and salivary glands of the insect. The fly becomes infective once the metacyclic trypomastigotes develop in the salivary glands. As the fly takes its next blood meal, saliva containing the trypanosomes is injected into the unsuspecting victim. The entire cycle within the insect takes about 3 weeks.

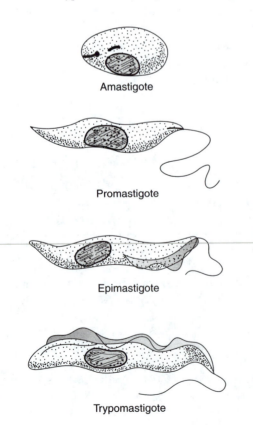

Amastigote

Promastigote

Epimastigote

Trypomastigote

FIG 8–1 Morphologic forms seen in hemoflagellates

TABLE 8-1 ▶ Human Trypanosome Infections

Organism	Disease	Vector	Transmission
Trypanosoma brucei gambiense	West African sleeping sickness	*Glossina* — tsetse fly	"Bite" — saliva
Trypanosoma brucei rhodesiense	East African sleeping sickness	*Glossina* — tsetse fly	"Bite" — saliva
Trypanosoma cruzi	American trypanosomiasis or Chagas' disease	Reduviid bug (kissing bug or cone nose bug)	Feces of infected reduviid bug into the "bite"
Trypanosoma rangeli	*T. rangeli* infection	Reduviid bug (kissing bug or cone nose bug)	"Bite" — saliva

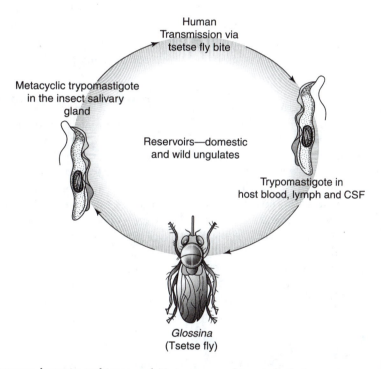

FIG 8–2 Life cycle of *Trypanosoma brucei gambiense* and *Trypanosoma brucei rhodesiense*

Once the parasite is passed to its new mammalian host, it begins to multiply locally in the tissues around the bite site. A **parasitemia** follows as the parasites gain entry to the bloodstream and lymphatic system. Eventually trypomastigotes invade the central nervous system and begin to proliferate, consequently leading to the associated signs and symptoms of the disease.

Trypomastigote forms continue to circulate in the bloodstream of the infected host and may be ingested by the next biting *Glossina*. Thus, the cycle continues. Humans serve as the main reservoir for *Trypanosoma brucei gambiense*, but domestic animals, as well as wild animals, may also serve as hosts.

Transmission and Pathogenesis

The typical mode of transmission of *Trypanosoma brucei gambiense* is through the bite of an infected tsetse fly. On rare occasions, the parasite has been acquired through blood transfusion, organ transplant or **congenital transmission** (from pregnant mother to fetus).

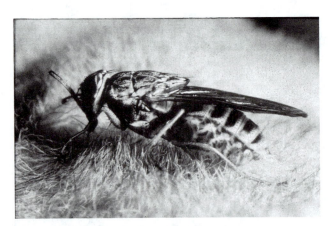

FIG 8–3 Tsetse fly feeding. (Courtesy of the World Health Organization, TDR Image Library, photograph by Douglas Fisher, 1991.)

Infection is characterized by three progressive stages. Following the bite of the infected insect vector, there is an asymptomatic incubation period, which may range from a few days to several weeks. The incubation period tends to be shorter for non-Africans than for African natives. During that time, the parasite begins to multiply locally. In many cases, the local inflammation leads to the development of a painful ulcerative lesion, called a trypanosomal **chancre** at the insect bite site (Figure 8–4). Even as the incubation period is ending, the patient may be without symptoms.

The second stage is marked by hematogenous spread of the parasites and the involvement of the lymphatic system. Trypomastigotes may be seen in the routine blood film examination. With the invasion of the lymph nodes, the patient experiences the first distinct symptoms: **febrile** (fever) attacks followed by afebrile periods. The fever is generally accompanied by headache, malaise, weakness, anorexia, and night sweats. Once the lymph nodes have become involved, it is uncommon to see trypomastigotes in the peripheral blood, except during febrile periods. Glandular

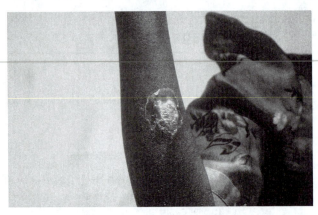

FIG 8–4 A patient with chancre, a primary symptom of sleeping sickness infection. (Courtesy of World Health Organization, TDR Image Library, photograph by Dr. P. de Raadt, Uganda, 1991.)

enlargement and **lymphadenopathy** (enlargement of the lymph nodes) are also quite common. One of the cardinal symptoms of this stage of disease is the enlargement of the postcervical chain of lymph nodes, which is known as **Winterbottom's sign**.

The glandular stage is also marked by bouts of **erythematous** (red) rash, **pruritus** (severe itching), localized joint **edema** (swelling) and delayed sensation to pain (**Kerandel's sign**). Trypomastigotes may be demonstrated in lymph node aspirations. In some cases, patients may experience a spontaneous recovery prior to the development of overt central nervous symptoms.

There is a gradual progression of symptoms to the meningoencephalitic stage of infection with *T. b. gambiense*. Frank expression of central nervous system involvement may take from six months to a year after the onset of first symptoms. The patient's health deteriorates with increased fatigue, mental dullness, apathy, diminished motor control, **somnolence** (excessive sleepiness) and emaciation. Trypomastigotes may be seen in the patient's spinal fluid. Sleepiness progresses to coma and eventual death. All symptoms are the result of damage within the CNS.

Laboratory Diagnosis

For patients with the correct history and exhibiting the characteristic symptoms, the diagnosis of West African sleeping sickness depends on the demonstration of trypomastigotes in blood, lymph node aspirates, bone marrow or spinal fluid specimens. Direct wet mounts can be examined for motile trypanosomes or fixed Giemsa stained smears may be examined for the presence of parasites (Figure 8–5). Concentration techniques, such as centrifugation, may increase the chance for early detection in spinal fluid analysis. For blood samples, trypanosomes concentrate in the buffy coat layer of a spun hematocrit specimen. Serologic techniques have been adapted for screening and epidemiologic surveys of *Trypanosoma brucei gambiense*. One such test is the Card Agglutination Trypanosomiasis Test (CATT)

Treatment and Prevention

Successful treatment of West African trypanosomiasis depends on early patient management. Once the central nervous system becomes involved the prognosis is poor. All the drugs that are currently available for the treatment of trypanosomiasis have some degree of toxicity. Generally, the least toxic drug is chosen for the primary treatment unless evidence exists for CNS invasion. The three drugs that are used most commonly are pentamidine, suramin and melarsoprol.

Pentamidine isothionate usually cures Gambian trypanosomiasis in the hemolymphatic stage of infection.

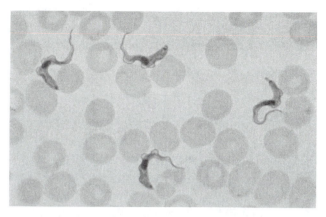

FIG 8–5 *Trypanosoma brucei gambiense* in a Giemsa stained blood smear. (Courtesy of the Centers for Disease Control and Prevention, Public Health Image Library.)

It is administered by intramuscular injection and is not effective for later stages of the illness because of its inability to cross the "blood-brain barrier."

Suramin is also effective only in the early stages of disease before central nervous involvement. It is administered intravenously and has more toxic side effects than pentamidine. One advantage is that suramin may be prescribed during pregnancy.

Melarsoprol, which is a trivalent arsenic compound, is much more toxic than pentamidine or suramin but is the drug of choice for the treatment of late stage Gambian sleeping sickness. It is administered intravenously and can effectively penetrate the blood-brain barrier.

Methods of prevention revolve around control, management, and avoidance of the insect vector. Clearing of the vegetation where tsetse flies breed and wide use of insecticides have met with some success in endemic areas. Political unrest in Africa, however, has made strict controls and continuous monitoring difficult.

Travelers to endemic areas are encouraged to wear long-sleeved protective clothing. Tsetse flies are attracted to bright and dark colors; therefore, thick khaki or olive drab clothing is preferred. The use of bed nets and insect repellant is also recommended.

TRYPANOSOMA BRUCEI RHODESIENSE

Morphology

Trypanosoma brucei rhodesiense is the cause of East African sleeping sickness. First isolated from a patient in Rhodesia, the organism has a geographical distribution over portions of Central and Eastern Africa. *Trypanosoma brucei rhodesiense*, like *T. b. gambiense*, is transmitted by the bite of an infected tsetse fly. Rhodesian trypanosomiasis has a similar clinical presentation to that of the Gambian form of the disease but is char-

acterized by a more fulminant course and severe symptoms. The incidence of Rhodesian sleeping sickness is far less than for Gambian disease but, if left untreated, death will ensue within several weeks to months rather than years.

Life Cycle

The life cycle of *Trypanosoma brucei rhodesiense* is similar to *Trypanosoma brucei gambiense* in man and its *Glossina* vector (Figure 8–2). The reservoir hosts are thought to be wild game animals, particularly antelope and domestic cattle.

Transmission and Pathogenesis

Trypanosoma brucei rhodesiense is transmitted between humans by the bite of an infected tsetse fly. The species of fly acting as vector in this part of Africa are *Glossina pallidipes*, *G. morsitans*, and *G. swynnertoni*.

In man, *T. b. rhodesiense* produces a more acute form of trypanosomiasis than *T. b. gambiense*. The stages of disease and symptomology parallel those of the Gambian infection; however, the disease progresses rapidly and has a much shorter clinical course. The incubation period for Rhodesian disease is shortened by the abrupt onset of febrile episodes. During periods of fever, trypomastigotes are found in the peripheral blood in large numbers. Lymphadenopathy and Winterbottom's sign are less pronounced in this form of the disease. Symptoms of **glomerulonephritis** (inflammation of the glomerulus of the kidney) and **myocarditis** (inflammation of the heart) may be evident. In untreated cases the patient typically dies before displaying the prolonged somnolence that characterizes "sleeping sickness" and indicates marked CNS involvement. The entire course of disease may take only 9 to 12 months.

Laboratory Diagnosis

The diagnosis of East African trypanosomiasis is made in the same manner as Gambian trypanosomiasis. The trypomastigotes are readily found in the peripheral blood during febrile episodes, and fixed, Giemsa stained blood smears effectively demonstrate the parasite. Lymph node aspirations and spinal fluid may also be diagnostic.

Treatment and Prevention

The same drug regimens are recommended for the treatment of both Rhodesian and Gambian sleeping sickness. If treatment is initiated early in the disease, suramin is effective and the patient's prognosis is usually good. Melarsoprol is prescribed for patients with more advanced disease. Pentamidine is used as a prophylaxis during epidemic outbreaks.

As with the Gambian infection, the key to prevention of *T. b. rhodesiense* infection lies with vector control. There is no vaccine available nor is there a recommended routine preventive drug.

TRYPANOSOMA CRUZI

Morphology

Trypanosoma cruzi is the cause of American trypanosomiasis or Chagas' disease, named for the Brazilian medical student, Carlos Chagas, who discovered the parasite in 1909. It is a zoonotic infection with a wide geographic distribution ranging from the southern portion of the United States, throughout Mexico, Central America and South America. The greatest incidence of disease is in Brazil. Unlike other trypanosomes that infect man, this organism has an intracellular amastigote stage that develops in cardiac, brain, and visceral tissues, in addition to the trypomastigotes in the peripheral circulation.

T. cruzi is transmitted by an insect that has a variety of names in the native population, including **reduviid bug**, **kissing bug**, or **triatomid bug** (Figure 8–6). Generally the vector is of the genus *Panstrongylus* or *Triatoma*. These insects have adapted to a life in close association with their human and mammalian hosts. By day, reduviid bugs live within the mud and thatch wall of dwellings and emerge at night to feed on human blood (Figure 8–7). The parasite develops within the gut of the insect and is subsequently passed as the insect defecates while feeding. The sleeping victim is often unaware, as the insect characteristically bites painlessly about the face. Young children have the highest rate of infection.

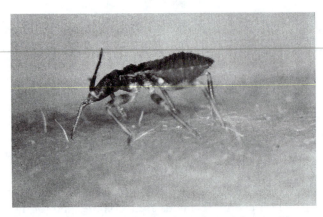

FIG 8–6 Triatomid bug biting. (Courtesy of the World Health Organization, TDR Image Library, photograph by Sinclair Stammers, 2000.)

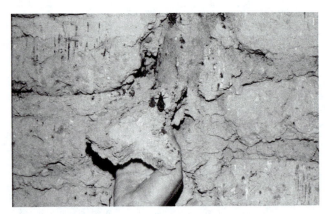

FIG 8–7 Mud walled dwelling. (Courtesy of the World Health Organization, TDR Image Library.)

Life Cycle

Trypanosoma cruzi has two phases in its life cycle, as seen in Figure 8–8. One phase takes place within the human or mammalian reservoir host and the other within the insect vector. Transmission to a human host most frequently occurs as an infected reduviid bug defecates during a blood meal and the infective metacyclic trypomastigotes, present in the feces, penetrate the skin as the bite wound is rubbed or scratched. In many cases the bite is near the eye or lip where cutaneous tissue transforms from keratinized to non-keratinized stratified squamous mucous membranes. The infective stage of the parasite gains entry easily through the mucous membranes. Less commonly, transmission via blood transfusion, transplacental route, or accidental ingestion of an infected insect has been documented.

The invading trypanomastigotes actively enter **histiocytes** (phagocytic cells of the reticuloendothelial system) and other tissue cells. Within these cells the parasites transform into amastigotes and multiply by binary fission. In Giemsa stained smears, the amastigote forms are round or ovoid, 1.5 to 4 micrometers in diameter, and contain a large red nucleus with a dark staining rod-shaped kinetoplast. The parasites may transitionally pass through a promastigote, epimastigote and trypomastigote form within the parasitized cell. The infected host cell eventually ruptures releasing new parasites to infect additional host cells. The repeating cycle of cell invasion and rupture activates a localized cellular inflammatory response with progression to the lymph nodes.

Trypomastigotes periodically appear in the peripheral circulation as the infection spreads beyond the regional lymph nodes. Giemsa stained blood films demonstrate "U" or "C" shaped trypomastigotes that average 20 micrometers in length (Figure 8–9). The nucleus is centrally located and the kinetoplast is large and positioned at the posterior end. A delicate slender undulating membrane runs the length of the organism and extends as a free flagellum at the anterior end. It is this trypomastigote form that is ingested by the reduviid bug when it takes a blood meal.

In the transmitting insect, *T. cruzi* is most commonly seen in the epimastigote stage in the mid-gut and transforms into the metacyclic trypomastigote which is excreted in the bug's feces. The metacyclic trypomastigotes are infective to humans or reservoir hosts when they are mechanically admitted to the bite wound or breaks in the skin. The complete life cycle of *Trypanosoma cruzi* is shown in Figure 8–8.

Transmission and Pathogenesis

The night feeding reduviid bug finds its next victim and takes a blood meal. Most commonly, the human victim is a child under the age of 5 years. As the insect bites, it deposits infective fecal material near the bite wound or onto nearby mucous membranes. The bite wound becomes intensely pruritic (itchy) and *T. cruzi* is scratched or rubbed into the bite wound. An average incubation period of 7 to 14 days ensues. An acute local inflammatory reaction results as the organism is carried by the lymphatics to the regional lymph nodes. The invading organisms enter fat cells and are ingested by histiocytes and macrophages where they transform into amastigotes and multiply.

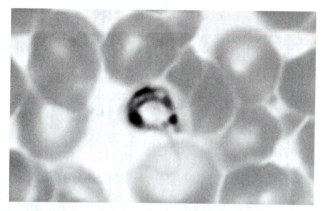

FIG 8–9 Trypomastigote of *Trypanosoma cruzi* in a Giemsa stained blood smear. (Courtesy of the Centers for Disease Control and Prevention, Public Health Image Library.)

At the site of infection, an acute inflammatory response blocks lymphatic flow and produces an erythematous primary lesion called a **chagoma**. Although the lesion can occur anywhere on the body, it usually is found on the face. This painful indurated lesion may take 2–3 months to resolve. Trypomastigotes and amastigotes may be aspirated from the chagoma. Many patients develop conjunctivitis and unilateral edema of the face and eyelids that is known as **Romana's sign**.

As the infection progresses beyond the regional lymph nodes, the symptoms of generalized infection

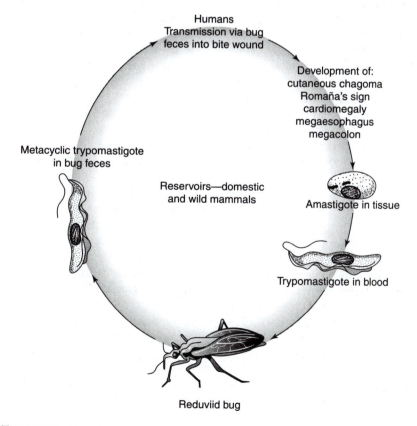

FIG 8–8 Life cycle of *Trypanosoma cruzi*

appear. This corresponds to the appearance of try-pomastigotes in the blood with systemic invasion of other organ systems. Acute Chagas' disease is characterized by bouts of fever and chills, generalized malaise, **myalgia** (muscles aches) and fatigue. Glandular enlargement and an abdominal rash may also occur. Acute symptoms appear in 4 days to 2 weeks following the insect bite.

The most severe symptoms are seen in very young children where the course of infection is abbreviated and the signs and symptoms of central nervous system involvement appear early in the infection. Amastigotes may be seen in meningeal tissues. Marked myocarditis and damage to the CNS lead to eventual death within a few days or weeks.

The progress and outcome of acute Chagas' disease is dependent on the age of the patient, and the virulence of the strain of *T. cruzi*. As previously stated, in young children the disease generally runs a more fulminant course ending in death. Other patients may experience complete recovery following the acute stage, but most will progress to the chronic Chagas' disease. Many of these cases will be asymptomatic for an extended period of time.

The symptoms of chronic Chagas' disease are dependent on the organ system affected and the extent of cellular damage. Myocardial cells are invaded and destroyed leading to **cardiomegaly** (enlargement of the heart), electro-cardiographic irregularities and peripheral signs of congestive heart failure (**dyspnea** or shortness of breath, ankle swelling and elevated central venous pressure). Destruction of ganglionic cells innervating the digestive tract leads to diminished peristaltic activity, and an inability to swallow with eventual gross enlargement of the esophagus (megaesophagus) and colon (megacolon). Central nervous system involvement causes signs of agitation, disorientation, **aphasia** (inability to coherently speak), and sometimes coma. The prognosis is poor if left untreated.

Laboratory Diagnosis

Trypanosoma cruzi infection should be suspected in any patient who has a history of being in an endemic area and who develops a clinical presentation which may include: febrile episodes, enlarged lymph nodes, chagoma, Romana's sign, myocarditis or CNS and digestive problems. The definitive diagnosis of Chagas' disease, however, does depend on the demonstration of the parasites in the blood or tissue or by positive serologic testing.

During the acute stage of infection, particularly in young children, trypomastigotes may be recovered from the peripheral blood during febrile episodes. Giemsa stained blood smears aid in the identification of the parasites. As the disease progresses, the organism is seen less frequently in the peripheral circulation. Blood cultures or animal inoculation may be helpful. Stained preparations of lymph node aspirates may demonstrate the amastigote form of *T. cruzi*.

Xenodiagnosis is a technique that has proven successful even later in the disease progression when blood films appear negative. Laboratory bred reduviid bugs are allowed to feed on the patient being tested. If organisms are present in the blood meal, they will multiply in the insect gut and be recovered from the gut contents.

A variety of serologic tests are also available for the diagnosis. The most commonly used methods include: complement fixation (CF), enzyme immunoassays (EIA), and indirect immunofluorescent assay (IIF). Polymerase chain reaction (PCR) testing procedures and an ELISA (enzyme-linked immunosorbant assay) that can detect *T. cruzi* antigen in urine have also been described.

Treatment and Prevention

The drug of choice for the treatment of *T. cruzi* infection is nifurtimox, also known as Lampit or Bayer 2502. This agent can be administered orally over a prolonged course of treatment but is not indicated during pregnancy. Allupurinol and benznidazole may also be prescribed.

The pathology or condition produced by this disease must be treated independently. Cardiac abnormalities may require diuretic treatment or the installation of a pacemaker. Megaesophagus and megacolon may respond to medication but usually require a surgical intervention.

The prevention of Chagas' disease requires a combination effort: the education of the endemic population and eradication of the triatomid vector. Socioeconomic conditions greatly affect the epidemiology of Chagas' disease. Generally, the poorest segments of the population are affected. Insect control involves the repeated application of insecticide to the roof and walls of thatched dwellings. The answer lies in the upgrading of home construction to eliminate cracks and crevices where the insect resides. Education programs designed to target individuals in endemic areas have helped to raise awareness about the disease, its mode of transmission (especially the role of the reduviid bug), and means of prevention. Additional research is ongoing for the development of an effective vaccine.

TRYPANOSOMA RANGELI

Morphology

Human infections with *Trypanosoma rangeli* have been reported with the same geographic range as *Trypanosoma cruzi*: namely Brazil, Venezuela, Columbia, Panama, El Salvador, Costa Rica, Honduras and Guatemala. Unlike *T. cruzi*, *Trypanosoma rangeli* produces asymptomatic infections with no evidence of pathological changes or disease. *Trypanosoma rangeli* is transmitted by the bite of the reduviid bug, *Rhodius prolixus*. The organisms are passed to the host in the insect's saliva. However, trypomastigotes may be identified in blood films throughout the course of the infection.

A definitive diagnosis of *T. rangeli* infections is based on the identification of trypomastigote forms in Giemsa stained blood smears. They average 30 micrometers in length and, in contrast to *T. cruzi*, have a small kinetoplast.

SUMMARY

The hemoflagellates are flagellated protozoa that are transmitted by blood-sucking arthropod vectors and infect the tissues and blood of man as well as other mammalian hosts. The *Trypanosoma* are hemoflagellates that have crescent or spindle-shaped cell structures with an undulating membrane and a unipolar flagellum. The medically important species are capable of causing trypanosomiasis.

African sleeping sickness is caused by organisms of the *Trypanosoma brucei-gambiense-rhodesiense* complex. These morphologically indistinguishable organisms are transmitted by the bite of the tsetse fly and invade the blood, lymphatics and the central nervous system of the human host. *T. b. gambiense*, the cause of West African or Gambian trypanosomiasis produces a chronic infection of the CNS. *T. b. rhodesiense*, the cause of East African or Rhodesian trypanosomiasis produces an infection with an acute or fulminant course. Clinical presentation includes fever, enlargement of the lymph nodes, joint swelling, fatigue, anorexia, somnolence and coma. Treatment with suramin or melarsoprol has varied success.

Trypanosoma cruzi is the etiologic agent of American trypanosomiasis or Chagas' disease. The infective stage is carried in the gut of the reduviid or kissing bug, and transmitted in the feces deposited on the skin or mucous membranes as the insect feeds. A local inflammatory response at the site of the infection leads to the development of a chagoma. As the organism disseminates, the heart, digestive organs and brain become involved. Acute and chronic forms of the illness exist. Treatment with nifurtimox is recommended.

REVIEW QUESTIONS

1. The tsetse fly (genus *Glossina*) serves as the vector for:
   a. *Leishmania donovani*
   b. *Trypanosoma brucei gambiense*
   c. *Trypanosoma cruzi*
   d. *Plasmodium falciparum*

2. Given the information: protozoan pathogen, spindle-shaped with flagellum, tsetse fly, progressive debilitation, and coma, one of the following applies:
   a. Chagas' disease
   b. toxoplasmosis
   c. trypanosomiasis
   d. malaria

3. The patient presents in the emergency room with a history of Peace Corps work in Brazil, cardiac arrhythmia, enlarged colon and esophagus. The most likely diagnosis is:
   a. Chagas' disease
   b. toxoplasmosis
   c. trypanosomiasis
   d. malaria

4. West African trypanosomiasis is caused by:
   a. *Trypanosoma rangeli*
   b. *Trypanosoma cruzi*
   c. *Trypanosoma brucei rhodesience*
   d. *Trypanosoma brucei gambiense*

5. All human hemoflagellate parasites are transmitted by:

a. tsetse flies

b. arthropod vectors

c. sand flies

d. mosquitos

6. The raised, red, primary lesion of *Trypanosoma cruzi* infection is called a/an:

a. granuloma

b. chancre

c. chagoma

d. ulcer

7. The drug of choice for the treatment of African sleeping sickness is:

a. Amphotericin B

b. Lampit

c. Nifurtimox

d. Melarsoprol

8. *Trypanosoma cruzi* is transmitted by the:

a. mosquito

b. reduviid bug

c. sandfly

d. tsetse fly

9. Chronic Chagas' disease is characterized by all of the following, *except*:

a. megacolon

b. megaesophagus

c. blindness

d. myocarditis

10. *Trypanosoma cruzi* and *Trypanosoma rangeli* infections have an overlapping geographic distribution. A differential diagnosis may be made based on symptomology and identification of the parasite. Infections with *Trypanosoma rangeli* are generally:

a. asymptomatic

b. acute

c. chronic

d. fatal

CASE STUDY

A 26-year old white male presents in the emergency room with general symptoms of malaise, anorexia, and intermittent bouts of low-grade fever. The patient's primary complaint was the occurrence of palpitations. A patient history revealed that the man had spent one year in missionary service for his church. He was responsible for teaching English in a small, remote village in the Amazon basin of Brazil.

Physical examination of the patient revealed a body temperature of 101 degrees F, a heart rate of 110 beats per minute (tachycardia) and a respiratory rate of 24 respirations per minute. The physician ordered an ECG, CBC, cardiac enzymes and a chest X-ray. The remarkable lab findings included an abnormal ECG with frequent premature ventricular complexes, enlarged cardiac silhouette on X-ray, and anemia. Giemsa stained blood films were ordered.

Questions

1. Based on the patient history and clinical findings, what parasite is suspected?

2. What is the name given to the infection?

3. Describe the form of the parasite that was found in the patient's blood.

4. Name the treatment of choice for this disease.

▶ BIBLIOGRAPHY

Beaver, P.C., Jung, R. C., & Cupp, E. W. (1984). *Clinical parasitology* (9th ed.). Philadelphia: Lea & Febiger.

Foulkes, J. R. (1981). The six diseases of WHO: Human trypanosomiasis in Africa. *British Medical Journal, 2,* 1172–1174.

Garcia, L. S. & Bruckner, D. A. (1993). *Diagnostic medical parasitology* (2nd ed.). Washington, DC: American Society of Microbiology.

Jordan, A. M. (1978). Principles of the eradication or control of tsetse flies. *Nature, 273,* 607–609.

Lanham, S. M. (1977). Field diagnosis of trypanosomiasis: protozoological methods in the field diagnosis of try-panosomiasis. *Transactions of the Royal Society of Tropical Medicine and Hygiene, 71,* 8–10.

Markell, E. K., John, D. K. & Krotoski, W. A. (1999). *Medical parasitology* (8th ed.). Philadelphia: W. B. Saunders.

Sousa, O. E. & Johnson, C. M. (1971). Frequency and distribution of *Trypanosoma cruzi* and *Trypanosoma rangeli* in the Republic of Panama. *American Journal of Tropical Medicine and Hygiene, 20,* 405–410.

Shimeld, L. A. (1999). *Essentials of diagnostic microbiology.* Albany, NY: Delmar Publishers.

CHAPTER NINE
Intestinal Sporozoa

OUTLINE

INTESTINAL *COCCIDIA*

Cryptosporidium parvum
(KRIP-to-spor-ID-ee-um PAR-vum)
Isospora belli (eye-SOS-por-a BELL-eye)
Sarcocystis species (SAR-ko-SIST-is)

Cyclospora cayetanensis
(SI-klo-SPOR-a KAY-et-an-EN-sis)
INTESTINAL *MICROSPORIDIA*
(MY-cro-SPOR-Id-ee-a)

LEARNING OBJECTIVES

After reading and studying this chapter, the student should be able to:

- List the clinically significant coccidia found in humans.
- List and describe characteristics used to identify coccidia of clinical significance.
- Describe the life cycles of *C. parvum, I. belli, Sarcocystis* species, and *C. cayetanensis*.
- Describe the transmission and pathogenesis of each coccidian parasite described.

- Discuss the laboratory diagnosis, treatment and prevention of the coccian protozoans described.
- Describe the morphology and life cycle of microsporidia of clinical significance.
- Describe the transmission and pathogenesis of the microsporidian protozoans of interest to man.
- Discuss the laboratory diagnosis, treatment and prevention of infection with microsporidian protozoans.

KEY TERMS

Macrogamete
(MA-kro-GAM-eet)
Merozoite (MER-o-ZO-ite)
Microgamete
(MY-kro-GAM-eet)

Oocyst (O-o-sist)
Polar tubule (PO-lar TOO-bul)
Sarcocyst (SAR-ko-sist)
Schizogony (skiz-OG-o-nee)
Schizont (SKY-zont)

Spore (SPOR)
Sporoblast (SPOR-o-blast)
Sporocyst (SPOR-o-sist)
Sporogony (Spor-OG-o-nee)
Sporozoite (SPOR-o-ZO-ite)

INTRODUCTION

The coccidia are in the phylum Apicomplexa and subphylum Sporozoa. These protozoans are nonmotile, obligate intracellular parasites, having complex life cycles, with alternating sexual and asexual phases (usually found in the definitive and the intermediate host, respectively). Although frequently found in a variety of animals, certain species are known to infect man. The encysted form of the zygote, called the **oocyst**, containing mature **sporozoites**, is usually the diagnostic form, and, in some cases, the infective form found in fecal specimens, and is characteristic for each parasite. The characteristic features of oocysts of intestinal coccidia are illustrated in Figure 9–1.

The **sporoblast** form is the immature precursor to the **sporocyst**, which is a sac within certain oocysts containing sporozoites.

Microsporidia are found in the phylum Microspora. These obligate intracellular parasites are widely distributed in nature, and have been identified in a variety of animals, especially invertebrates. Of the five genera identified as causing human infection, three have only been identified in patients suffering from the Acquired Immunodeficiency Syndrome (AIDS).

INTESTINAL COCCIDIA

The coccidia, which lack any obvious organelles of locomotion, may be recognized and identified by the observation of characteristic morphologic forms of the parasite in fecal preparations. Ingestion of infective oocysts in food and water is the most common mode of transmission. Knowledge of the life cycles is essential to predict the diagnostic stage passed in the stool.

Cryptosporidium parvum

Morphology

Oocyst: The round to slightly oval oocyst of *Cryptosporidium parvum* measures four to six micrometers (Figure 9–2). When mature, the oocyst contains four sporozoites, which are not always visible, and is surrounded by a thick double-layered wall. No sporocysts are visible; dark-staining granules are usually apparent.

Schizonts and gametocytes: Small schizonts and gametocytes (two to four micrometers) are produced during the life cycle of *C. parvum*, but are rarely seen in human specimens.

Life Cycle

Following ingestion of oocysts, sporozoites are released in the upper gastrointestinal tract, and invade the epithelial cells of the small intestine. Further development occurs on the brush border of host intestinal epithelial cells. The parasites are intracellular but extracytoplasmic, being surrounded by host-derived membranes. Asexual reproduction, or **schizogony**, results in the formation of **schizonts**, containing **merozoites**, which are cells produced during schizogony (Figure 9–3). Schizonts undergo **sporogony**, which is a cycle of sexual reproduction. In the sexual cycle, **microgametes** and **macrogametes** (male and female sex cells, respectively) develop and unite to form zygotes. The zygotes develop into environmentally-resistant thick-walled oocysts, containing sporozoites. These oocysts

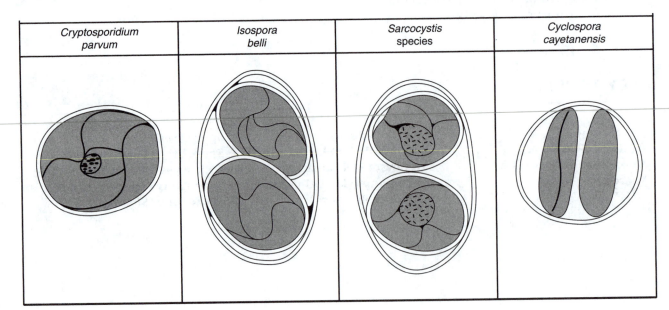

Cryptosporidium parvum	*Isospora belli*	*Sarcocystis* species	*Cyclospora cayetanensis*

FIG 9–1 Oocysts of intestinal coccidia

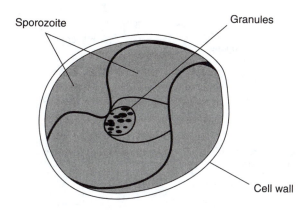

FIG 9–2 *Cryptosporidium parrum* oocyst 4–6 μm

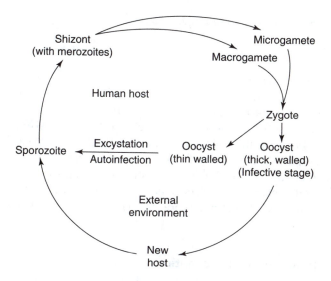

FIG 9–3 Life cycle of *Cryptosporidium parvum*

may remain intact, pass through feces, and serve as the infective stage for a new host. Thin-walled oocysts are also formed, and are considered to be responsible for autoinfection, releasing invasive sporozoites to parasitize other intestinal cells reinitiating the life cycle.

Transmission and Pathogenesis

The mature resistant thick-walled oocyst, passed in the feces of man or animals, is the infective form for new hosts. Transmission of infection with *C. parvum* mainly occurs by ingestion of food or water contaminated with infective oocysts, although person-to-person contact may transmit disease. Several water-borne outbreaks have occurred. Oocysts are distributed worldwide, being present in most untreated water supplies. They are difficult to remove physically, and are resistant to many chemicals, including chlorine.

Cryptosporidiosis is a known zoonosis, and cattle may act as reservoirs of infection. *C. parvum* causes self-limited diarrhea in immunocompetent individuals, follow-

ing an incubation period of one to several weeks. Symptoms include nausea, fever, vomiting, anorexia, abdominal cramps, and watery diarrhea, often alternating with constipation. Recovery from this illness is dependent on the immune status of the host. This illness is especially serious in infants, probably being a significant cause of morbidity and mortality. Immunocompromised individuals often suffer severe, intractable diarrhea.

In patients with AIDS, and other severely immunocompromised individuals, the illness often becomes progressively worse, does not respond to treatment, and may cause death. Body sites other than the gastrointestinal tract, such as the respiratory tract, may also be infected.

Laboratory Diagnosis

Examination of fecal specimens or intestinal biopsy specimens for oocysts characteristic of *C. parvum* is often diagnostic. Use of a modified acid-fast stain is recommended; the oocysts stain reddish-pink using this method (see Chapter 2). When Sheather's sugar flotation method is used, refractile oocysts are seen microsopically, especially when using phase-contrast microscopy. Oocysts may also be seen by the examination of formalin-fixed, Giemsa stained Smears. Immunodiagnostic assays, an enzyme linked immunosorbent assay (ELISA), and fluorescent antibody detection methods, are available, and are considered to be more sensitive and specific than available microscopic methods (see Chapter 3).

Treatment and Prevention

Most antiparasitic agents have proven to be ineffective against *C. parvum*. The infection appears to be self-limited in immunocompetent individuals. The macrolide, spiramycin, shows some promise of being useful in treatment, and has been given to AIDS patients, with limited success. Proper water treatment and adherence to good sanitary practices should prevent infection with *C. parvum*. It is imperative that water supplies are treated with filtration techniques, as well as chemicals. Zoonotic transmission may be prevented by reducing or eliminating contact, especially of immunocompromised individuals, with animals.

Isospora belli

Morphology

Oocyst: The elliptical or oval oocysts of *Isospora belli* measure 25 to 30 micrometers by 10 to 17 micrometers (Figure 9–4). When passed, the noninfective oocyst is immature, containing a single central mass. After further maturation, the oocyst develops two sporoblasts, which develop into two sporocysts, each

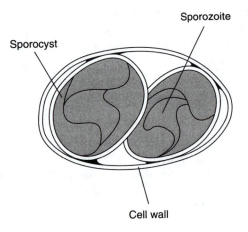

FIG 9–4 *Isospora belli* oocyst (mature) 25–30 μm by 10–17 μm

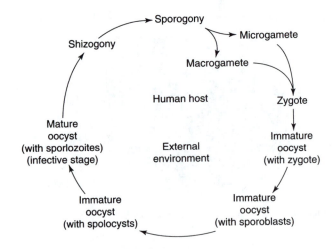

FIG 9–5 Life cycle of *Isospora belli*

containing four cigar-shaped sporozoites. A clear, double-layered wall surrounds the oocyst. This is the mature cyst which is the infective form.

Life Cycle

I. belli is the only coccidian protozoan not shown to have an intermediate host. The human acts as the definitive host, in which sexual and asexual reproduction occurs. The life cycle is similar to other coccidia (Figure 9–5). After ingestion of the mature, infective oocyst in food or water, sporozoites are released, and development occurs within the epithelial cells of the duodenum and jejunum. After schizogony (asexual reproduction) occurs, with formation of merozoites, macro- and microgametes are formed during the sexual stage, which also takes place in the intestine. The gametes unite to form the immature oocyst, which is passed in the feces. In the environment, the immature oocyst develops into the mature, sporulated form, infective for man.

Transmission and Pathogenesis

Transmission occurs by ingestion of water or food containing infective oocysts of *I. belli*. Zoonotic transmission does not occur. Transmission through unprotected homosexual activity, such as anal-oral sexual contact has been reported. Although cases of isosporiasis have occurred worldwide, infection is often asymptomatic and self-limited. When present, symptoms include diarrhea, abdominal pain, weight loss and anorexia. An increase in cases of infection in AIDS patients has been reported in recent years.

Laboratory Diagnosis

Examination of fecal specimens for mature and immature oocysts is the method of choice for detection of parasites. Methods are similar to those used to detect *C. parvum*. The modified acid-fast stain shows pink organisms, similar to, but larger than, *C. parvum*. As previously discussed for the diagnosis of *C. parvum*, the Entero-test and Sheather's sugar flotation method may also be used in the diagnosis of this infection. An ocular micrometer is essential to accurately measure oocysts. Duodenal contents may be examined. Intestinal biopsies may also be used in diagnosis.

Treatment and Prevention

Asymptomatic individuals may not require treatment. Those having more serious symptoms may be treated with trimethoprim-sulfamethoxazole. Metronidazole, tetracycline, and pyrimethamine-sulfadiazine may also be used. Prevention of infection involves good personal hygiene, and sanitary conditions. Unprotected homosexual contact should be avoided.

Sarcocystis species

Morphology

Oocyst: The oval oocyst of *Sarcocystis* species *S. bovihominis* (BO-vee-HOM-in-is) in cattle and *S. suihominis* (SOO-ee-HOM-in-is) in pigs contains two sporocysts and measures 25 to 33 micrometers (Figure 9–6). It resembles *Isospora belli*, with which it was previously classified. The oocyst frequently releases the two sporocysts, each of which contains four cigar-shaped sporozoites. The sporocyst is similar to the oocyst of *C. parvum*, but larger, at 9 to 16 micrometers. A clear, double-layered wall surrounds the oocyst.

Sarcocystis "*lindemanni*" is the term given to those organisms that may potentially parasitize humans.

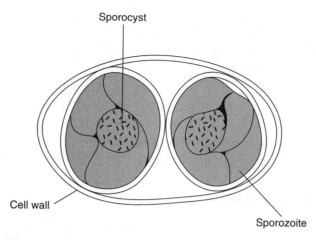

FIG 9–6 *Sarcocystis* species oocyst 25–33 μm

Life Cycle

Humans may act as definitive or intermediate hosts. After ingestion by humans (definitive host) of uncooked meat (cattle or pigs) containing **sarcocysts** (the cyst form of *Sarcocystis* found in muscle), sexual reproduction of the parasite occurs in intestinal cells, with the production of gametes. Gametes unite to produce oocysts, which subsequently release sporocysts.

Asexual reproduction occurs in the intermediate host. When humans ingest the oocyst stage in feces of animals other than cattle or pigs, asexual reproduction occurs, and cysts develop in human muscle.

Transmission and Pathogenesis

As noted above, transmission of *Sarcocystis* infection may occur by ingestion of improperly cooked meat (containing the sarcocyst form in muscle), or ingestion of animal feces-contaminated food or water (oocyst stage in stool).

Symptomatic illness is found rarely in immunocompromised individuals. Symptoms such as diarrhea, abdominal pain, and weight loss, similar to symptoms of infection with *I. belli*, may occur. Muscle pain may be associated with the presence of sarcocysts in human striated muscle, although most cases are asymptomatic.

Laboratory Diagnosis

Fecal specimens should be examined for the presence of characteristic oocysts and sporocysts, by routine methods. Wet preparations are preferred. Muscle biopsies may be stained by routine histological methods.

Treatment and Prevention

There is no treatment for the muscle form of *Sarcocystis* infection. Therapy for symptomatic infection in humans acting as the definitive host are similar to that for *I. belli*. Trimethoprim-sulfamethoxazole or pyrimethamine-sulfadiazine may be used.

Infection of humans as definitive hosts may be prevented by adequate cooking of meat. Avoidance of contact with animal feces prevents infection of humans as intermediate hosts.

Cyclospora cayetanensis

Morphology

Oocyst: The spherical oocysts of *Cyclospora cayetanensis* are remarkably similar to those of *C. parvum*, but can be distinguished by their larger size at 8 to 10 micrometers (Figure 9–7). The oocyst contains two sporocysts, each containing two sporozoites.

Life Cycle

The life cycle of *C. cayetanensis* is not well-understood. It appears to be similar to that of *I. belli*. After ingestion of infective oocysts, sporozoites are released in the gastrointestinal tract. The sporozoites enter and multiply in the epithelial cells of the intestinal tract. Unsporulated oocysts are passed in the stool. Sporulation occurs within 13 days.

Transmission and Pathogenesis

This parasite was initially thought to be a member of the cyanobacteria (blue-green algae). Clinical symptoms of cyclosporiasis are similar to those of cryptosporidiosis. After an incubation period of two to seven days, clinical manifestations develop. These include diarrhea, myalgia, anorexia, weight loss, fatigue, vomiting, and other "flu-like" symptoms. Periods of diarrhea

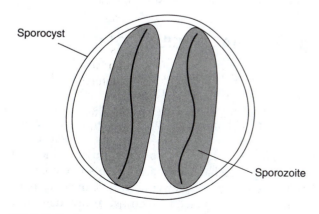

FIG 9–7 *Cyclospora cayetanensis* oocyst 8–10 μm

alternating with periods of constipation may occur. Remission may occur within a few days, but relapse is common. Symptoms in patients with AIDS may persist for several months.

Although water-borne transmission occurs, food-borne illness has been responsible for most serious outbreaks. The largest outbreak of cyclosporiasis was attributed to ingestion of contaminated raspberries.

Laboratory Diagnosis

When cyclosporiasis is suspected, special studies should be added to the routine examination of fecal specimens for ova and parasites. The organisms are acid-fast variable, with some cells staining light pink to dark red; some cells remain unstained, with a glassy, wrinkled appearance. In wet mounts, the oocysts appear as nonrefractile, slightly wrinkled spheres, and will autofluoresce bright green using a 450–490 DM excitation filter, and intense blue using a 365 DM excitation filter. When using the formalin-ethyl acetate concentration procedure (see Chapter 2), centrifugation should be performed at 500 X g for ten minutes. The modified acid-fast procedure may reveal oocysts, ranging from unstained wrinkled spheres to light pink or dark red structures containing granules, or having a bubbly appearance.

Flotation methods followed by examination using phase-contrast microscopy are also useful in diagnosing cyclosporiasis. Electron microscopy is often used to make a diagnosis of cyclosporiasis.

Treatment and Prevention

The drug of choice is trimethoprim-sulfamethoxazole, although relapses following therapy are common. Although specific preventive measures are not recommended at this time, good hygiene and sanitation practices, as well as adequate water treatment methods, may be useful in controlling this infection. Thorough washing of fruits and vegetables may reduce contamination of these food items.

INTESTINAL MICROSPORIDIA

Microsporidia infections are newly-recognized opportunistic infections found in immunocompromised individuals, especially in AIDS patients. Microsporidians that infect humans produce **spores** which are tiny and difficult to identify using conventional microscopic techniques. Spores contain **polar tubules**, which act as extrusion mechanisms to introduce spore contents into the new host cell. Newer diagnostic methods have recently been introduced which aid in the identification of these parasites.

Five genera of microsporidians have been reported: *Encephalitozoon*, *Enterocytozoon*, *Pleistophora*, *Nosema*, and *Microsporidia*. *Encephalitozoon*, *Pleistophora* and *Nosema* have been found in patients with AIDS. *Microsporidia* is the genus name for a varied group of microsporidia with no other assigned genus. Criteria for classification include characteristics which vary among genera and species, such as the size of the spores, configuration of the nuclei in the spores, and the number of polar tubule coils within the spore.

Morphology

Spore: The spores of the microsporidia measure 1.5 to 4.0 micrometers. The spores contain polar tubules, which are the extrusion mechanisms for delivery of sporoplasm to the host (Figure 9–8).

Life Cycle

The life cycle of microsporidia begins with the characteristic spore. The means by which the polar tubule is used to infect host cells is the same for all microsporidia. The ingested spore is stimulated by the gastrointestinal environment to evert its coiled tube, which penetrates a host cell and injects the spore contents into the host cell cytoplasm. After introduction of sporoplasm into the host cell, extensive multiplication of the microsporidia occurs in the cytoplasm of the host cell. Repeated cell divisions occur, by the processes of binary fission (merogony), multiple fission (schizogony), and spore production (sporogony). During this latter process, a thick spore wall forms, and is protective against harmful environmental effects. This stage disseminates within host tissues, or passes into the environment, usually in feces or urine, and is infective for the next host.

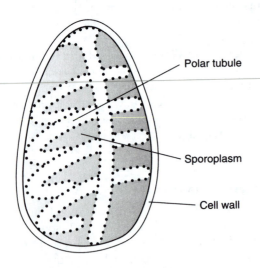

FIG 9–8 *Microsporidium* spore 1.5–4.0 µm

Transmission and Pathogenesis

Initially considered to be invertebrate animal parasites, microsporidia are now known to be important opportunistic parasites in AIDS patients. *Enterocytozoon bieneusi* (EN-ter-o-si-to-ZO-an bay-NU-see) is an intestinal pathogen. Many gastrointestinal infections with this parasite have been reported in HIV-infected patients. Symptoms include intractible diarrhea, fever, weight loss, nausea, and anorexia. Symptoms of microsporidiosis resemble those of cryptosporidiosis; both infections may coexist within an affected patient. *Encephalitozoon intestinalis* (en-SEF-a-lit-o-ZO-an intes-tin-AL-is) also causes intestinal infection in humans.

Other species of *Encephalitozoon* have caused human infections of the eye and central nervous system. *Nosema* (no-SEEM-a) species has been reported to cause a fatal, systemic infection in an immunodeficient infant, as well as several cases of keratoconjunctivitis. *Pleistophora* (PLY-sto-FOR-a) is a rare cause of infection in AIDS patients.

Although not known with certainty, transmission of microsporidiosis is thought to be by person-to-person, or animal-to-animal contact. Infection may result from ingestion or inhalation of spores from the environment or from animals (zoonotic transmission.).

Laboratory Diagnosis

Tissue examination using electron microscopy methods is recommended for the diagnosis of microsporidiosis. Other recently-introduced techniques include modifications of the trichrome stain, a routine stain used in the routine examination of fecal specimens for ova and parasites (see Chapter 2). Chemofluorescent agents, such as Calcofluor, may also be used. When stained by the Gram stain technique, microsporidia are Gram positive.

These parasites may be grown in tissue culture. Histological staining methods may be useful in making a diagnosis of microsporidiosis. Antigen detection methods may soon be available (see Chapter 3).

Treatment and Prevention

No acceptable therapy exists for most microsporidian infections, including *Enterocytozoon bieneusi*. However, albendazole has been reported to be effective in treating disseminated infections with *Encephalitozoon intestinalis*.

Although no specific recommendations exist for prevention of infection, good personal hygiene and careful infection control practices can prevent some infections.

SUMMARY

Coccidia and microsporidia have recently been recognized as newly-emerging opportunists causing human infection. Although many affected individuals are immunocompromised, such as those having AIDS, some individuals are immunocompetent. Transmission of infection may be via the fecal-oral route, from animals (zoonotic infections) or man, or may be by contact. Most coccidian parasites have complex life cycles, involving stages of asexual and sexual reproduction, and usually involving more than one host. Detection of characteristic oocysts in feces is the most common means of diagnosis. Key characteristics of intestinal coccidia are listed in Table 9–1.

Table 9–1 ▶ Key Characteristics of Intestinal Coccidia

ORGANISM	OOCYSTS
Cryptosporidium parvum	4–6 µm Infective on passage Round to slightly oval Mature oocyst contains 4 sporozoites Acid-fast
Isospora belli	25–30 µm Immature oocyst noninfective on passage Elliptical or oval Mature oocyst contains 2 sporocysts, each containing 4 sporozoites Acid-fast

(continues)

Table 9–1 (continued)

ORGANISM	OOCYSTS
Sarcocystis species	25–33 μm Elliptical or oval Similar in structure to *I. belli* Mature oocyst contains 2 sporocysts, each containing 4 sporozoites Sporocysts usually released from oocyst and seen singly
Cyclospora cayetanensis	8–10 μm Round Similar in structure to *C. parvum*, but larger Mature oocyst contains 2 sporocysts, each containing 2 sporozoites Nonrefractile, glassy, wrinkled spheres Variably acid-fast Autofluorescent

Microsporidia are increasingly being reported as infectious agents, particularly in HIV-infected patients. *Enterocytozoon bieneusi* is the most common microsporidian protozoon known to infect humans, causing intestinal infection. Diagnostic procedures adaptable to the clinical laboratory are still being developed.

REVIEW QUESTIONS

1. The oocysts of _____ are immediately infective when passed in the feces.
   a. *Isospora belli*
   b. *Cryptosporidium parvum*
   c. *Cyclospora cayetanensis*
   d. none of the above

2. Which protozoan parasite requires no intermediate host?
   a. *Cryptosporidium parvum*
   b. *Cyclospora cayetanensis*
   c. *Isospora belli*
   d. none of the above

3. The modified acid-fast procedure may be used to diagnose which of the following parasites?
   a. *Cryptosporidium parvum*
   b. *Cyclospora cayetanensis*
   c. *Isospora belli*
   d. all of the above

4. No sporocysts are found in the oocysts of the coccidian parasite
   a. *Cryptosporidium parvum*
   b. *Cyclospora cayetanensis*
   c. *Isospora belli*
   d. *Sarcocystis* species

5. Which of the following parasites does not belong to the phylum Microspora?
   a. *Enterocytozoon bieneusi*
   b. *Encephalitozoon* species
   c. *Nosema* species
   d. *Cyclospora cayetanensis*

6. Humans may act as either the intermediate or the definitive host for
   a. *Cryptosporidium parvum*
   b. *Cyclospora cayetanensis*
   c. *Isospora belli*
   d. *Sarcocystis* species

7. This parasite was once considered to be a blue-green alga (cyanobacterium).

   a. *Cryptosporidium parvum*

   b. *Cyclospora cayetanensis*

   c. *Isospora belli*

   d. *Sarcocystis* species

8. Spores containing polar tubules are characteristic of all

   a. coccidia

   b. microsporidia

   c. sporozoa

   d. acid-fast organisms

9. _____ sporozoite(s) are found in each sporocyst of *Cyclospora cayetanensis*

   a. One

   b. Two

   c. Three

   d. Four

10. The most common microsporidian parasite found in cases of human intestinal infection belongs to the genus

    a. *Enterocytozoon*

    b. *Encephalitozoon*

    c. *Nosema*

    d. *Pleistophora*

CASE STUDY

A patient presented to his primary care physician suffering from diarrhea of 10 days duration, intense fatigue, abdominal cramps, malaise, myalgia, vomiting, and anorexia. Diarrheal stool specimens were collected and submitted to the laboratory for routine ova and parasite testing, as well as culture for enteric bacterial pathogens. Tests for bacterial and parasitic pathogens were negative, and the patient was sent home. His symptoms disappeared for about one week, then relapse occurred. The patient's periods of diarrhea alternated with constipation.

The physician ordered special studies to be performed on the patient's stool specimens, including a modified acid-fast stain, and use of ultraviolet epifluorescence. On microscopic examination, spherical, wrinkled structures showing a range of staining intensity were noted. The cells were fluorescent when viewed using epifluorescence.

Questions

1. What intestinal protozoan parasite might you suspect from these findings?

2. Why were the initial tests negative?

3. What other test should be ordered on this patient?

4. What other protozoan parasite is similar in appearance, but smaller? How would you distinguish the two?

5. Should the patient be treated? With what agent?

► **BIBLIOGRAPHY**

Bryan, R.T., Cali, A., Owen, R.L., & Spencer, H.C. (1991). In Sun, Y. (Ed) *Progress in clinical parasitology* (pp.1–26). Philadelphia: Field and Wood.

Garcia, L.S. & Bruckner, D.A. (1997). *Diagnostic medical parasitology* (3rd ed.) (pp. 54–81). Washington, DC: ASM Press.

Koneman, E. W., Allen, S.D., Janda, W.M., Schreckenberger, P.C., & Winn, Jr, W.C. (1997). *Color atlas and textbook of diagnostic microbiology* (5th ed). Philadelphia: Lippincott.

Shimeld, L., & Rodgers, A. T. (1999). Intestinal and atrial protozoans. In Shimeld, L. (Ed). *Essentials of diagnostic microbiology*. (pp. 572–589). Albany, NY: Delmar Publishers.

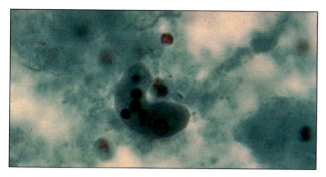

PLATE 1 *Entamoeba histolytica* trophozoite. (Courtesy of the CDC Public Health Image Library)

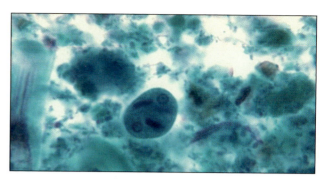

PLATE 2 *Entamoeba histolytica* cyst. (Courtesy of the CDC Public Health Image Library)

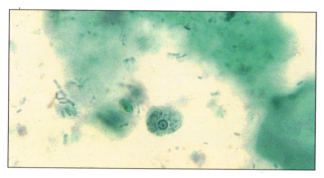

PLATE 3 *Entamoeba hartmanni* trophozoite. (Courtesy of the CDC Public Health Image Library)

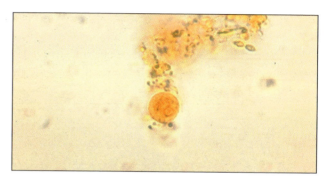

PLATE 4 *Entamoeba hartmanni* cyst. (Courtesy of the CDC Public Health Image Library)

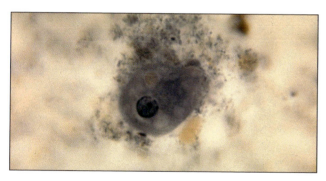

PLATE 5 *Entamoeba coli* trophozoite. (Courtesy of the CDC Public Health Image Library)

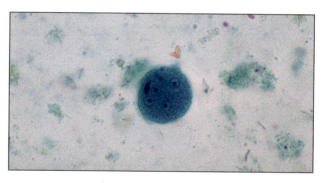

PLATE 6 *Entamoeba coli* cyst. (Courtesy of the CDC Public Health Image Library)

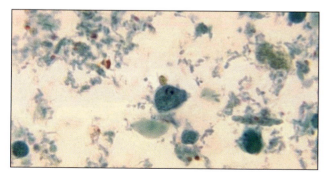

PLATE 7 *Endolimax nana* trophozoite. (Courtesy of the CDC Public Health Image Library)

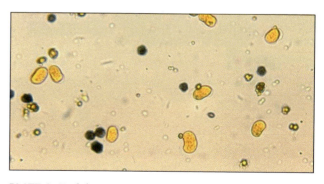

PLATE 8 *Endolimax nana* cyst—iodine stain. (Courtesy of the CDC Public Health Image Library)

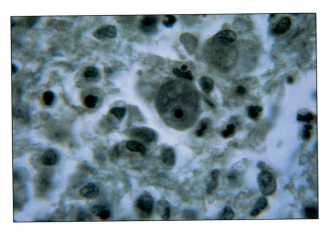

PLATE 9 *Iodamoeba butschlii* amebiasis of brain. (Courtesy of the CDC Public Health Image Library)

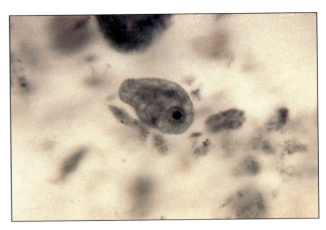

PLATE 10 *Iodamoeba butschlii* cyst. (Courtesy of the CDC Public Health Image Library

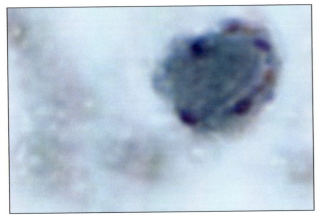

PLATE 11 *Blastocystis hominis*—trichrome stain. (Courtesy of the CDC, National Center for Infectious Diseases, Division of Parasitic Diseases Image Library)

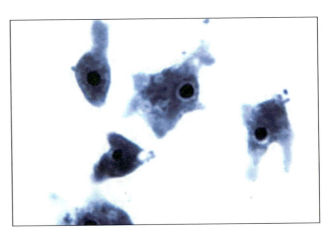

PLATE 12 *Naegleria fowleri* amebic trophozoite cultured from CSF—trichrome stain. (Courtesy of the CDC, National Center for Infectious Diseases, Division of Parasitic Diseases Image Library)

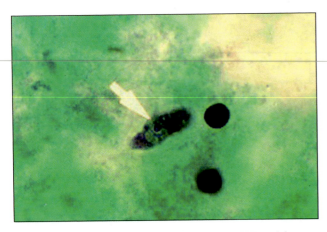

PLATE 13 *Naegleria fowleri* trophozoite in CSF—trichrome stain. (Courtesy of the CDC, National Center for Infectious Diseases, Division of Parasitic Diseases Image Library)

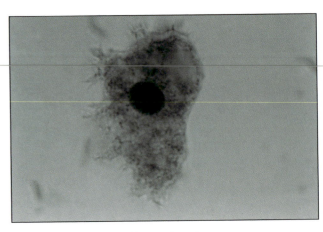

PLATE 14 *Acanthamoeba* trophozoite.

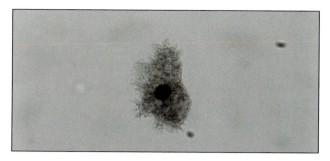

PLATE 15 *Acanthamoeba* cyst.

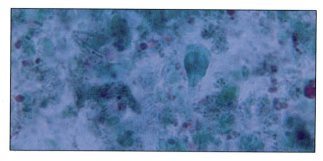

PLATE 16 *Giardia lamblia* trophozoite—trichrome stain. (Courtesy of the CDC Public Health Image Library)

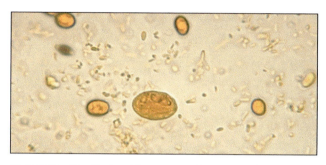

PLATE 17 *Giardia lamblia* cyst—iodine stain. (Courtesy of the CDC Public Health Image Library)

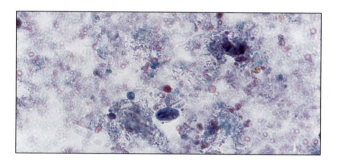

PLATE 18 *Giardia lamblia* cyst at 10x.

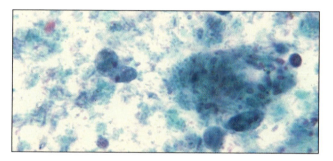

PLATE 19 *Dientamoeba fragilis* trophozoite—trichrome stain. (Courtesy of the CDC Public Health Image Library)

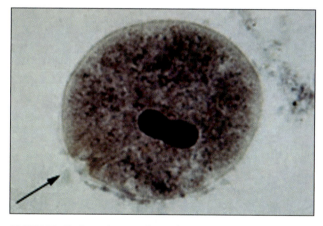

PLATE 20 *Balantidium coli* trophozoite—trichrome stain. (Courtesy of the CDC, National Center for Infectious Diseases, Division of Parasitic Diseases Image Library)

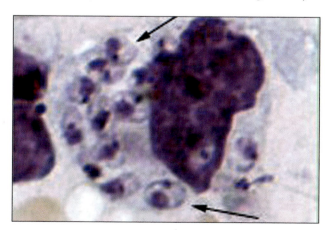

PLATE 21 *Leishmania tropica* amastigotes within an intact macrophage from a skin touch preparation. The arrows demonstrate organisms with clearly visible nucleus and kinetoplast. (Courtesy of the CDC Public Health Image Library)

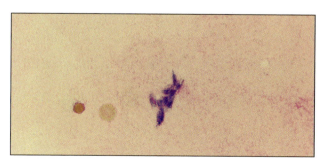

PLATE 22 Giemsa stain of promastigote stage of *Leishmania* species from NNN media at 100x (low power objective)

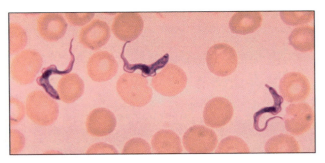

PLATE 23 *Trypanosoma brucei gambiense* blood smear. (Courtesy of the CDC Public Health Image Library)

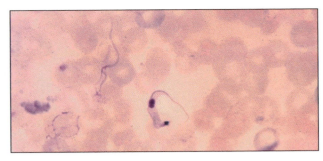

PLATE 24 *Trypanosoma cruzi.* (Courtesy of the CDC Public Health Image Library)

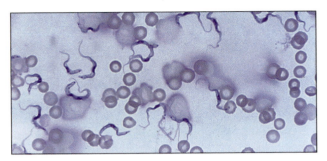

PLATE 25 *Trypanosoma cruzi*, a tryptomastigote in blood.

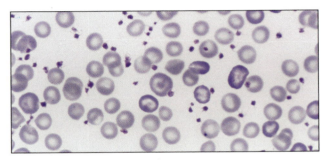

PLATE 26 *Trypanosoma cruzi*, an amastigote in blood.

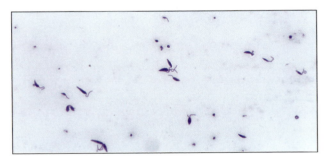

PLATE 27 Amastigotes and tryptomastigotes in blood.

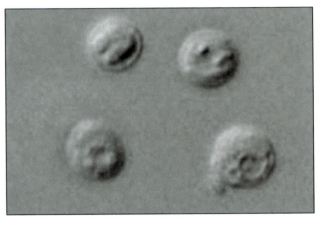

PLATE 28 *Cryptosporidium parvum* oocysts—wet mount. (Courtesy of the CDC, National Center for Infectious Diseases, Division of Parasitic Diseases Image Library)

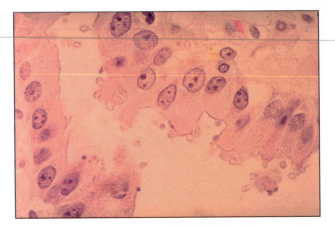

PLATE 29 Cryptosporidiosis of gallbladder. (Courtesy of the CDC Public Health Image Library)

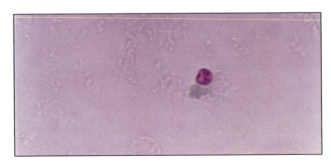

PLATE 30 *Cryptosporidium parvum* stained by the modified acid-fast method.

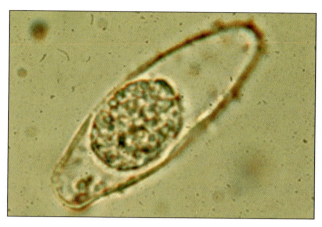

PLATE 31 *Isospora belli* oocyst—wet mount. (Courtesy of the CDC, National Center for Infectious Diseases, Division of Parasitic Diseases Image Library)

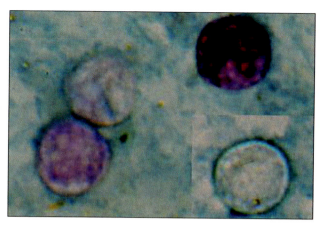

PLATE 32 *Cyclospora cayetanensis* oocysts—acid-fast stain. (Courtesy of the CDC, National Center for Infectious Diseases, Division of Parasitic Diseases Image Library)

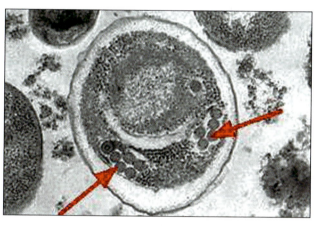

PLATE 33 *Enterocytozoon bieneusi* spore—electron micrograph. (Courtesy of the CDC, National Center for Infectious Diseases, Division of Parasitic Diseases Image Library)

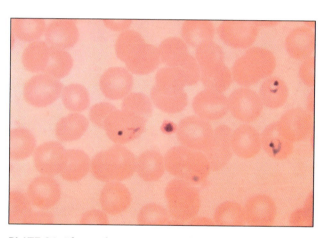

PLATE 34 *Plasmodium vivax* ring forms. (Courtesy of the CDC Public Health Image Library)

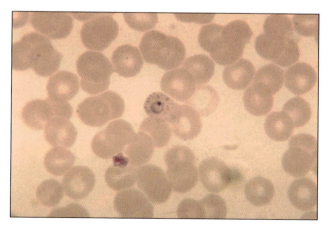

PLATE 35 Late ring form in RBC with Schüffner's dots. (Courtesy of the CDC Public Health Image Library)

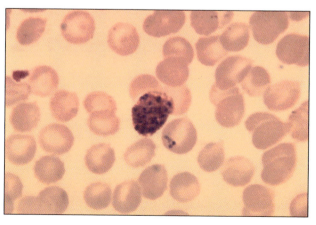

PLATE 36 *Plasmodium vivax* schizont in a Giemsa stained blood smear. (Courtesy of the CDC Public Health Image Library)

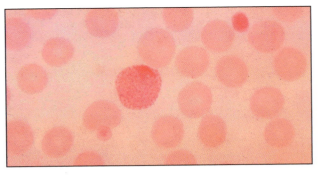

PLATE 37 *Plasmodium vivax* macrogametocyte in blood smear. (Courtesy of the CDC Public Health Image Library)

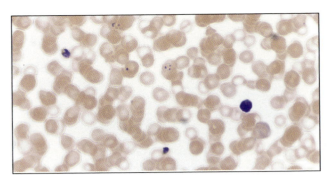

PLATE 38 *Plasmodium vivax* ring stage.

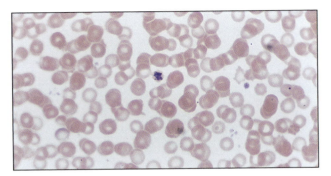

PLATE 39 *Plasmodium vivax* ameboid atage.

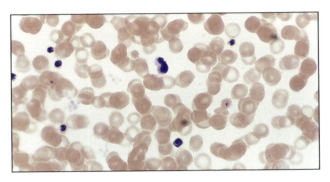

PLATE 40 *Plasmodium vivax* schizonts.

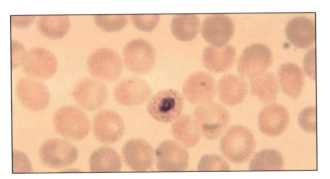

PLATE 41 *Plasmodium ovale* trophozoite. (Courtesy of the CDC Public Health Image Library)

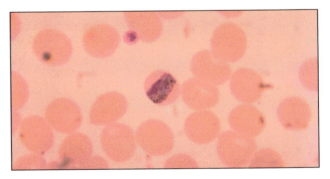

PLATE 42 *Plasmodium malariae* band form trophozoite in blood smear. (Courtesy of the CDC Public Health Image Library)

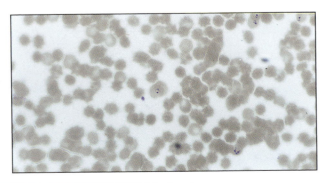

PLATE 43 *Plasmodium malariae* ring stage.

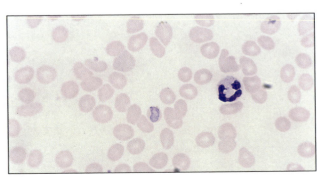

PLATE 44 *Plasmodium malariae* banded schizonts.

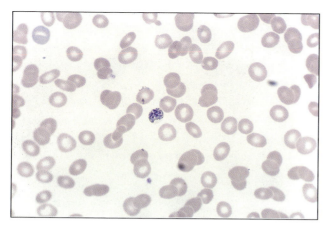

PLATE 45 *Plasmodium malariae* gametocytes.

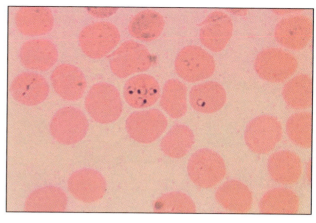

PLATE 46 *Plasmodium falciparum* ring form. (Courtesy of the CDC Public Health Image Library)

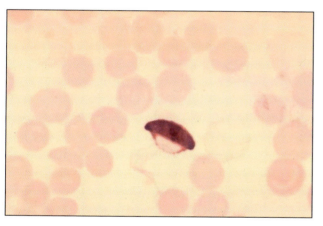

PLATE 47 *Plasmodium falciparum* mature gametocyte. (Courtesy of the CDC Public Health Image Library)

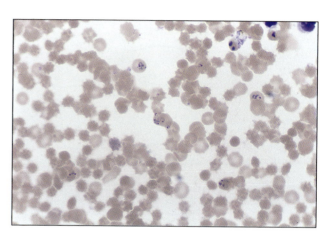

PLATE 48 *Plasmodium falciparum* ring stage.

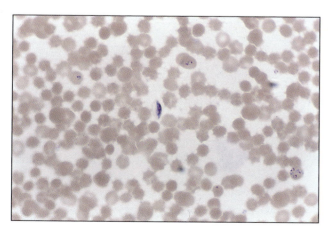

PLATE 49 *Plasmodium falciparum* schizonts.

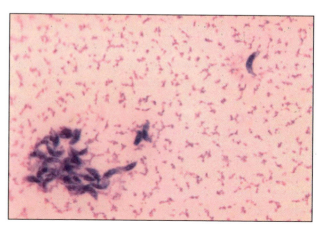

PLATE 50 *Toxoplasma gondii* trophozoites. (Courtesy of the CDC Public Health Image Library)

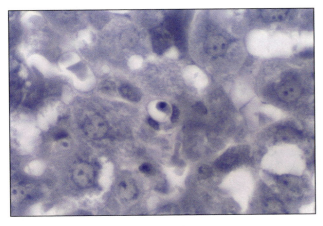

PLATE 51 *Toxoplasma gondii* in liver section.

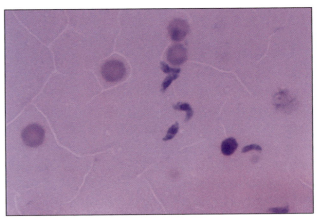

PLATE 52 *Toxoplasma gondii* trophozoite in blood smear.

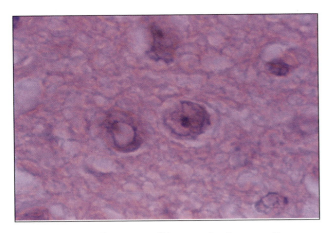

PLATE 53 *Toxoplasma gondii* oocyst in tissue section.

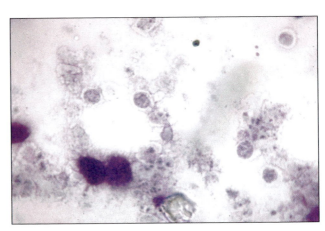

PLATE 54 *Pneumocystis carinii* smear in Giemsa stain. (Courtesy of the CDC Public Health Image Library)

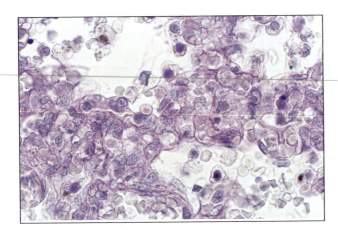

PLATE 55 *Pneumocystis carinii*, tissue section.

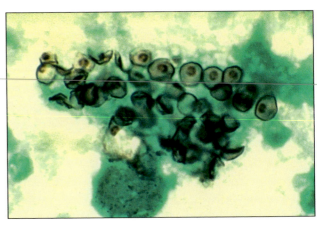

PLATE 56 *Pneumocystis carinii* cysts in a broncho-alveolar lavage (BAL) specimen stained with methanamine silver stain. (Courtesy of the CDC Public Health Image Library)

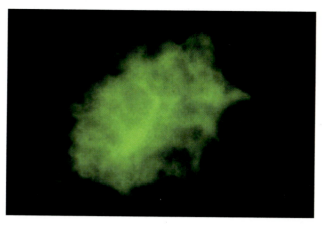

PLATE 57 Indirect immunoflourescence using monoclonal antibody against *Pneumocystis carinii*. (Courtesy of the CDC, National Center for Infectious Diseases, Division of Parasitic Diseases Image Library)

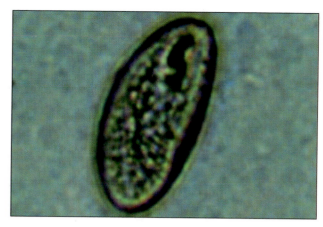

PLATE 58 *Enterobius vermicularis* egg. (Courtesy of the CDC, National Center for Infectious Diseases, Division of Parasitic Diseases Image Library)

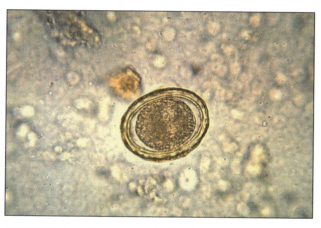

PLATE 59 *Ascaris lumbricoides* fertilized egg. (Courtesy of the CDC Public Health Image Library)

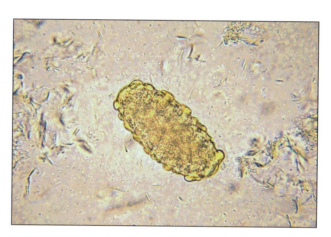

PLATE 60 *Ascaris lumbricoides* unfertilized egg. (Courtesy of the CDC Public Health Image Library)

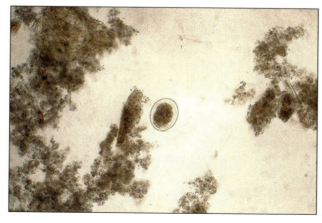

PLATE 61 *Ascaris lumbricoides* unfertilzed egg (decorticated). (Courtesy of the CDC Public Health Image Library)

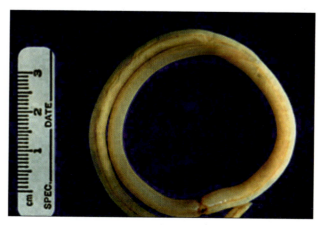

PLATE 62 *Ascaris lumbricodes* adult worm. (Courtesy of the CDC, National Center for Infectious Diseases, Division of Parasitic Diseases Image Library)

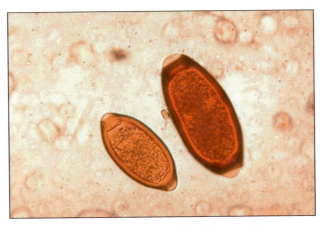

PLATE 63 *Trichuris trichiura* and *trichuris vulpis* eggs. (Courtesy of the CDC Public Health Image Library)

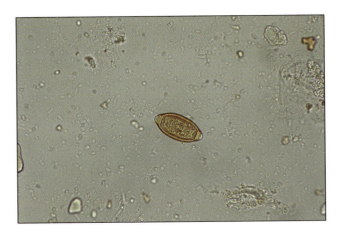

PLATE 64 *Trichuris trichiura* ova.

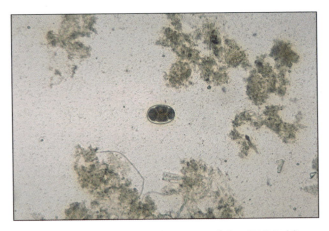

PLATE 65 Hookworm egg. (Courtesy of the CDC Public Health Image Library)

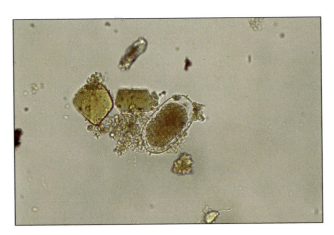

PLATE 66 Hookworm ova at 40x.

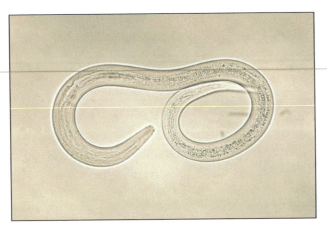

PLATE 67 Hookworm filariform larva. (Courtesy of the CDC Public Health Image Library)

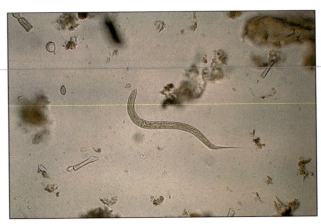

PLATE 68 Hookworm rhabditiform larva. (Courtesy of the CDC Public Health Image Library)

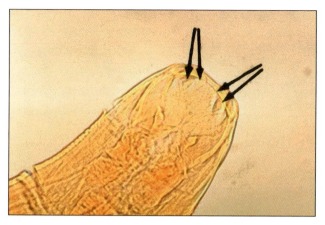

PLATE 69 *Ancylostoma duodenale* mouth parts. (Courtesy of the CDC Public Health Image Library)

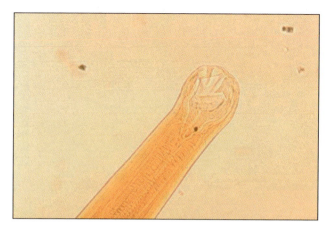

PLATE 70 *Ancylostoma braziliense* mouth parts. (Courtesy of the CDC Public Health Image Library)

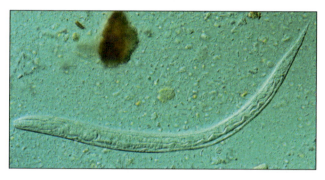

PLATE 71 *Strongyloides stercoralis* larva. (Courtesy of the CDC Public Health Image Library)

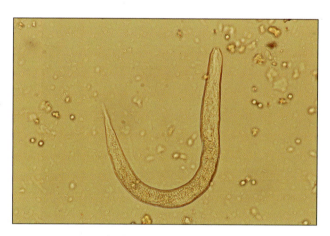

PLATE 72 *Strongyloides stercoralis* in lung tissue.

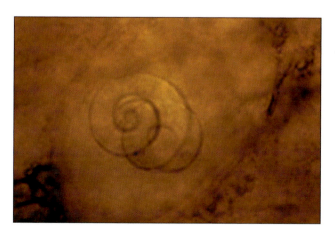

PLATE 73 *Trichinella spiralis* larvae encysted in muscle tissue. (Courtesy of the CDC, National Center for Infectious Diseases, Division of Parasitic Diseases Image Library)

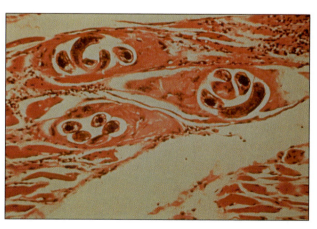

PLATE 74 Muscle biopsy of *Trichinella spiralis*. A single-coiled *Trichinella spiralis* larva in striated muscle at 300x. (Courtesy of the Armed Forces Institute of Pathology [AFIP]).

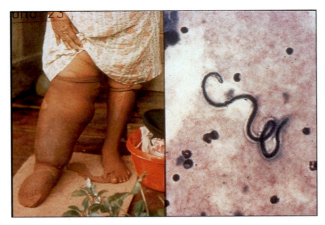

PLATE 75 Bancroftian filariasis: On the right an adult *Wuchereria bancrofti*, the parasite that causes the disease. On the left elephantiasis of the lower leg, one of the visible symptoms of the disease. (Courtesy of the WHO/TDR/TALC).

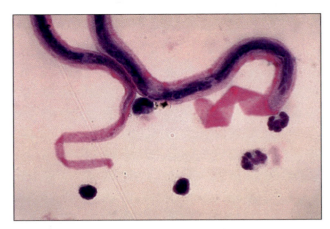

PLATE 76 *Brugia malayi*. (Courtesy of the CDC Public Health Image Library)

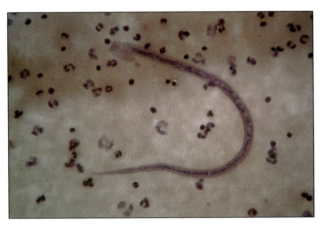

PLATE 77 *Brugia malayi* microfilaria from peripheral blood via Knott's concentration method, stained with Delafield's hematoxylin at 350x. (Courtesy of the Armed Forces Institute of Pathology [AFIP]).

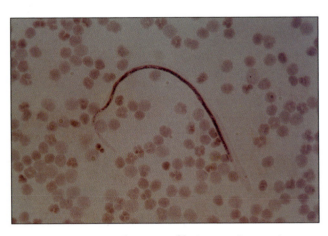

PLATE 78 *Brugia malayi* microfilaria, anterior portion.

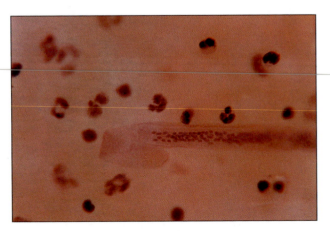

PLATE 79 *Brugia malayi* microfilaria, posterior portion.

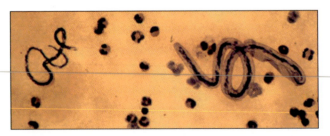

PLATE 80 Microfilariae of *Loa loa* (right) and *Mansonella perstans* (left) in a blood smear stained with iron hematoxylin.

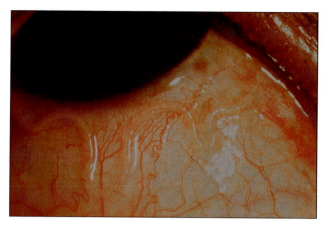

PLATE 81 Ocular *Loa loa* microfilaria. Adult *L. loa* beneath the eye conjunctiva. (Courtesy of the Armed Forces Institute of Pathology [AFIP]).

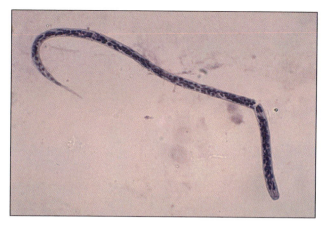

PLATE 82 Microfilaria of *Onchocerca volvulus*. (Courtesy of the CDC Public Health Image Library)

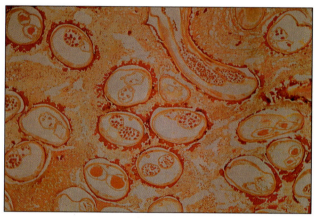

PLATE 83 *Onchocerca volvulus* microfilaria, anterior portion.

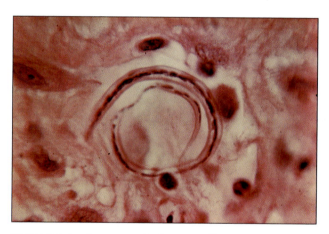

PLATE 84 *Onchocerca volvulus* microfilaria, posterior portion.

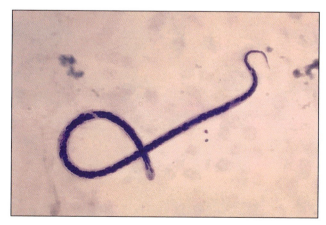

PLATE 85 Microfilaria of *Mansonella ozzardi* stained with Giemsa. The microfilaria is unsheathed and the nuclei do not extend to the end of the tapered hooked tail. (Courtesy of the CDC Public Health Image Library)

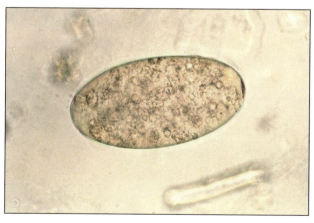

PLATE 86 *Fasciolopsis buski* egg. (Courtesy of the CDC Public Health Image Library)

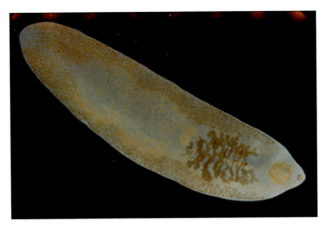

PLATE 87 *Fasciolopsis buski* adult worm. (Courtesy of the CDC, National Center for Infectious Diseases, Division of Parasitic Diseases Image Library)

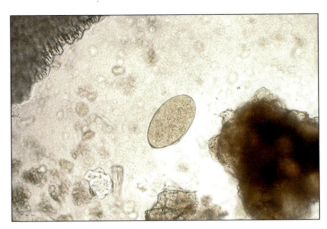

PLATE 88 *Fasciola hepatica* egg. (Courtesy of the CDC Public Health Image Library)

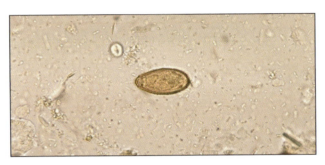

PLATE 89 *Clonorchis sinensis* egg. (Courtesy of the CDC Public Health Image Library)

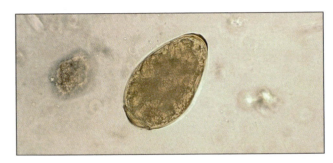

PLATE 90 *Paragonimus westermani* egg. (Courtesy of the CDC Public Health Image Library)

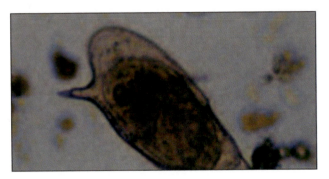

PLATE 91 *Schistosoma mansoni* egg. (Courtesy of the CDC Public Health Image Library)

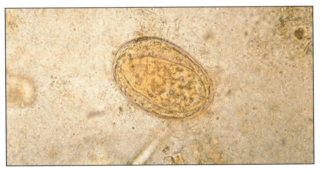

PLATE 92 *Schistosoma japonicum* egg. (Courtesy of the CDC Public Health Image Library)

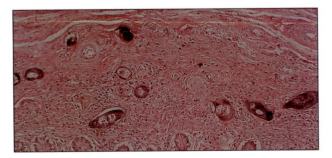

PLATE 93 *Schistosoma japonicum* eggs in colonic submucosa at 87x. (Courtesy of the Armed Forces Institute of Pathology [AFIP]).

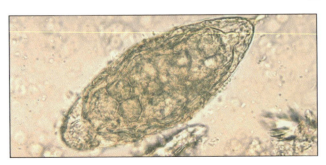

PLATE 94 *Schistosoma haematobium* egg. (Courtesy of the CDC Public Health Image Library)

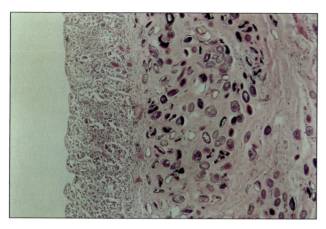

PLATE 95 *Schistosoma haematobium* ova from tissue sample.

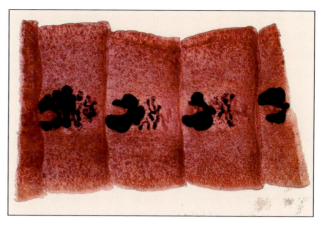

PLATE 96 Proglottids of *Diphyllobothrium latum*. (Courtesy of the CDC Public Health Image Library)

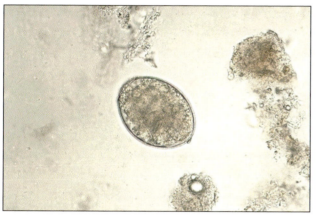

PLATE 97 Egg of *Diphyllobothrium latum*. (Courtesy of the CDC Public Health Image Library)

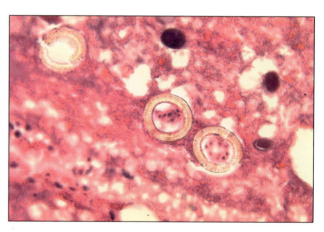

PLATE 98 Histopathology of *Taenia saginata* in appendix. (Courtesy of the CDC Public Health Image Library)

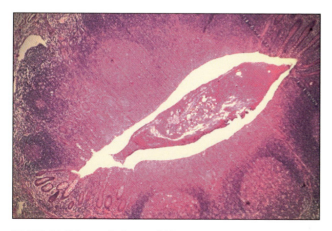

PLATE 99 Histopathology of *Taenia saginata* in appendix. (Courtesy of the CDC Public Health Image Library)

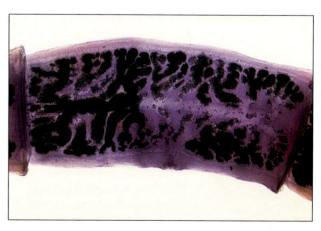

PLATE 100 Proglottid of *Taenia solium*. (Courtesy of the CDC Public Health Image Library)

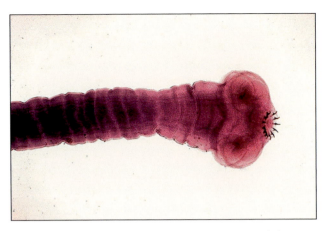

PLATE 101 Scolex of *Taenia solium*. (Courtesy of the CDC Public Health Image Library)

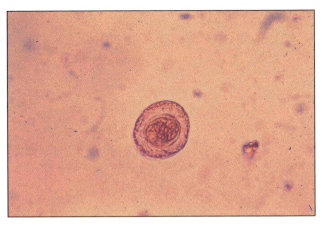

PLATE 102 Egg of *Hymenolepis nana*. (Courtesy of the CDC Public Health Image Library)

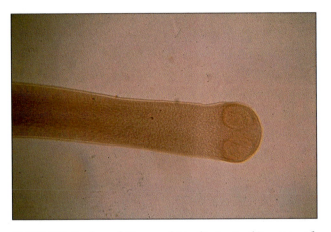

PLATE 103 Scolex of *Hymenolepis diminuta*. (Courtesy of the CDC Public Health Image Library)

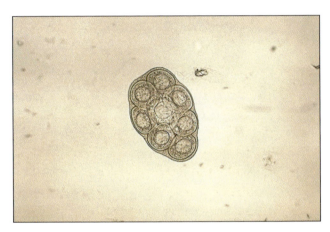

PLATE 104 Egg packet of *Dipylidium caninum*. (Courtesy of the CDC Public Health Image Library)

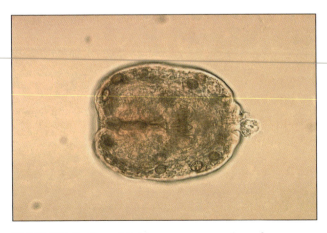

PLATE 105 Scolex of *Echinococcus granulosus* from a hydatid cyst. (Courtesy of the CDC Public Health Image Library)

CHAPTER TEN
Blood and Tissue Sporozoa

LEARNING OBJECTIVES

After reading and studying this chapter, the student should be able to:

- Define the key terms.
- For each organism cited, state the geographic distribution.
- Describe the morphologic characteristics of the parasites listed in this chapter.
- Briefly describe the life cycle of each organism cited.
- Identify the vector for each organism and the infective stage.
- Describe the mechanism of pathogenesis for each organism.
- Discuss the clinical presentation of each disease.
- Name the specimen of choice for the diagnosis and/or recovery of each parasite.
- Identify means of treatment and prevention for each parasite.

KEY TERMS

Accolè (ak-oh-lay)
Benign tertian malaria
  (bee-nine/ter-shun)
Blackwater fever
Bradyzoite (brad-ee-zoh-ite)
Encephalomyelitis
  (en-sef-ah-loh-my-el-i-tis)
Erythrocytic cycle
  (e-rith-roh-sit-ik)
Exoerythrocytic cycle
  (exo-e-rith-roh-sit-ik)

Gametocytogenesis
  (gam-ee-toh-cyto-jen-e-sis)
Hemoglobinuria
  (hemo-glo-bin-ur-ia)
Hyphozoite
Ischemia (isk-ee-mee-ah)
Macrogametocyte
  (macro-gam-ee-toh-cyte)
Malarial paroxysm
  (par-ox-siz-em)
Malarial pigment

Malignant jaundice
  (mah-lig-nant/jon-dis)
Malignant tertian malaria
Maurer's dots or clefts
  (mow-erz/dots)
Merozoite (mer-oh-zoh-ite)
Microgametocyte
  (micro-gam-ee-toh-cyte)
Oocyst (oh-oh-cyst)
Ookinete (oh-oh-kin-ate)

(continues)

INTRODUCTION

Malaria and babesiosis are diseases caused by protozoan, obligate intracellular parasites of the phylum Apicomplexa. The causative organisms are vectored by blood sucking insects and belong to the genera *Plasmodium* and *Babesia*, respectively. They have complex life cycles, including an intermediate and definitive host, and although they have different geographic distributions, both produce febrile hemolytic anemias. Characteristics of the various morphological forms are summarized in Figure 10–1.

MALARIA

Throughout the course of human history, malaria has been responsible for untold morbidity and mortality. To this day, malaria remains the world's most notorious tropical parasitic disease, threatening some 2,400 million people—40% of the world population. According to the World Health Organization, there are an estimated 300–500 million new cases of malaria each year and over 1 million deaths, most of whom are African children.

Morphology

The agents of human malaria are four species of the genus *Plasmodium*: *Plasmodium vivax*, *Plasmodium malariae*, *Plasmodium ovale*, and *Plasmodium falciparum*. *P. vivax* accounts for the vast majority of malarial infections, mainly because of the wide distribution of the parasite. *P. vivax* is the only one of the four species that extends through tropical, subtropical and temperate regions. *P. falciparum*, which causes falciparum malaria, is confined to the tropics and subtropics and is probably the most lethal form of malaria. Pockets of *P. malariae* infection are distributed throughout the subtropics and tropics, while

P. ovale is primarily confined to tropical West Africa, South America and Asia.

These parasites have complex life cycles involving both sexual and asexual phases and are transmitted primarily by the female *Anopheles* mosquito. Of the approximate 1,200 cases of malaria reported in the United States each year, most are immigrants or travelers returning from malaria endemic areas. One should also consider, however, that malaria may be contracted through the sharing of contaminated hypodermic needles (as in drug abuse and tatooing), through blood transfusion, congenital transmission, or by the bite of a domestic mosquito that has previously bitten an individual with an imported infection.

Life Cycle

The life cycle of the malarial parasite is divided into two distinct phases: asexual development, or **schizogony**, which takes place in the human host and sexual development, or **sporogony**, which takes place in the mosquito. As noted, the mosquito is considered the definitive host and man is the intermediate host.

Human infection with *Plasmodium* spp. begins with the bite of an infected *Anopheles* mosquito. A variety of *Anopheles* species are known to harbor the parasite, but only the females bite. As the mosquito draws its blood meal, saliva and spindle-shaped **sporozoites** are injected into the capillary wound. Infective sporozoites make their way into the general circulation and are carried throughout the body.

Within an hour, circulating sporozoites have made their way to the liver and have taken up residence in the parenchymal cells. It is here that asexual division (schizogony) begins. This portion of development within the liver cells, is called the pre-erythrocytic or **exoerythrocytic cycle** and may last from 5 to 16 days depending on the species of *Plasmodium*.

Within the parenchymal cells, the sporozoites become round or oval and begin to divide. The liver

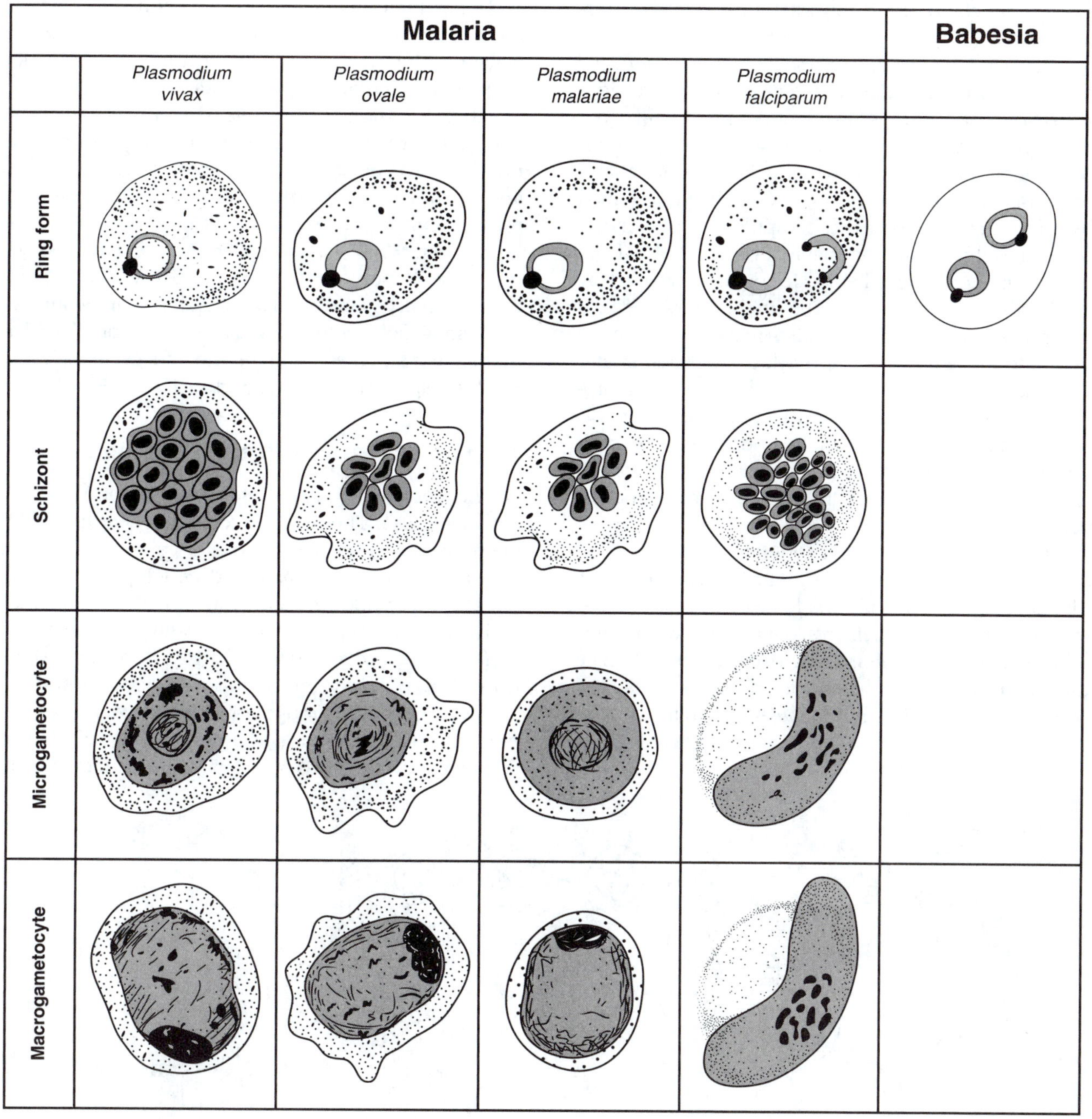

Malaria				Babesia
Plasmodium vivax	*Plasmodium ovale*	*Plasmodium malariae*	*Plasmodium falciparum*	
Ring form				
Schizont				
Microgametocyte				
Macrogametocyte				

FIG 10–1 Characteristics of malarial and babesiosis parasites.

cells carry a heavy burden as thousands of exoerythrocytic **merozoites** are produced. As the infected cells rupture, merozoites are free to leave the liver, enter the circulation, invade red blood cells and initiate the **erythrocytic cycle** of development.

All four *Plasmodium* species undergo asexual multiplication within liver cells, but animal research models have shown that the course of events may be somewhat different for *P. vivax* and *P. ovale*. As the infective sporozoites of these species enter the parenchymal cells, only a portion begin to actively multiply. The remainder enter a latency period or resting state. The resting form of the parasite is called a **hypnozoite**. The reactivation of these dormant forms, weeks or months after the original erythrocytic infection has been cleared, accounts for the instances of true clinical relapse seen in *P. vivax* and *P. ovale* infection.

Circulating merozoites invade red blood cells and reticulocytes and begin to grow as young trophozoites, also known as ring forms. The developing parasites are uninucleate and vacuolated and feed on hemoglobin. The remaining byproducts of hemoglobin metabolism combine to form what we now call **malarial pigment**.

The trophozoite continues to enlarge until its nucleus begins to divide, at which point it is called a **schizont**. The mature schizont undergoes erythrocytic schizogony, forming multiple merozoites. The number of merozoites produced is species dependent and has diagnostic value when observed in Giemsa stained blood smears. Infected red cells rupture releasing merozoites into the circulation to infect new red blood cell and complete yet another cycle, or be destroyed by the host's immune system. The liberation of the parasites from the red cells is also marked by a mass dumping of parasitic waste products and debris into the bloodstream. This toxic material is thought to provoke the onset of the **malarial paroxysm** which is characterized by shaking chills and fever. The periodicity of these symptoms is determined by the length of the erythrocytic cycle (48–72 hours) and is species dependent.

After several erythrocytic generations, some of the erythrocytic merozoites undergo **gametocytogenesis** (the development of male and female sex cells). Rather than maturing into schizonts containing merozoites, they develop into male **microgametocytes** or female **macrogametocytes**. If these circulating gametes happen to be ingested by an *Anopheles* mosquito, the sexual cycle of development, sporogony, is initiated within the mosquito.

The maturation of gametocytes continues within the gut of the mosquito. Through the process of exflagellation, the nucleus of the microgametocyte divides to produce multiple spindle-shaped microgametes, which erupt from the red blood cell to fertilize the mature macrogamete. The union of the two sex cells produces a **zygote** which elongates, becomes motile and is known as an **ookinete**. This stage penetrates the mosquito's gut wall, rounds up, and grows into an **oocyst**. When maturation is complete, the oocyst gives rise to hundreds of sporozoites, which migrate to the salivary glands and are capable of infecting the next individual that the mosquito bites. A complete diagrammatic representation of the life cycle of *Plasmodium* species is seen in Figure 10–2.

Transmission and Pathogenesis

The *Anopheles* mosquito serves as the primary vector for malaria. The risk of infection is determined by the number and species of mosquito present in a given area as well as the climate and geography. In many parts of the world, transmission of malaria coincides with the rainy season when mosquitoes thrive and there is increased agricultural activity. Population shifts caused by political unrest, climatic events, and environmental changes brought on by urbanization, deforestation and forced irrigation have all contributed to the increased incidence of malaria. Ease of international

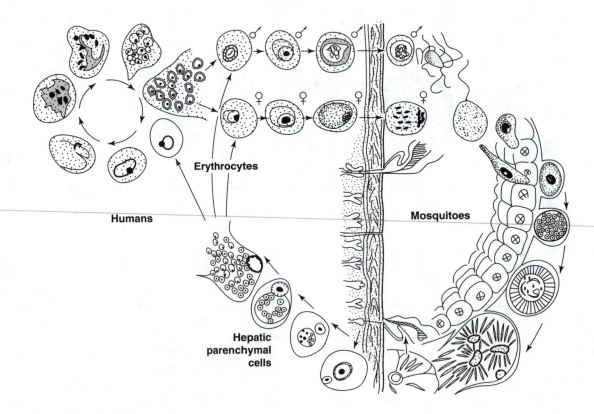

FIG 10–2 Life cycle of *Plasmodium* spp.

travel has raised the frequency of imported cases and brought about the phenomenon of "airport malaria." A small number of airport workers, with no other apparent risk, have contracted malaria from the bite of accidentally imported infected mosquitos.

Each year in the United States, a few cases of malaria result from a situation not involving an infected mosquito. Cases have been reported of patients becoming infected following a blood transfusion, after sharing contaminated hypodermic needles, or through congenital transmission.

In all cases, once acquired, the patient remains asymptomatic for more than a week while the parasite goes through the exoerythrocytic cycle in the liver. The incubation period varies by species and may last from ten days to a month or longer. The onset of clinical disease may be marked by nonspecific prodromal symptoms, such as headache, myalgia, and gastrointestinal disturbance. The simultaneous rupture of large numbers of infected RBCs and the resulting release of erythrocytic merozoites, red cell debris, and toxic waste byproducts, triggers the malarial paroxysm. Patients experience a period of shaking chills or **rigor** which lasts 10 to 15 minutes or more, followed by 2 to 6 hours or more of fever, body aches and disorientation. As the fever subsides, the patient starts to sweat profusely and returns to normal until the onset of the next paroxysm. After several erythrocytic cycles, the episodes become synchronous and develop a 48 or 72 hour periodicity, depending on the species of parasite.

The principal clinical symptoms of malaria are anemia and splenomegaly. Anemia is caused by the direct lysis of infected red blood cells during the erythrocytic cycle or by splenic removal of infected antibody coated red cells. Red cell production may also be diminished because of bone marrow suppression.

The extent of the infection and the resulting anemia is somewhat limited by the parasite itself. *P. vivax* and *P. ovale* only invade reticulocytes (young red blood cells) which constitute only about 2% of the red blood cell population. *P. malariae* primarily infects senescent (older) RBCs, an even smaller portion of all circulating red blood cells. *P. falciparum* invades RBCs of all ages without discrimination, and the parasitemia affects a high percentage of available cells. Consequently, the degree of anemia with *P. falciparum* infection can be quite severe.

Untreated primary vivax attacks may last 3 weeks to 2 months; relapses are common and may persist for 5 to 8 years. The initial attacks of ovale malaria last from 2 to 3 weeks and often end with spontaneous recovery. Relapse is possible, but seldom occurs after one year. Primary infection with *P. malariae* lasts from 3 weeks to as long as 24 weeks. The patient may have complete recovery or maintain a low grade parasitemia, which results in a series of **recrudescenses** (re-

occurrences) over the next two decades. An untreated primary attack of *P. falciparum* malaria typically has a duration of 2 to 3 weeks but may be marked by a variety of complications, coma, or even death. Recrudescence can occur, but is seldom seen after a year.

Complications of malarial infection, particularly falciparum malaria, are generally caused by the obstruction of capillaries by parasitized red cells and/or red cell debris. The symptoms vary with the level of tissue hypoxia and the organ involved. Renal complications, such as glomerulonephritis, nephrotic syndrome, and renal failure, may be life-threatening. Central nervous system involvement may produce severe headaches, cortical blindness, stroke, and death.

It should also be noted that there are certain genetic conditions affecting changes to the red blood cell that confer degrees of natural immunity against malaria. Increased resistance to malaria, particularly *P. falciparum* malaria, is seen in individuals with inherited hemoglobinopathies. In malaria endemic areas, mortality rates for malaria are significantly decreased among individuals with sickle cell trait (hemoglobin S). The presence of hemoglobin C, hemoglobin E, or beta thalassemia, also offers resistance to falciparum malaria, as does glucose 6-phosphate dehydrogenase (G6PD) deficiency.

Duffy blood group negativity has been shown to afford resistance to *P. vivax* infection. Erythrocytes that are Duffy antigen negative, lack the surface receptors for the attachment and invasion of *P. vivax* merozoites. This accounts for the prevalence of *P. ovale* malaria and not *P. vivax* in West Africa where a large percentage of the local population is Duffy negative.

Specific characteristics and signs and symptoms are discussed by organism in the following sections.

Plasmodium vivax

Of the four malaria species that infect man, *P. vivax* has the greatest geographic distribution, ranging from the tropics to temperate zones. The incubation period ranges from 10 to 17 days and may be followed by a series of prodromal, flu-like, symptoms before the organism is seen in the peripheral blood.

In early infection, paroxysms may not be synchronous. Later, a regular 48 hour periodicity is established, marking the erythrocytic cycle of the parasite. The three day interval between clinical episodes, beginning with the first symptoms and ending with the onset of the next paroxysm, gave *P. vivax* the name **benign tertian malaria**.

A review of Giemsa stained blood films may reveal a variety of asexual forms of the parasite and gametocytes, depending on the timing of the specimen collection. As the paroxysm begins, merozoites are released from infected RBCs to invade new red cells. It is important to note that only reticulocytes are infected. Within hours, early trophozoites or ring forms (Figure 10–3A) can be seen in the infected cells. On occasion, the parasites are first seen as crescent shapes at the edge of the RBC known as accolè or appliquè-form. As the parasite grows, Giemsa stain shows that a vacuole forms within the blue cytoplasm and the red dot-like chromatin moves to one side, giving a classic signet ring configuration. By 24 hours, the parasite contains brownish malarial pigment and the infected cell appears pale and enlarged. It may contain reddish colored granules known as **Schüffner's dots** (Figure 10–3B). These granules are a diagnostic feature of *P. vivax* and *P. ovale*. Once mature, the trophozoite chromatin divides and becomes a mature schizont which will contain 14–22 individual merozoites (Figure 10–3C). At 44–48 hours, the cycle is completed with the rupture of infected cells. After several erythrocytic cycles, gametocytes (Figure 10–4) are also seen in the peripheral blood.

Untreated primary attacks may persist for 3 weeks to 2 months or more. Hypnozoites that lay dormant in liver cells are responsible for relapses months to years following the initial infection. Vivax malaria generally subsides spontaneously but prognosis may depend on the presence of any intercurrent infections or the patient's prior state of health. Rapid diagnosis and treatment produces excellent results and complications are rare.

Plasmodium ovale

Epidemiologically, *Plasmodium ovale* is widely distributed throughout tropical Africa, with a heavy concentration in coastal West Africa, and occasional outbreaks in parts of Asia and South America.

Morphologically and clinically, *P. ovale* is remarkably similar to *P. vivax*. The asexual cycle of both species approximates 48 hours (**tertian**), and all developmental stages may be seen in peripheral blood films depending on the timing of the draw. Both species only invade reticulocytes and are prone to relapse caused by dormant hypnozoites. However, unlike *P. vivax*, clinical symptoms tend to be less severe with *P. ovale* and, even with relapses, the untreated patient usually demonstrates spontaneous recovery within 12 to 20 months.

Several morphologic characteristics may be helpful in the differentiation of *P. ovale* from other malaria species. As its name may indicate, red cells infected with *P. ovale* have an ovoid appearance when smears are properly dried and stained. Infected RBCs are larger than normal, pale, contain Schüffner's dots in early trophozoite stages, and may have ragged margins (Fig-

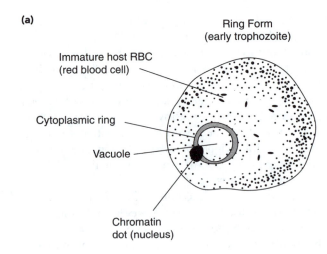

(a) Ring Form (early trophozoite)

- Immature host RBC (red blood cell)
- Cytoplasmic ring
- Vacuole
- Chromatin dot (nucleus)

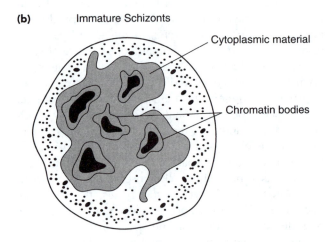

(b) Immature Schizonts

- Cytoplasmic material
- Chromatin bodies

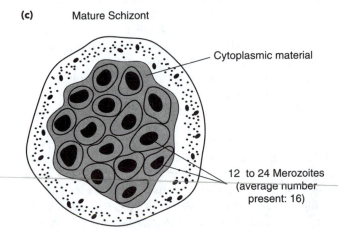

(c) Mature Schizont

- Cytoplasmic material
- 12 to 24 Merozoites (average number present: 16)

FIG 10–3 Commonly seen morphologic forms of *Plasmodium vivax*.

ure 10–5A). *P. ovale* tends to be smaller and less ameboid than *P. vivax* but a definitive diagnosis may depend on finding a mature schizont (Figure 10–5B). The mature schizont of *P. ovale* contains 4 to 12 merozoites, with an average of eight.

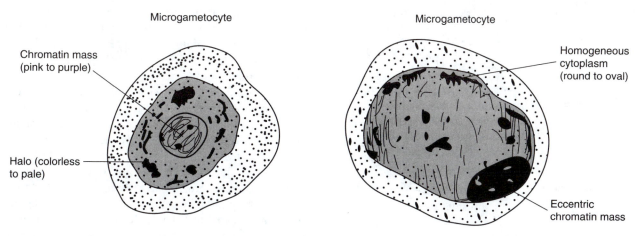

Microgametocyte

Chromatin mass
(pink to purple)

Halo (colorless
to pale)

Microgametocyte

Homogeneous
cytoplasm
(round to oval)

Eccentric
chromatin mass

FIG 10–4 Commonly seen morphologic forms of *Plasmodium vivax.*

Plasmodium malariae

Although less frequent in occurrence, *Plasmodium malariae* malaria overlaps the distribution of *P. vivax* and *P. falciparum* in subtropical and temperate regions.

Patients infected with *P. malariae* experience an incubation period that typically lasts 18 to 40 days and is followed by prodromal symptoms that resemble those of vivax malaria. The initial paroxysm may be moderate to severe in nature and marks the beginning

(a)

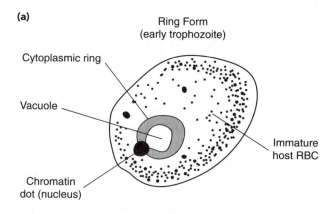

Ring Form
(early trophozoite)

Cytoplasmic ring

Vacuole

Chromatin
dot (nucleus)

Immature
host RBC

(b)

Mature Schizont

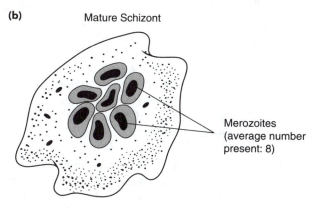

Merozoites
(average number
present: 8)

FIG 10–5 Commonly seen morphologic forms of *Plasmodium ovale.*

of a series of asexual cycles that will have a regular 72 hour periodicity (**quartan malaria**).

Merozoites of *P. malariae* predominantly invade mature red blood cells. Trophozoites grow quickly and assume an elongated "band" form (Figure 10–6A) characteristic of *Plasmodium malariae*. Developing trophozoites are non-ameboid. Infected red blood cells do not appear enlarged but may contain a fine, pink, cytoplasmic stippling known as **Ziemann's dots**. As the schizont matures, 6 to 12 merozoites (average 8) can be seen in a rosette or irregular pattern surrounding dark staining malarial pigment (Figure 10–6B). Gametocytes are non-remarkable.

Clinical symptoms of an untreated primary attack may last 3 weeks to 6 months. The initial infection may end in spontaneous recovery or patients may experience chronic low-grade parasitemia leading to recrudescence for 20 or more years.

Plasmodium falciparum

Although once common in southern regions of the United States, along the Mediterranean and other temperate zones, falciparum malaria is now fairly limited to the tropics and subtropics. The severity of its symptoms, pathogenicity, and complications have won it the title: **malignant tertian malaria**. *Plasmodium falciparum* infection typically produces the greatest morbidity and mortality of all the *Plasmodium* species.

Morphologically, there are certain characteristics that help to differentiate *P. falciparum* as well. Schizogony generally occurs in the capillaries and blood sinuses of internal organs (spleen, liver, bone marrow) rather than in the peripheral blood. Infected RBCs containing developing parasites plug small vessels, leading to **ischemia** (insufficient blood supply) and complications to be discussed later. Only early trophozoites (ring forms) and gametocytes are seen in peripheral blood smears. *Plasmodium falciparum* will invade any red

(a)

Developing Trophozoite

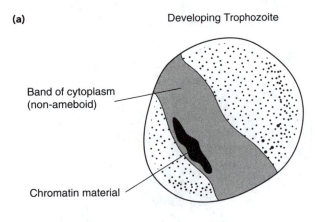

Band of cytoplasm
(non-ameboid)

Chromatin material

(b) Mature Schizont

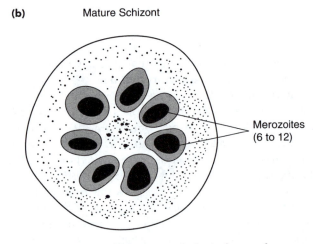

Merozoites
(6 to 12)

FIG 10–6 Commonly seen morphologic forms of *Plasmodium malariae.*

blood cell, young or old, and the proportion of infected cells may be as high as 50% or more.

After an incubation period of 8 to 12 days, the patient experiences prodromal symptoms which are followed by the onset of fever, severe headache and gastrointestinal upset. Cyclic paroxysms are established at 36–48 hour intervals (tertian). Untreated, the primary attack may last 2–3 weeks. Hypnozoites are not produced and true relapses do not occur.

Giemsa stained peripheral blood smears reveal small, ring form trophozoites or **accolè** forms along the periphery of the red blood cell. Young trophozoite rings may have two small chromatin dots giving a "headphone" configuration (Figure 10–7A). Red blood cells may be multiply infected, with two or more merozoites invading the same cell. Although the infected cells do not appear enlarged or distorted, they may contain dark red irregular markings known as **Maurer's clefts** or dots. If the mature schizont is seen, it will contain 8–36 merozoites (average 24) (Figure 10–7B). Larger numbers may be the result of two parasites dividing within a single cell. Gametocytes of *P. falciparum* appear in the peripheral circulation and

have a characteristic crescent or sausage shape (Figure 10–7C). The pale staining red cell is stretched lengthwise to accommodate a crescent shaped parasite. Identification of this stage is diagnostic for *P. falciparum* malaria.

Complications of *P. falciparum* malaria are related to the heavy parasite load and the plugging of blood vessels resulting in deprivation of oxygen to organs and tissues. Anemia is a common and often severe consequence of the heavy parasitemia. Cerebral malaria, however, is the most serious and often fatal complication of falciparum malaria. Symptoms include disorientation, headache, extreme fevers exceeding 107 degrees F, coma and death. Gastrointestinal invasion leads to diarrhea or dysentery. Kidney involvement may result in acute renal failure, tubular necrosis or nephrotic syndrome. Although rare, **Blackwater fever** is a complication of falciparum malaria brought on by sudden intravascular hemolysis. The massive outpouring of hemoglobin results in marked **hemoglobinuria** and a dark brown to black urine color. It is thought that Blackwater fever may be associated with quinine treatment in some patients.

Laboratory Diagnosis

Thick and thin Giemsa stained peripheral blood smears are the specimens of choice for the diagnosis of malaria, although in many cases the presence of the parasite is first noted in hematologic Wright stained smears. The diagnosis of malaria can only be confirmed by demonstration of the causative *Plasmodium* species.

Laboratory requests for malarial blood smear examination should always be done *stat* because of the possible life threatening nature of the infection. Laboratories should be supplied with patient information regarding malarial risk factors: travel history, transfusion, and possible needle transmission (IV drug abuse).

Collection of blood samples for malarial studies must be carefully timed to successfully recover plasmodia. Blood drawn immediately after the onset of a paroxysm will contain free merozoites which, if seen in stained blood smears, are difficult to identify by species. The greatest number of parasites are present late in the febrile episode. All asexual stages, including gametocytes, may be found in the peripheral blood smears of *P. vivax, P. ovale,* and *P. malariae* infections. In *P. falciparum* infections, only ring forms and gametocytes are found.

Multiple Giemsa stained blood films (thick and thin) should be prepared and examined under oil immersion (100x) in order to rule out malaria. Thick smears are used for screening purposes while thin blood films are thoroughly examined for species identification.

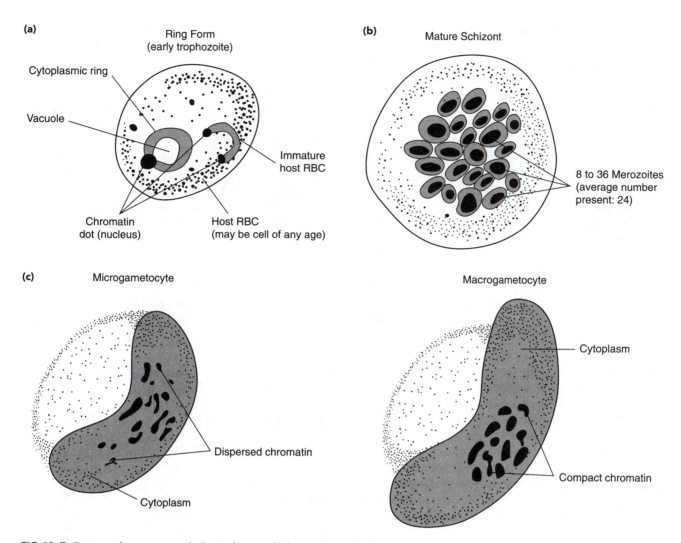

(a) Ring Form (early trophozoite)

Cytoplasmic ring

Vacuole

Immature host RBC

Chromatin dot (nucleus)

Host RBC (may be cell of any age)

(b) Mature Schizont

8 to 36 Merozoites (average number present: 24)

(c) Microgametocyte

Dispersed chromatin

Cytoplasm

Macrogametocyte

Cytoplasm

Compact chromatin

FIG 10–7 Commonly seen morphologic forms of *Plasmodium falciparum*.

Therapeutic management is determined by the species of *Plasmodium* detected. A diagnosis of malaria can not be excluded with a single set of negative smears. This is particularly true of patients who have taken a partial course of antimalarial prophylactic therapy. It is suggested that multiple blood specimens be collected over a 48 hour period before considering the patient negative for malarial parasites.

Serologic testing procedures and DNA probes are also available for the diagnosis of malaria. Although not used routinely, these tests are quite useful in epidemiological studies and for ruling out malaria in patients with fever of unknown origin.

Treatment and Prevention

The treatment of malaria has become somewhat of a challenge because of the sheer adaptive nature and tenacity of both the parasite and the *Anopheles* mosquito. Prior to World War I, only quinine, a derivative of the bark of the *cinchona* tree, was available as an antimalarial therapy. By World War II, several synthetic drugs had been developed, of which chloroquine became the drug of choice. Standard use of antimalarial drugs and incomplete courses of therapy selected for drug-resistant strains of malaria, particularly, *P. falciparum*. After years of spraying in endemic areas, the *Anopheles* vector has also developed resistance to the most common insecticides.

Ideally, malarial treatment should destroy all forms of the parasite, from sporozoite to gametocyte, without being toxic to the patient. Unfortunately, each of the available chemotherapeutic agents acts on specific morphologic stages of the malarial life cycle. Combination drug therapy may be required to prevent relapse or recrudescence.

Current treatment regimes generally include some form of quinine or quinine derivative. Chloroquine is the least toxic drug that effectively eliminates nonresistant forms of the parasite.

In parts of the world where resistant strains of *P. falciparum* and *P. vivax* predominate, mefloquine or quinine may be the drug of choice. Managing infections of *P. vivax* or *P. ovale* may require long-term treatment with primaquine, which is known to eliminate hypnozoites from the liver and prevent "true relapse."

The key to the control and prevention of malaria is long-term mosquito abatement and human treatment and prophylaxis. Elimination of standing water and mosquito breeding sites and the broadcast use of environmental insecticides should drastically reduce the vector population. Early diagnosis and treatment of existing cases is also fundamental to breaking the human-mosquito-human cycle.

Humans can reduce their risk of infection: by wearing long-sleeve protective clothing and using insect repellant (with DEET) to prevent bites; by remaining indoors at night when mosquitoes bite; by using screens and bed-netting soaked in pyrethrum; by avoidance of shared IV drug needles; and by maintaining compliance with prophylactic drugs. Care should also be taken to screen and protect the donor blood supply.

The development of an effective malaria vaccine would be a powerful weapon in the arsenal for malaria control. The World Health Organization reports that more than a dozen vaccines are in developmental stages worldwide. Potential vaccines target particular areas of the parasite life cycle—the sporozoite, the merozoite, and the developmental forms in the mosquito. With continued success in clinical trials, it is hoped that an effective vaccine will be available within the next 7–15 years.

BABESIOSIS

Like *Plasmodium* species, *Babesia* species are blood parasites. Members of the genus *Babesia* are known as tick-borne parasites of domestic animals and wild rodents, and are responsible for causing **Texas cattle fever** and **malignant jaundice** of dogs, both of which have economic significance. Human infections are rare but have been documented worldwide. Like other mammals, man is an accidental host.

Morphology

In North America, the most common cause of human babesiosis is *Babesia microti*. The greatest concentration of cases in the United States occurs in the southern New England area: Long Island, Shelter Island, Nantucket, Martha's Vineyard and Connecticut. These areas are also endemic for the hard tick vector, genus *Ixodes*. Most cases occur in the late summer and early fall when ticks are prevalent.

Babesiosis closely mimics malaria in morphology, pathology and symptomology. In most instances, however, babesiosis is a self-limited, non-fatal infection. Asplenic patients have a higher mortality rate.

Life Cycle

The life cycle of *Babesia* (Figure 10–8) is remarkably similar to *Plasmodium* species, with the asexual cycle taking place in the mammalian host and sexual reproduction taking place in the arthropod vector. The vector for *Babesia* is one of a number of species of *Ixodes* ticks. The infective forms (sporozoites) are introduced into the human host as the tick takes a blood meal. The organisms invade red blood cells and undergo asexual reproduction, appearing as intracellular ring forms that resemble early trophozoites of *Plasmodium* species. Unlike malaria, gametocytes are not seen in the peripheral blood.

Ticks acquire the parasite by feeding on *Babesia* infected mammals, generally rodents or domestic livestock. More often, ticks acquire the infection from their mothers through transovarian passage of the parasite. Within the tick, the sexual reproduction cycle takes place and infective sporozoites are formed.

Transmission and Pathogenesis

Babesia species are transmitted by a number of species of ixodid ticks, including *Ixodes scapularis* which is also the vector of Lyme disease. As the tick takes a blood meal, the pathogens are passed to a new host. As with Lyme disease, evidence suggests that the tick must feed for 12 hours or more before transmit-

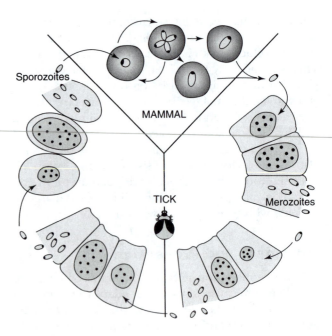

FIG 10–8 Life cycle of *Babesia*

ting the infective organisms. Early detection and removal of the infected tick can prevent transmission. Concurrent infections (babesiosis and Lyme disease) are possible.

Babesiosis is a febrile hemolytic anemia characterized by an incubation period of 1 to 4 weeks. Most infections are self-limited, with a gradual onset of malaise, fever, headache, muscle aches, chills, sweating and fatigue. Unlike malaria, there is no periodicity associated with the fever. Patients may experience a mild hepatosplenomegaly and jaundice. Babesiosis is rarely fatal, except in the asplenic or immunocompromised patient. Transfusion associated infections have been documented.

Laboratory Diagnosis

Diagnosis of babesiosis in humans is made by demonstration of the parasite in thick and thin Giemsa stained peripheral blood smears. Only ring forms will be seen in infected red blood cells. Care must be taken to differentiate *Babesia* species form *Plasmodium falciparum*.

Red blood cells infected with *Babesia* may contain multiple ring forms as is characteristic of *P. falciparum* infection. Ring forms measure 1.0 to 5.0 micrometers and may have one or more chromatin dots depending on the maturity of the trophozoite (Figure 10–9). They often appear in pairs or tetrads within infected red blood cells, commonly know as the "Maltese" cross arrangement. Unlike cells infected with malarial parasites, erythrocytes infected with *Babesia* will not contain malarial pigment or stippling and will not appear enlarged as might be seen with *P. vivax* or *P. ovale* infection.

Serologic testing procedures, including the indirect immunofluorescence assay (IFA), as well as polymerase chain reaction (PCR) tests are also available. These tests are particularly helpful in diagnosis when the parasitemia is low.

Treatment and Prevention

Babesiosis is typically a self-limited infection in humans. When treatment is necessary, a combination of clindamycin and quinine is effective in eliminating the parasite. Chloroquine phosphate treatment offers symptomatic relief but parasites tend to persist in the blood.

Prevention of human babesiosis is dependent on avoidance of tick bites in endemic areas. Individuals who frequent these areas for work or recreation should wear protective clothing, use an effective insect repellent, and examine their body for ticks immediately following suspected exposure.

Methods that have been proven effective at killing the deer tick vector of Lyme disease (*Ixodes scapularis*) have also decreased the incidence of babesiosis. Mice serve as the principal reservoir host of both diseases. In one such eradication method, insecticide treated cotton balls were distributed in wooded areas to be used as nesting material by the rodents. Those ticks that attached to the mouse were killed when the mouse returned to its nest, thus interrupting the transmission of the pathogen.

TOXOPLASMA GONDII

Toxoplasma gondii is an apicomplexan parasite of worldwide distribution that can infect most warm blooded vertebrates, including man, causing the disease **toxoplasmosis**. The organism was first described in the early 1900s as an infection of a small rodent from North Africa called a gundi, from which it got its name. Members of the cat family (Felidae) serve as the definitive hosts, and a variety of birds and mammals may serve as intermediate hosts in the life cycle. Human disease is relatively rare but serologic evidence indicates that toxoplasmosis may be one of the most common human infections worldwide. Most exposures result in asymptomatic cases. Those at greatest risk of clinical disease are the immunocompromised and pregnant women and their developing fetuses.

Life Cycle

Cats are the main reservoir of infection for *Toxoplasma gondii*. The entire life cycle of the parasite may be completed within the feline host. Cats become infected by eating infected prey. Trophozoites encysted within the contaminated meat are released in the

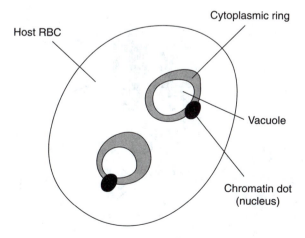

FIG 10–9 *Babesia microti* ring form.

cat's gut and an asexual and sexual cycle of reproduction takes place in the epithelial cells lining the small intestine.

Within 2 to 3 weeks of ingestion of the parasite, the cats begin to pass unsporulated **oocysts** in its feces. These oocysts take 1 to 5 days in the environment to become infective (sporulate). Oocysts are 9–11 micrometers wide by 11–14 micrometers long and contain two **sporocysts**, each with four **sporozoites** (Figure 10–10).

In moist soil, oocysts can remain viable for more than a year. Grazing animals such as cattle, sheep and pigs acquire the oocyst while feeding. Rodents become infected while foraging. All these animals are common intermediate hosts.

Human infections are accidental and can be acquired in several ways. Infection may occur by ingesting infective *Toxoplasma* oocysts through the fecal-oral route. Commonly, contact is made while cleaning the cat's litter box or while gardening in contaminated soil. Toxoplasmosis may also be acquired by eating raw or poorly cooked meat, or through transfusion, organ transplantation and transplacental passage.

In human infections, only the non-intestinal forms of the parasite are found. Early in the infection, actively proliferating trophozoites called **tachyzoites** may be seen as intracellular parasites of many tissues throughout the body. Crescent shaped tachyzoites ranging in size from 2 to 3 micrometers wide by 4 to 8 micrometers long may be seen in Giemsa stained smears of heart, lung, lymph node and central nervous system tissue. One end of the trophozoite is more rounded than the other and accommodates a single spherical nucleus.

In chronic infections, the resting forms called **tissue cysts** are found in brain and muscle tissue (Figure 10–11). These forms contain large numbers of slow growing trophozoite **bradyzoites**. Cysts are thought to form in response to host defense mechanisms. Upon microscopic examination, bradyzoites have the same morphologic appearance as tachyzoites. Cysts, how-

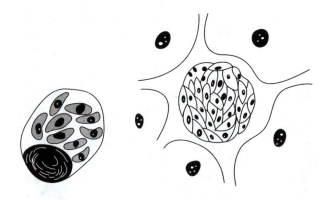

FIG 10–11 *Toxoplasma gondii* tissue cyst

ever, can measure 12 to 100 μm in diameter. A diagrammatic representation of the life cycle of *T. gondii* can be seen in Figure 10–12.

Transmission and Pathogenesis

Human infection with *Toxoplasma gondii* may be acquired in one of the following ways: fecal-oral transmission of the oocysts; ingestion of raw or undercooked meat containing encysted *T. gondii*; transplacental passage; blood transfusion; or organ transplantation. In the

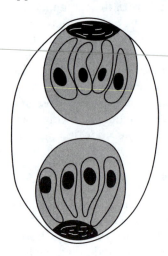

FIG 10–10 *Toxoplasma gondii* oocyst

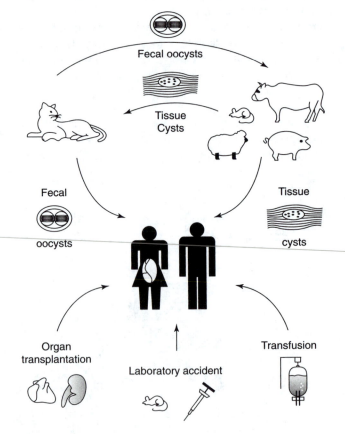

FIG 10–12 Life cycle of *Toxoplama gondii*

human host, rapidly multiplying tachyzoites are responsible for the tissue damage that may occur in active infection. As the patient mounts an immune response, tissue cysts containing bradyzoites are formed in the heart, brain and skeletal muscle. Cysts may remain in the host indefinitely.

The clinical features of toxoplasmosis are also widely varied. As evidenced by the large number of individuals who are seropositive for *T. gondii*, the majority of human infections are asymptomatic and benign. In a small number of *Toxoplasma* infections, symptoms may occur. The clinical presentation generally mimics infectious mononucleosis with headache, fever, chills, lymphadenitis, myalgia and fatigue as characteristics. On rare occasions, severe symptoms may ensue, with the development of maculopapular rash and/or myocarditis, hepatitis, **encephalomyelitis** (inflammation of the brain and spinal cord) or **retinochoroiditis** (inflammation of the retina and the choroid) which may progress to blindness. The most severe symptoms are documented in cases of congenital toxoplasmosis and infections of the immunocompromised host.

Fetal mortality resulting from transplacental passage of *T. gondii* occurs at a rate of approximately 2 to 6 of every 1,000 pregnancies in the United States. Transmission occurs when expectant mothers develop an acute but asymptomatic case of toxoplasmosis during pregnancy. The severity of resulting disease is dependent on the gestational age of the fetus at the time of infection. Infections acquired during the first or second trimester of pregnancy have the greatest consequences. The congenitally infected newborn may demonstrate symptoms of retinochoroiditis, encephalomyelitis, calcifications in the brain, hydrocephalus or microcephaly, and psychomotor dysfunction. The future of these infants is often marked by mental retardation and blindness. When infection occurs in the last trimester, the fetus may appear normal at birth but has a significant risk of developing retinochoroiditis or central nervous system involvement later in life through reactivation.

Reactivation of toxoplasmosis is also a problem for individuals who become medically immunosuppressed or otherwise compromised. Patients being treated for neoplastic diseases, such as Hodgkin's disease, non-Hodgkin's lymphoma, leukemia, as well as solid tumors, collagen-vascular disorders, organ transplant and AIDS are all at risk of reactivation of latent infection. In these patients, the presentation is most commonly cerebral toxoplasmosis with associated diffuse encephalopathy, meningoencephalitis or cerebral mass lesions. MRI and CT scans of the brain show characteristic "ring- enhanced" lesions. Patients may experience headache, motor disorders, altered mental status, and other neurologic sequelae.

Serum antibody tests are not reliable for the diagnosis of *Toxoplasma* encephalitis in immunocompromised patients. IgM antibodies are not present with reactivation of latent infection and IgG titers are usually low.

Microscopic analysis of spinal fluid reveals diagnostic tachyzoite forms and stained histologic sections of brain biopsy tissue demonstrate minute necrotic foci containing *Toxoplasma* organisms. Clinical improvement is seen in greater than 85% of cases treated with anti-*Toxoplasma* therapy, although AIDS patients require a prolonged course of treatment to maintain a clinical response. *Toxoplasma* encephalitis remains one of the most common causes of encephalitis in the United States.

Laboratory Diagnosis

Most cases of *Toxoplasma gondii* infections elude diagnosis because they are either asymptomatic or mimic common viral infections. The routine method of diagnosis for suspected toxoplasmosis is serologic testing. Detection of IgM anti-*Toxoplasma* antibodies may be diagnostic of acute infection, particularly in congenital infections, because IgM appears early in the infection. A variety of testing procedures are currently available including: the indirect fluorescent antibody test (IFA), the Sabin-Feldman dye test, the indirect hemagglutination test, complement fixation and ELISA. Antigen detection tests are also available.

Stained histologic slide preparations are used to demonstrate trophozoites or cysts containing bradyzoites in tissue biopsy samples. Observation of parasites in bronchoalveolar lavage or CSF may be effective in immunocompromised patients. Animal inoculation and tissue culture techniques offer limited value and may be cumbersome for most laboratories.

Treatment and Prevention

It is generally accepted that an otherwise healthy, asymptomatic, infected person will not require treatment. For patients with clinically active toxoplasmosis, AIDS patients and other immunocompromised individuals, a month long course of combination therapy with pyrimethamine and trisulfapyrimidines is recommended. These drugs are not without their side effects. Pyrimethamine has been associated with bone marrow suppression and may require supplemental folic acid administration. Clindamycin has also been used in the treatment of *Toxoplasma* encephalitis in AIDS patients and in patients with a history of allergy to sulfa-based medication. Pyrimethamine is not recommended for use in pregnant women. An alternative drug, Spiramycin, which has been used in France for a number of years, is now available in the United

States through the FDA. In patients with retinochoroiditis, the administration of corticosteroids aids in the reduction of inflammation.

The majority of human infections with *Toxoplasma gondii* are acquired through ingestion or handling of contaminated meat or from contact with infected cat feces. Therefore, preventive measures should surround these activities. The populations at greatest risk of serious consequence are pregnant women and the immunocompromised.

Meat should be thoroughly cooked before eating to prevent ingestion of viable *T. gondii* tissue cysts. Careful hand washing is also necessary when handling raw meat. Cutting boards and utensils used during meat preparation should be sanitized.

The transmission of *T. gondii* may also be prevented by wearing disposable gloves when gardening in possibly contaminated soil or changing the litter box. Cats that have access to the outdoors are likely to be infected. They pass oocysts in their feces that become infective in several days. For this reason, the litter box should be cleaned and disinfected daily. Children's sandboxes should be covered when not in use to prevent contamination with cat feces. Indoor cats that feed solely on dry or canned cat food are less likely to carry the parasite.

PNEUMOCYSTIS CARINII

First reported in 1909 by Chagas, *Pneumocystis carinii* has long had an uncertain taxonomic status. Once considered a rather obscure protozoan parasite of animals, it instantly rose in clinical significance when identified as the agent of **Pneumocystis carinii pneumonia (PCP).** Although most recent nucleic acid and biochemical studies have determined that *Pneumocystis carinii* is a fungus, it is briefly discussed for the sake of completeness.

Life Cycle

The life cycle and epidemiology of *Pneumocystis* are still incompletely understood. *Pneumocystis carinii* has a widespread distribution. It is found in the environment as well as the lungs and upper respiratory tract of healthy humans and animals. Serologic evidence indicates that the majority of the population is exposed to the organism before age five.

Pneumocystis carinii is known to have two distinct stages, a trophozoite stage and a cyst stage. The trophozoites are ovoid or ameboid in shape, contain one nucleus, measure less than 5 micrometers, and probably multiply by binary fission. The rounded cyst form measures 5 to 8 micrometers in diameter and when mature, contain 6 to 8 intracystic bodies, also referred to in some sources as developing trophozoites. Both stages may be recovered from clinical material obtained from the lungs of infected individuals. Neither stage appears to be intracellular.

It is suggested that *Pneumocystis carinii* is transmitted from person-to-person via respiratory droplets. Once inside the respiratory tract, *P. carinii* settles into the alveolar spaces. Mature cysts rupture, releasing actively growing and multiplying trophozoites. Eventually, the trophozoites develop into new, mature cysts and the cycle is complete (Figure 10–13).

Transmission and Pathogenesis

Pneumocystosis is the most frequent opportunistic infection in immunosuppressed patients and a leading cause of death in AIDS patients. Prior to the AIDS epidemic, the incidence of symptomatic *P. carinii* infection was rare, being reported only in the occasional premature, malnourished infant or immunocompromised adult.

The organism is thought to be transmitted from person-to-person by respiratory droplets. The lungs are the primary site of infection. In the immunocompetent patient, the infecting cyst is usually inactivated by the host's immune defenses and the patient remains asymptomatic. However, in the compromised host, *P. carinii* multiplies unchecked on the surface of epithelial cells and the alveolar spaces begin to fill with a foamy exudate. Chest X-ray demonstrates characteristic diffuse, bilateral infiltrates. Pulmonary function becomes deficient and the patient shows signs of hypoxia.

The clinical symptoms of *Pneumocystis carinii* pneumonia are nonspecific and typically include a history of fever, labored breathing, a dry, nonproductive cough and cyanosis. Extrapulmonary infections are rare but may involve the spleen, liver, lymph nodes and bone marrow. The prognosis for untreated cases is poor, ranging from 50% to 100% mortality. For approximately 60% of patients with HIV, PCP is the initial AIDS defining diagnosis. Prophylactic treatment is recommended.

Laboratory Diagnosis

A specific diagnosis is based on identification of *Pneumocystis carinii* in clinical specimens. Since the organism tends to fill the alveolar spaces, the specimen of choice is induced (nebulized) sputum or bronchoalveolar lavage (BAL) material or, in some cases, lung biopsy tissue.

Smears are prepared and stained with Giemsa or iron hematoxylin for demonstration of trophozoite nuclei and intracystic stages. Histologic preparations

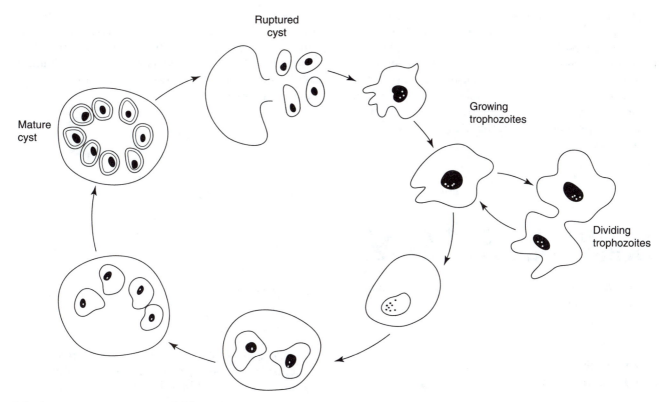

FIG 10–13 *Pneumocystis carinii* life cycle

stained with Gomori's methenamine silver stain are recommended for the demonstration of cysts in tissue. Immunofluorescent techniques that utilize monoclonal antibodies may identify *P. carinii* with a high degree of sensitivity and specificity.

Treatment and Prevention

Traditional antifungal drugs are ineffective. The treatment of choice for *Pneumocystis carinii* infection is trimethoprim/sulfamethoxazole (TMP/SMX or Bactrim) given IV or orally over a 21 day period. Recommended alternative therapy, particularly for patients with sulfa allergy, is pentamidine, atovaquone or trimethoprim plus dapsone.

Because the true life cycle is still uncertain, there are no preventive measures available. It is thought that *Pneumocystis carinii* is spread between humans by inhalation of infected droplet nuclei. Patients with immunodeficiency should be monitored for disease and promptly treated.

SUMMARY

The apicomplexans (sporozoans) are small, intracellular parasites transmitted to humans via the bite of a blood-sucking arthropod. They have complex life cycles, including sexual and asexual phases.

Malaria remains the world's most significant tropical parasitic disease, threatening 40% of the world population. Four species of *Plasmodium* cause human malaria: *Plasmodium vivax*, *Plasmodium ovale*, *Plasmodium malariae*, and *Plasmodium falciparum*. All are vectored by the female *Anopheles* mosquito. Sporozoites serve as the infective stage for humans.

Malaria is a febrile hemolytic anemia characterized by periodic episodes of chills, fever, and sweating, called paroxysms. Diagnosis is made by demonstration of the parasite in Giemsa stained blood smears. Therapy is generally chloroquine, quinine, or primaquine.

Babesiosis is a tick-borne, malaria-like, disease of humans caused most frequently in the United States by *Babesia microti*. The majority of cases are concentrated in the southern New England area and are vectored by species of *Ixodes* ticks. Diagnosis is made by demonstration of the organism in Giemsa stained blood smears. The disease is usually self-limited.

Toxoplasma gondii is an apicomplexan parasite of worldwide distribution that can infect most warm blooded vertebrates, including man. Members of the cat family serve as the primary reservoir and man is generally accidentally infected.

Human toxoplasmosis is acquired by ingestion of raw or poorly cooked meat containing the tissue cyst, or by ingestion of oocysts, or by the congenital route. Infections are typically mild, with flu-like symptoms, except in the immunocompromised patient or the developing fetus where the infection may be life-threatening. Combination therapy of pyrimethamine and trisulfapyrimidines is recommended for clinically active disease.

Pneumocystis carinii is a widely distributed opportunistic fungus of the respiratory tract that causes a severe and sometimes fatal pneumonia in premature infants and patients with AIDS and immunodeficiency. The treatment of choice is trimethoprim-sulfamethoxazole.

REVIEW QUESTIONS

1. Sexual reproduction of *Plasmodium vivax* takes place in the:
   a. human gut
   b. red blood cells
   c. mosquito
   d. parenchymal cells of the liver

2. During the exoerythrocytic phase of infection, *Plasmodium* merozoites develop within:
   a. liver cells
   b. red blood cells
   c. the salivary glands
   d. macrophages

3. A self-limited apicomplexan infection that is characterized by a gradual onset of headache, chills, sweating and fatigue following tick bite is caused by:
   a. *Borrelia burgdorferi*
   b. *Babesia microti*
   c. *Plasmodium vivax*
   d. *Plasmodium ovale*

4. *Plasmodium* species are vectored by members of the genus:
   a. *Ixodes*
   b. *Anopheles*
   c. *Culex*
   d. *Glossina*

5. The drug of choice for the treatment of uncomplicated malaria is most commonly:
   a. Penicillin
   b. Chloroquine
   c. Aspirin
   d. Clindamycin

6. The infective stage of the *Plasmodium* parasite for humans is the:
   a. merozoite
   b. trophozoite
   c. gametocyte
   d. sporozoite

7. This species of *Plasmodium* is characterized by crescent shaped gametocytes and multiple ring forms within red blood cells:
   a. *Plasmodium vivax*
   b. *Plasmodium ovale*
   c. *Plasmodium falciparum*
   d. *Plasmodium malariae*

8. Giemsa stained blood smears demonstrate normal size blood cells containing ring form trophozoites in tetrads, without pigment or stippling. The most likely parasite is:
   a. *Babesia microti*
   b. *Plasmodium falciparum*
   c. *Plasmodium vivax*
   d. *Plasmodium malariae*

9. A malarial infection characterized by a 72-hour periodicity of paroxysms and stained blood films with normal size red cells containing band form trophozoites and Ziemann's dots is most likely caused by:
   a. *Plasmodium vivax*
   b. *Plasmodium ovale*
   c. *Plasmodium falciparum*
   d. *Plasmodium malariae*

10. The dormant parasite forms found in patients with vivax malaria are called:
    a. trophozoites
    b. sporozoites
    c. hypnozoites
    d. gametocytes

11. The definitive host for *Toxoplasma gondii* is the:

    a. mosquito

    b. dog

    c. cat

    d. human

12. The infective stage for this parasite is transmitted in cat feces and presents the greatest risk to the immunocompromised patient and the unborn fetus:

    a. *Toxoplasma gondii*

    b. *Pneumocystis carinii*

    c. *Plasmodium ovale*

    d. *Trypanosoma cruzi*

13. *Pneumocystis carinii* is the common cause of:

    a. hemolytic disease of the newborn

    b. interstitial pneumonia in AIDS patients

    c. hemolytic anemia in compromised hosts

    d. disseminated intravascular coagulation

14. Toxoplasmosis can be acquired by:

    a. eating tissue cysts in raw meat

    b. cleaning the cat litter box

    c. transplacental passage of the parasite

    d. all of the above

15. The treatment of choice for *Pneumocystis carinii* pneumonia is:

    a. Penicillin

    b. Amphotericin B

    c. Bactrim

    d. Quinine

16. The infective form of *Toxoplasma gondii* that is commonly found in cat feces is the:

    a. oocyst

    b. tachyzoite

    c. bradyzoite

    d. zygote

17. The tissue cyst of *Toxoplasma gondii* contains slow growing trophozoites called:

    a. tachyzoites

    b. bradyzoites

    c. sporozoites

    d. oocysts

18. Reactivation of cerebral toxoplasmosis is a major cause of encephalitis in patients with:

    a. ear infections

    b. cardiac arrhythmia

    c. AIDS

    d. osteoporosis

CASE STUDY

A 38-year old man presents at the emergency room with a 10 day history of headache, fever, chills, sweats and myalgias. A patient history also reveals that the man is employed as a consulting oil geologist and has just returned from a 2 month assignment in Ethiopia, Sudan and Thailand. He had been immunized against hepatitis A and B, poliomyelitis, and typhoid. He admits to having been non-compliant with malarial prophylaxis (chloroquine). Physical exam reveals a fever of 103 degrees F, a rapid pulse rate and generalized sweating. All other findings were not remarkable. A complete blood count was ordered and demonstrated intra-erythrocytic organisms.

Questions

1. What is the most likely diagnosis?

2. Which of the following laboratory studies would be most helpful in narrowing a diagnosis:

    a. blood smears for malaria studies
    b. stool for ova and parasites
    c. stool culture for *Salmonella*
    d. serum glucose level

3. How would you explain the discrepancy between the clinical findings and the patient history of immunization and prophylaxis?

▶ BIBLIOGRAPHY

Anderson, J. F., Mintz, E. D., Gadbaw, J. J., & Magnarelli, L. A. (1991). *Babesia microti*, human babesiosis, and *Borrelia burgdorferi* in Connecticut. *Journal of Clinical Microbiology, 29*, 2779–2783.

Beaver, P.C., Jung, R. C., & Cupp, E. W. (1984). *Clinical parasitology* (9th ed.). Philadelphia: Lea & Febiger.

Berkow, R., & Fletcher, A. J. (1992). *The Merck manual of diagnosis and therapy* (16th ed.). Whitehouse Station, NJ: Merck Research Laboratories.

Bottone, E. J. (1991). Diagnosis of acute pulmonary toxoplasmosis by visualization of invasive and intracellular tachyzoites in Giemsa stained smears of bronchoalveolar lavage fluid. *Journal of Clinical Microbiology, 29*, 2626–2627.

Centers for Disease Control and Prevention (1997). Probable locally acquired mosquito transmitted *Plasmodium vivax* infection—Georgia, 1996. *Morbidity and Mortality Weekly Report, 46*, 264–267.

Centers for Disease Control and Prevention. (1999). *Parasites and health*, Pneumocystis carinii *infection*. Division of Parasitic Diseases.

Centers for Disease Control and Prevention. (1999). *Parasites and health, Toxoplasmosis*. Division of Parasitic Diseases.

Frenkel, J. K. (1985). Toxoplasmosis. *Pediatric Clinics of North America, 32*, 917–932.

Frenkel, J. K. (1990). Toxoplasmosis in human beings. *JAVMA, 196*, 240–248.

Garcia, L. S., & Bruckner, D. A. (1993). *Diagnostic medical parasitology* (2nd ed.). Washington, DC: American Society of Microbiology.

Garnham, P. C. C. (1966). *Malaria parasites and other Haemosporidia*. Oxford: Blackwell Scientific Publications.

Garnham, P. C. C. (1977). The continuing mystery of relapses in malaria. *Protozoology Abstracts, 1*, 1–12.

Healy, G. R., & Ruebush, T. K., II. (1980). Morphology of *Babesia microti* in human blood smears. *American Journal of Clinical Pathology, 73*, 107.

Homer, K. S., Wiley, E. L., Smith, A. L., Mccollough, L., Clark, D., Nightengale, S. D., & Vuitch, F. (1992). Monoclonal antibody to *Pneumocystis carinii*—comparison with silver stain in bronchial lavage specimens. *American Journal of Clinical Pathology, 97*, 619–624.

Isaacson, M. (1989). Airport malaria: A review. *W. H. O. Bulletin, 67*, 737–743.

Jones, T. C., Kean, B. H., & Kimball, A. C. (1969). Acquired toxoplasmosis. *New York State Journal of Medicine, 69*, 2237–2242.

Krick, J. A., & Remington, J. S. (1978). Toxoplasmosis in the adult—an overview. *New England Journal of Medicine, 298*, 550–553.

Markell, E. K., John, D. K. & Krotoski, W. A. (1999). *Medical parasitology* (8th ed.). Philadelphia: W. B. Saunders.

Marshall, E. (1991). Malaria parasite gaining ground against science. *Science, 254*, 190.

Panisko, D. M., & Keystone, J. S. (1990). Treatment of malaria—1990. *Drugs, 39*, 160–189.

Richards, F. O., Kovacs, J. A., & Luft, B. J. (1995). Preventing toxoplasmosis encephalitis in persons infected with human immunodeficiency virus. *Clinical Infectious Diseases, 21*, (Suppl 1), S49–56.

Ruebush, T. K., II, Juranek, D. D., Chisholm, F. S., et al. (1977). Human babesiosis in Nantucket Island: Evidence of self limited and subclinical infections. *New England Journal of Medicine, 297*, 825–827.

Shimeld, L.A. (1999). *Essentials of diagnostic microbiology*. Albany, NY: Delmar Publishers.

Siddiqui, W. A. (1991). Where are we in the quest for vaccines for malaria? *Drugs, 41*, 1–10.

Talaro, K. P., & Talaro, A. (1999). *Foundations in microbiology* (3rd ed.). Boston: WBC McGraw-Hill.

Wiest, P. M., Opal, S. M., Romulo, R. L., & Olds, G. R. (1991). Malaria in travelers in Rhode Island: A review of 26 cases. *American Journal of Medicine, 91*, 30–36.

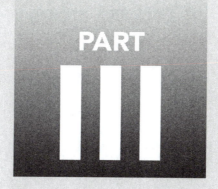

PART

III

Helminths

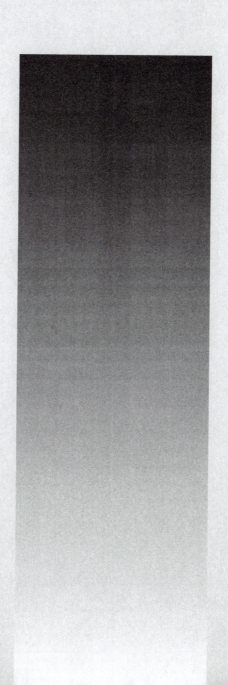

CHAPTER ELEVEN
Intestinal Nematodes

OUTLINE

INTESTINAL NEMATODES
Enterobius vermicularis
(en-ter-O-bee-us ver-mik-u-LAR-is)
Ascaris lumbricoides
(as-KAR-is lum-bri-KOY-dees)

Trichuris trichiura (tri-KUR-is tri-KUR-a)
Necator americanus (ne-KAY-tor a-mer-i-KAN-us)/*Ancylostoma duodenale* (AN-si-LOS-to-ma DOO-o-den-AL-ee)
Strongyloides stercoralis
(STRON-gee-LOY-dees STER-kor-AL-is)

LEARNING OBJECTIVES

After reading and studying this chapter, the student should be able to:

- List the clinically significant intestinal nematodes which cause human disease.

- List and describe characteristics used to identify intestinal nematodes.

- Describe and compare life cycles of intestinal nematodes, and identify the stage of development which is infective for man.

- Compare the morphological characteristics of intestinal nematode ova, larvae and adult forms;

determine which stage of development is usually diagnostic for human infection.

- Describe the pathogenesis of human intestinal nematode infections.

- Describe the treatment and prevention of infection with intestinal nematodes.

- Define the hyperinfection syndrome, and identify which parasite is apt to cause this phenomenon.

KEY TERMS

Buccal capsule
(BUK-al kap-sul)
Buccal cavity (BUK-al cav-IT-E)
Decorticated
(dee-KOR-ti-ka-ted)

Embryonated
(EM-bree-o-na-ted)
Filariform larva
(fil-AR-i-form Lar-va)
Gravid (GRA-vid)
Helminth (HELL-minth)

Larva (LAR-va)
Nematode (NEM-a-toad)
Parthenogenic
(PAR-then-o-JEN-ik)
Rhabditiform larva
(rab-DIT-i-form LAR-va)

INTRODUCTION

The diagnosis of infections caused by worms **(helminths)** of the intestinal tract is usually made by observing the characteristic eggs (ova), **larvae** (immature forms), adults, or other structures in feces or other bodily material. The ova of a helminth are usually characteristic of that species. The eggs are much larger than protozoan parasites, and easier to observe. Diagnostic features of helminth ova include size, shape, and the color and thickness of the eggshell. An embryo may develop within the egg; the egg is then described as being **embryonated**. The stage of development of the parasite within the egg may be useful in the identification of the helminth. The eggshell may be colorless, or yellowish or brown because of bile staining. Thickness varies among species.

INTESTINAL NEMATODES

Nematodes (roundworms) are members of the phylum Aschelminthes and the class Nematoda. Round-worms are the most common helminths which infect humans. They have a cylindrical shape, covered by a tough outer covering called a cuticle, and a complete digestive system, including a mouth and an anus. Separate sexes exist, with the females typically being larger than the males. Most adult nematodes are not found in human feces; ova and larvae are the most common diagnostic forms. The size and shape of intestinal nematode ova are constant for a given species. Ova may be round or oval, and the shape may vary in fertilized and unfertilized eggs. The characteristic features of intestinal nematode ova are illustrated in Figure 11–1.

The stage of development of the parasite within an ovum is characteristic for a given species of nematode. Infertile eggs tend to contain unorganized masses of material within the eggshell. Nematode eggs left at room tempereature may develop embryos, which may hatch, displaying larvae in the stool.

Most intestinal nematodes which cause human infection have direct life cycles, being transmitted from person-to-person, with no intermediate hosts. The life cycles of all nematodes include four larval stages,

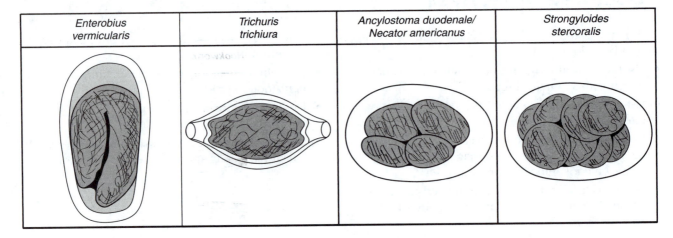

Enterobius vermicularis	*Trichuris trichiura*	*Ancylostoma duodenale/ Necator americanus*	*Strongyloides stercoralis*

Ascaris lumbricoides

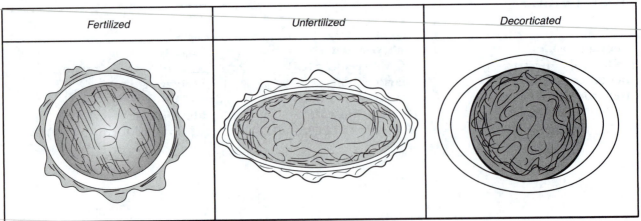

Fertilized	*Unfertilized*	*Decorticated*

FIG 11–1 Ova of intestinal nematodes

undergoing three molts, and one adult stage. Transmission of infection occurs by ingestion of ova or via the larval stage. The characteristic features of significant intestinal nematode larvae are illustrated in Figure 11–2.

Enterobius vermicularis

Morphology

Enterobius vermicularis is called the pinworm, because of the long, pointed tail (resembling a pin) found on the adult worm. The female worm, larger than the male, measures 7–13 mm long (Figure 11–3); adult males are smaller, and usually go unnoticed. The ovum of *E. vermicularis* is oval, flattened on one side, and has a thick, colorless shell (Figure 11–4). It measures 50–60 µm in length by 20–30 µm in width. Larvae may be visible within the embryonated eggs.

Life Cycle

The direct life cycle of *E. vermicularis* begins with the deposition of partially embryonated eggs, when the **gravid** (egg-bearing) female migrates, usually at night, from the intestine to the perianal folds of the infected individual. The female worm is highly prolific. The ova develop to the infectious stage within six hours. After ingestion of the embryonated egg, maturation to the adult stage occurs in the intestine in about 30 days.

Transmission and Pathogenesis

Enterobiasis, a very common parasitic infection, is transmitted directly by the fecal-oral route, by ingestion or inhalation of embryonated ova, from contaminated fingers or fomites, such as bed linen, toilet seats or clothing. Infection is found worldwide, but especially in temperate climates. It occurs most commonly in children, and is frequently spread in families. The ova of *E. vermicularis* have been associated with transmission of infection with the protozoan parasite, *Dientamoeba fragilis* (see Chapter 6).

Although anal itching is common, and insomnia and irritability have been reported, infections are often asymptomatic. Eosinophilia has been reported. In rare cases, migration of worms into the vagina has occurred, with subsequent vaginal discharge.

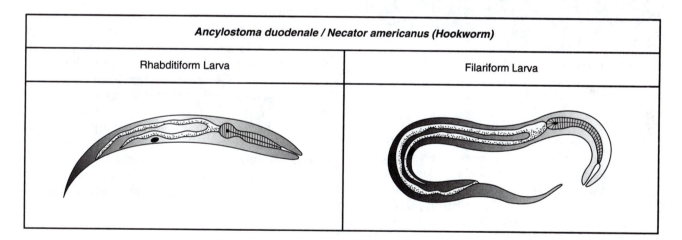

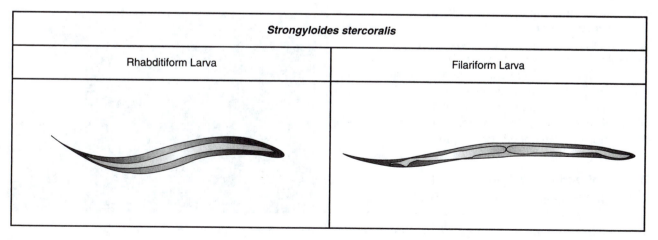

FIG 11–2 Larvae of intestinal nematodes

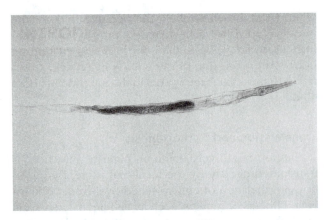

FIG 11–3 Adult worm of *E. vermicularis*

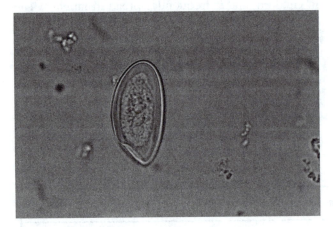

FIG 11–4 Embryonated eggs of *E. vermicularis*

Laboratory Diagnosis

The diagnosis of enterobiasis is best accomplished using the "scotch tape test." The specimen should be taken before the child has a bowel movement, and is collected by applying transparent cellophane tape ("scotch tape") to the perianal area late at night, or in the morning, after female worm migration has occurred. The tape is then pressed onto a clean microscope slide. The slide is examined microscopically for the presence of typical ova. Four to six slides should be examined to rule out infection. A commercially available device called a "Swoop Tube" (see Chapter 2) provides a more convenient method of specimen collection for the examination for pinworm. The adult worm may occasionally be found in stool specimens; however, the routine examination for ova and parasites is not recommended for diagnosis.

Treatment and Prevention

The antihelminthic agent, mebendazole, or piperazine may be used to treat enterobiasis in symptomatic individuals. Asymptomatic individuals are rarely treated. Although total prevention of infection is usually not possible, good hygiene, as well as prompt and thorough laundering of contaminated linens, should reduce the spread of infection.

Ascaris lumbricoides

Morphology

Ascaris lumbricoides, known as the large intestinal roundworm, is the largest of the intestinal nematodes, with the adult female often measuring more than 30 cm (Figure 11–5). The male worm is about half this length.

The fertilized egg is broadly oval, and measures 45–75 μm in length and 35–50 μm in width. The egg usually has a thick, transparent shell, surrounded by a yellow/brown bile-stained mammillated outer covering. When the mammillated outer covering is absent, the ovum is said to be **decorticated**. Eggs passed in the feces are usually in the one-cell stage. Infertile eggs are more elongated (80–90 μm long), showing disorganized globular internal contents. Mammilations may be prominent and scattered irregularly, or altogether absent. Figure 11–6 shows the variations in the ova.

Life Cycle

Ingested embryonated eggs containing second-stage larvae hatch in the small intestine. Larvae penetrate the intestinal wall, and migrate by means of the hepatic portal circulation to the liver, right heart, pulmonary vessels and lungs, eventually reaching the trachea and pharynx (Figure 11–7). The larvae are swallowed and pass into the small intestine, where they mature and mate. About two months after infection, egg deposition occurs. Fertilized eggs, passed in feces, become infective in warm, moist soil, within two weeks. Females produce infertile eggs in the absence of males.

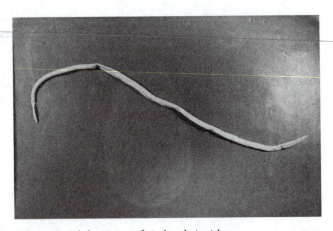

FIG 11–5 Adult worm of *A. lumbricoides*

(A)
Fertile egg

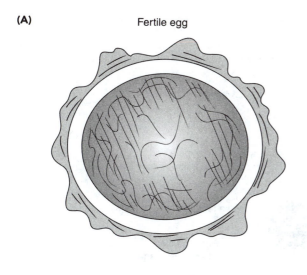

(B)
Infertile egg

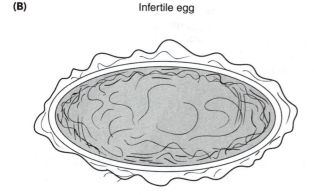

(C)
Decorticated egg

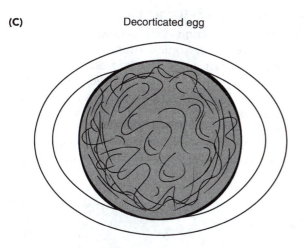

FIG 11–6 *Ascaris lumbricoides*

Transmission and Pathogenesis

Ascariasis occurs worldwide, and is transmitted by the fecal-oral route. Humans become infected by ingesting embryonated eggs from contaminated soil. Eggs passed in feces usually contain first stage larvae. Maturation occurs in the soil, particularly in the hard clay type of soil, with formation of the second stage larvae within approximately two weeks. Transmission of the protozoan parasite, *Dientamoeba fragilis*, has been associated with *Ascaris* ova (see Chapter 6). Infection with *Trichuris trichiura* may occur simultaneously with *Ascaris* infection.

Most infections are asymptomatic. In heavy infections, nutritional deficiencies may develop, especially in children. Larval migration may elicit intense tissue reactions. Migrating worms may lead to obstruction, such as intestinal blockage.

Infections caused by ascarid parasites of dogs and cats, esecially *Toxacara canis*, primarily a dog ascarid, occur occasionally, especially in children. The disease visceral larva migrans is caused by the migration of parasitic larval stages through body viscera. Since the human is an abnormal host for this parasite, larvae do not mature and produce eggs.

Laboratory Diagnosis

The diagnosis of infection with *A. lumbricoides* is made by the identification of fertilized or unfertilized eggs in human feces. The zinc sulfate flotation method is not recommended for processing these specimens. Adult worms, which produce extremely large numbers of eggs, may sometimes be passed in feces, or may pass out of a body orifice, such as anus, nose, or mouth. Larvae may also be found in sputum or gastric washings.

Visceral larva migrans caused by dog and cat ascarid parasites is diagnosed by serologic means, or by histologic demonstration of larvae in tissue, since typical diagnostic stages are not found in feces.

Treatment and Prevention

Treatment with antihelminthic agents, such as mebendazole or piperazine, is effective in eliminating adult worms. However, larvae may not be so affected. Prevention of infection requires the maintainance of adequate sanitary facilities to prevent contamination of the soil with human feces. The practice of using human feces as fertilizer (as in many developing countries) should be avoided.

Trichuris trichiura

Morphology

Trichuris trichiura is referred to as the whipworm because of the resemblance of the adult worm to a whip, having a long, slender, thread-like anterior portion, and a thicker posterior portion (Figure 11–8), with the appearance of a whip handle. The length of the adult worm is in the range of 30–50 mm. The adult male has a coiled tail, and is smaller than the female.

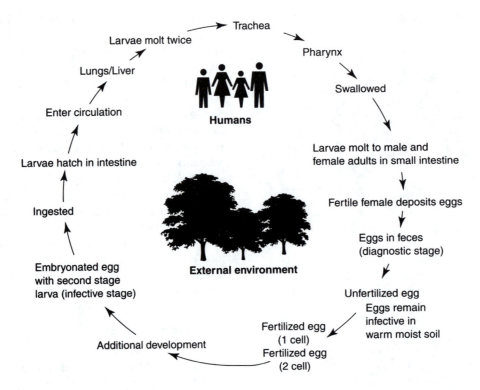

FIG 11–7 *Ascaris lumbricoides,* life cycle

The eggs of *T. trichiura* are bile-stained and oval or barrel-shaped, with a thick, smooth shell, and a clear, prominent polar plug at each end. The eggs measure 45–55 μm in length by 20–23 μm in width (Figure 11–9).

Life Cycle

The life cycle of *T. trichiura* is direct. After passage in the feces, the eggs take approximately two weeks to mature and become infective. Embryonated eggs containing the first stage larvae are ingested from contaminated hard clay soil. Development occurs in the duodenum and cecum. The worm attaches by its ante-rior end to the intestinal mucosa. It takes about three months before the adult worm begins to lay eggs.

Transmission and Pathogenesis

Whipworm infection occurs worldwide, but especially in developing tropical countries and the rural southwestern part of the United States. Infection occurs after ingestion of embryonated eggs in contaminated food or water, or directly from soil. Most infections are asymptomatic. With a heavy worm burden, nausea, diarrhea, abdominal pain, and weight loss may occur. Blood loss in serious infections may result in anemia, and serious infections may lead to

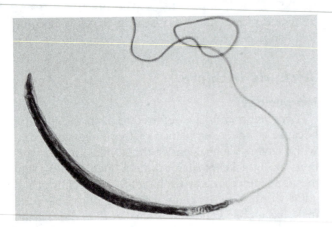

FIG 11–8 Adult worm of *T. trichiura*

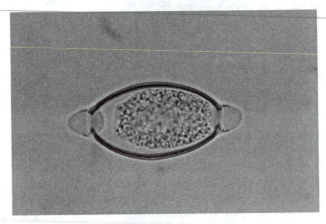

FIG 11–9 Embryonated egg of *T. trichiura*

rectal prolapse. Simultaneous infections with *Ascaris* are common.

Laboratory Diagnosis

The diagnosis of infection is usually made by the identification of typical, oval eggs, displaying the prominent polar plugs at each end. The routine concentration methods (see Chapter 2) for detection of ova and parasites are recommended. Distorted eggs may be present in patients receiving antihelminthic treatment. Adult worms are rarely seen in feces.

Treatment and Prevention

The drug of choice is mebendazole. Prevention requires adherence to good personal hygiene, and avoidance of contaminated food or water. Avoidance of the use of human feces as fertilizer is necessary to prevent infection.

Necator americanus/ Ancylostoma duodenale

Morphology

The adult stages of the hookworms *Necator americanus* and *Ancylostoma duodenale* are rarely seen, and are similar in appearance. Characterized by a hooklike anterior end (thus the name "hookworm"), the male is somewhat smaller than the female, which measures 10–12 mm. The **buccal capsules** (which are primitive mouths) of the two hookworms differ in structure. That of *A. duodenale* is characterized by teeth, while the mouth parts of *N. americanus* consist of cutting plates (Figure 11–10A and B). These well-developed structures account for the firm attachment of the adult worms to the intestinal mucosa, with the scarcity of their appearance in feces. Differentiation

of the two genera of hookworms requires the examination of the mouthparts of the adult worms.

The ova of the two hookworms, although slightly different in size, are essentially identical, and are usually not used to distinguish them. The egg of the slightly larger *N. americanus* measures 55–75 μm long by 35–40 μm wide (Figure 11–11). A thin, clear, smooth, colorless shell encloses the embryonated contents of the egg. A clear space is apparent between the eggshell and the developing embryo. After passage, the first-stage larva hatches in soil.

The first stage **rhabditiform larva** (the noninfective free-living form), which measures about 270 μm, is characterized by a prominent primitive mouth called a **buccal cavity**, and a small genital primordium (Figure 11–12A). These characteristics help to distinguish the hookworm larva from the larva of *Strongyloides stercoralis* (described in the next section). The **filariform larva** is not capable of living independently and must find a host. This form is characterized by an esophagus, notably shorter than that of the rhabditiform larva, and by the presence of a long, pointy tail (Figure 11–12B).

Life Cycle

The life cycles of *N. americanus* and *A. duodenale* are identical. The infection is initiated with the penetration of the skin by the filariform (third stage) larvae from the soil (Figure 11–13). The larvae enter the circulation, migrate to the lungs, trachea and pharynx, and are swallowed. Maturation to the adult stage occurs in the intestine, when the worm attaches to the intestinal mucosa, by means of well-developed mouth parts previously described. Eggs are produced in the intestine, and are passed in the feces, usually in the early cleavage stage. The egg hatches to produce a rhabditiform larva, which develops into the third stage

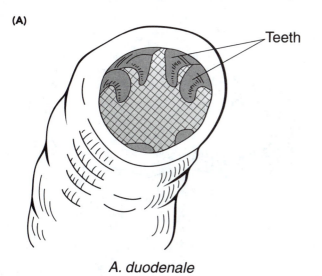

(A)

Teeth

A. duodenale

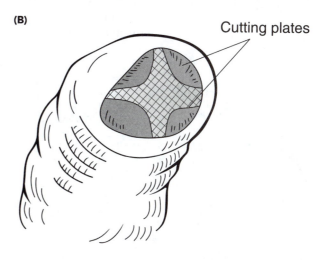

(B)

Cutting plates

N. americanus

FIG 11–10 Hookworm buccal capsules

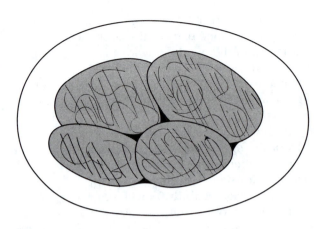

FIG 11–11 Hookworm egg

(infective stage) filariform larva after two molts in the soil.

Transmission and Pathogenesis

Hookworm infection is acquired when the filariform larvae penetrate the skin, usually hands or feet, from contaminated soil. Although the pathogenesis of hookworm infection is similar for both agents, geographical distributions differ. *N. americanus* is known as "New-world hookworm," causing infection predominantly in North and South America. *A. duodenale* is called "Old-world hookworm," because of its prevalence in Africa, India, China, southern Europe, and Japan. Today, since widespread international travel is commonplace, infections with either agent may be encountered worldwide.

Laboratory Diagnosis

The diagnosis of hookworm infection is made by identifying typical hookworm eggs in human feces.

Because of the similarity of the ova of both agents, a report of "hookworm ova" is sufficient to make a diagnosis. Occasionally the egg hatches in feces, producing a rhabditiform larva. It is then necessary to distinguish the hookworm larva from the larvae of *Strongyloides stercoralis*, which requires different therapy.

Treatment and Prevention

Some hookworm infections are asymptomatic, and require little treatment other than adequate nutrition. Patients with more severe infections suffer from symptoms including nausea, fatigue, vomiting, abdominal pain, anorexia, and diarrhea. Mebendazole and piperazine are recommended for treatment of symptomatic infection. Severe cases of anemia may require iron replacement therapy.

Recommendations for prevention of infection are similar to those for *Ascaris*, including proper sanitation practices, and the avoidance of using human feces as fertilizer.

Strongyloides stercoralis

Morphology

Adult worms, known as threadworms, reside in the intestine. The adult female is **parthenogenic** (self-fertilizing), rarely seen in feces, and is approximately 2 mm in length. It has a short buccal cavity, and a long, thin esophagus.

The thin-shelled eggs of *Strongyloides stercoralis* are slightly smaller than those of hookworms, but are otherwise virtually indistinguishable. The eggs generally release the noninfective rhabditiform larvae in the intestine, and are not often detected in stool specimens.

The first stage rhabditiform larva (diagnostic stage), usually passed in feces, is approximately 200–400 μm

(A)

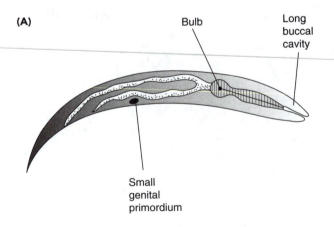

Bulb

Long buccal cavity

Small genital primordium

Rhabditiform

(B)

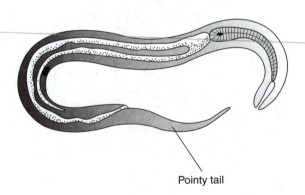

Pointy tail

Filariform

FIG 11–12 Hookworm larvae

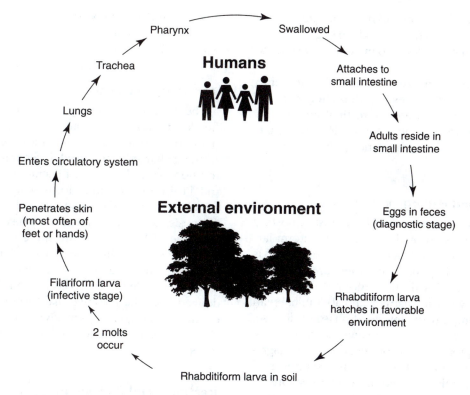

FIG 11-13 Hookworm life cycle

long, and 15–20 μm wide (Figure 11–14A). The larva is characterized by having a short buccal cavity, and a prominent genital primordium. These features distinguish it from the hookworm larva, with a long buccal cavity, and a small genital primordium (see Figure 11–12A)

The third stage filariform larva (infective stage) develops from the rhabditiform larva, usually in soil. It is larger than the rhabditiform larva, measuring up to 680 μm in length (Figure 11–14B). It has a longer esophagus than the hookworm, and a notched, rather than a pointy, tail (see Figure 11–12B).

Life Cycle

The infective filariform larvae, usually in the soil, penetrate the skin (Figure 11–15). The larvae then pass into the circulation and migrate to the right heart, to the lungs, trachea, and pharynx, where they are swallowed, and mature to adult worms in the intestine in approximately two weeks. The female adult worms produce eggs, which usually hatch, releasing rhabditiform larvae in the intestine. These noninfective larvae are often passed in the feces. In the soil, they develop into infective filariform larvae, ready to penetrate the skin of a new host. In the indirect cycle, the

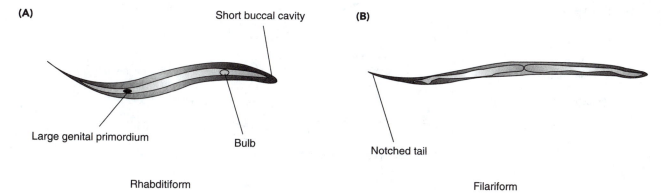

(A)

Short buccal cavity

Large genital primordium

Bulb

Rhabditiform

(B)

Notched tail

Filariform

FIG 11-14 *Strongyloides* larvae

rhabditiform larvae develop into free-living adult male and female worms, which may produce eggs and non-infective larvae that develop into infective larvae in the soil.

The rhabditiform larvae may also develop into filariform larvae in the intestine; the latter infective forms may then penetrate the intestinal mucosa, or the perianal skin to result in autoinfection. These larvae may then enter the circulation, and begin the cycle again.

Transmission and Pathogenesis

Strongyloidiasis is transmitted from host to host by penetration of the skin by the infective filariform larvae in contaminated soil. Although some itching is common during skin penetration, there are few other symptoms associated with this stage of disease; allergic reactions may occur. Diarrhea and abdominal pain frequently accompany the intestinal phase of disease. Other symptoms may include vomiting and weight loss. Pulmonary symptoms may be present during the migratory phase in the lungs. Coughing and shortness of breath are frequently reported in heavy infections.

Autoinfection may lead to the hyperinfection syndrome, which may occur years after the initial infection. Sepsis and meningitis, often polymicrobial, may develop, with the spreading of enteric bacteria from intestine to blood. Disseminated infection occurs especially in immunocompromised individuals. During autopsy, larvae may be found in many organs, such as lungs, liver, and heart.

Laboratory Diagnosis

The diagnosis of strongyloidiasis is usually made by the identification of rhabditiform larvae in human feces. Filariform larvae may sometimes be seen. Distinguishing characteristics used to separate strongyloides and hookworm larvae are illustrated in Figures 11–12 and 11–14. Ova or adult forms may occasionally be found. The Entero-test may also be used to make a diagnosis. Duodenal contents may be examined for the presence of larvae. Ova are more apt to be seen in these specimens. In disseminated infections, larvae have been identified in sputum specimens.

Antibody detection assays should use antigens derived from the infective filariform larvae of *S. stercoralis* for the greatest sensitivity and specificity (see chapter 3). Cross-reactions with other nematodes may occur.

Treatment and Prevention

The treatment of choice for strongyloidiasis is thiabendazole, although complete helminth eradication does not always occur. Prevention of disease is accomplished by the practice of wearing shoes, as well as

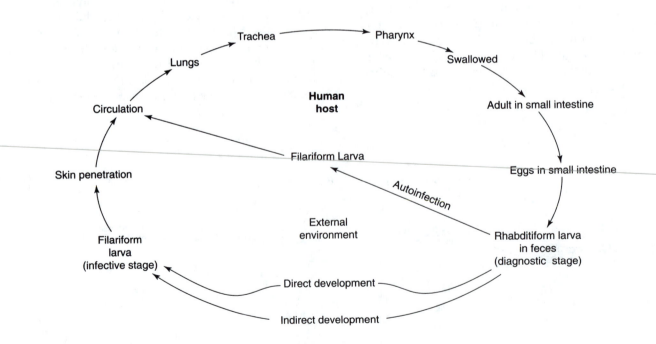

FIG 11–15 Life cycle of *Strongyloides stercoralis*

by the avoidance of contaminated soil. Patients should be screened for threadworm infection before receiving immunosuppressive agents.

SUMMARY

Intestinal nematodes cause human diseases ranging from self-limited, asymptomatic infections to disseminated, life-threatening syndromes. The life cycles of nematodes vary, depending on the parasite. The direct life cycle of the pinworm contrasts greatly with the highly complex life cycle of the threadworm.

Diagnosis of infection is usually based upon the recovery and identification of the ova, larvae, or adult forms of the helminth in human feces, following a standardized examination for ova and parasites. Table 11–1 summarizes the characteristic features of intestinal nematodes.

The diagnostic stage of development varies, depending on the life cycle of the parasite. Great care must be taken to avoid confusion among intestinal nematode infections, since treatments vary. Prevention of infection generally requires employment of safe sanitary practices, as well as good personal hygiene. The use of human feces as fertilizer should be avoided

Table 11–1 ▶ Key Characteristics of Intestinal Nematodes

NEMATODE	CHARACTERISTIC FEATURES
Enterobius vermicularis	Smooth, thick-shelled, football-shaped eggs, flattened on one side Scotch tape test recommended for diagnosis Adult worm is white with pointy tail; may be seen in feces Transmission is usually by ingestion of infective eggs
Ascaris lumbricoides	Mammillated, thick-shelled eggs, fertilized (1-cell stage), or unfertilized (exaggerated bumpy mammilated shell) eggs may be found Decorticated eggs may be present Adults may be seen in feces, or crawl out of mouth, anus, or nares Transmission is usually by ingestion of infective eggs
Trichuris trichiura	Barrel-shaped thick-shelled egg with 2 polar plugs Adult worm with whiplike shape rarely seen in feces Transmission is usually by ingestion of infective eggs
Ancylostoma duodenale/ Necator americanus	Oval, thin-shelled eggs in 4 to 8-cell stage; a clear space exists between the shell and the developing embryo Larvae may develop from eggs left at room temperature Adult worms rarely seen in feces Transmission is usually by skin penetration
Strongyloides stercoralis	First stage rhabditiform larva, having a short buccal capsule, and a large genital primordium Thin-shelled eggs are not usually found in feces Transmission is usually by skin penetration

REVIEW QUESTIONS

1. The following statement regarding intestinal nematodes is false:
   a. The stage of development within the ovum is characteristic for the species
   b. Infertile eggs tend to contain unorganized masses of material within the eggshell
   c. The male adult worm is usually larger than the female
   d. Most intestinal nematodes have direct life cycles

2. Intestinal nematodes having thin eggshells include
   a. *Ascaris lumbricoides*
   b. *Enterobius vermicularis*
   c. *Trichuris trichiura*
   d. *Necator americanus*

3. The largest intestinal roundworm is
   a. *Ascaris lumbricoides*
   b. *Enterobius vermicularis*
   c. *Trichuris trichiura*
   d. *Necator americanus*

4. The whipworm is the name given to
   a. *Ascaris lumbricoides*
   b. *Enterobius vermicularis*
   c. *Trichuris trichiura*
   d. *Necator americanus*

5. The "scotch tape test" is used to diagnose infection with
   a. whipworm
   b. threadworm
   c. hookworm
   d. pinworm

6. Visceral larva migrans is associated with infections with the dog or cat
   a. hookworm
   b. ascarid
   c. threadworm
   d. whipworm

7. The antihelminthic agent, thiabendazole, is recommended to treat
   a. *Ascaris lumbricoides*
   b. *Enterobius vermicularis*
   c. *Necator americanus*
   d. *Strongyloides stercoralis*

8. Which of the following intestinal roundworms is transmitted by ingestion of eggs?
   a. *Necator americanus*
   b. *Ascaris lumbricoides*
   c. *Strongyloides stercoralis*
   d. *Ancylostoma duodenale*

9. Mammillated outer coats are common on the ova of which parasite?
   a. *Necator americanus*
   b. *Ascaris lumbricoides*
   c. *Strongyloides stercoralis*
   d. *Ancylostoma duodenale*

10. Which parasite is capable of autoinfection, which may lead to the hyperinfection syndrome?
    a. *Strongyloides stercoralis*
    b. *Ascaris lumbricoides*
    c. *Enterobius vermicularis*
    d. *Necator americanus*

CASE STUDY

The patient was a 66-year old Hispanic male from Puerto Rico who was admitted to the hospital several years earlier, suffering from diarrhea, dyspnea and abdominal pain. The patient's pulmonary complaint was diagnosed as chronic obstructive pulmonary disease (COPD), and he was treated with high dose intravenous steroids, and inhaled bronchodilators. Abdominal CT scans were unrevealing.

Two years later, the patient was re-admitted with eosinophilia, as well as continued dyspnea. He continued to receive intravenous glucocorticoids for what was considered to be exacerbations of his existing pulmonary disease. One year later the patient was re-admitted with fever and wheezing. He was diagnosed with COPD exacerbation and congestive heart failure. Blood cultures grew enterococci and *E. coli*. Although treated aggressively with antibiotics for bacteremia, the patient's condition deteriorated, and he expired on the thirtieth hospital day.

A complete autopsy was performed, and histological studies showed nematode larvae present in the heart, liver, and lungs.

Questions

1. What intestinal parasite would you consider to be responsible for the patient's condition?

2. What laboratory test should have been ordered to make a diagnosis of the patient's illness?

3. What aspects of the patient's illness should act as clues to the etiology of infection?

4. How does the life cycle of this parasite relate to the patient's disease?

5. What role do intravenous steroids play in this syndrome?

▶ BIBLIOGRAPHY

Ash, L. R. & Orihel, C. (1999). Intestinal helminths. In Murray, P. R., Baron, S. J., Pfaller, M. A., Tenover, F. C., & Yolken, R. H. (Eds.) *Manual of clinical microbiology* (7th ed.). (pp. 1421–1435). Washington, DC: ASM Press.

Garcia, L. S. & Bruckner, D. A. (1997). *Diagnostic medical parasitology* (3rd ed.). Washington, DC: ASM Press.

Koneman, E. W., Allen, S. D., Janda, W. M., Schreckenberger, P. C., & Winn, Jr, W.C., (1997). *Color atlas and textbook of diagnostic microbiology* (5th ed.). Philadelphia: Lippincott.

Shimeld, L. & Rodgers, A. T. (1999). Intestinal helminths. In Shimeld, L. (Ed.) *Essentials of diagnostic microbiology*. (pp. 603–615). Albany, NY: Delmar Publishers.

Zeibig, E. A. (1997). *Clinical parasitology*. Philadelphia: W. B. Saunders.

CHAPTER TWELVE

Blood/Body Fluid/ Tissue Nematodes

OUTLINE

TRICHINELLA SPIRALIS AND OTHER TRICHINELLA SPECIES
(TRICK -i- NELL - ah/ SPIR - al - is)

DRACUNCULUS MEDINENSIS
(drah- KUNK - you- lus/ MED - i - NEN - sis)

THE FILARIA

WUCHERERIA BANCROFTI
(VOO - ker - EE - ree - ah/ ban - CROF - tee)

BRUGIA MALAYI AND BRUGIA TIMORI
(BREW - gia/ ma - LAY -eye) (ti - MOR - eye)

LOA LOA
(Lo - ah/ LO - ah)

ONCHOCERCA VOLVULUS
(ON - ko - SIR - kah/ VOL - view - lus)

MANSONELLA OZZARDI
(MAN - so - NELL - ah/ oh - ZAR - dee)

MANSONELLA PERSTANS
(MAN - so - NELL - ah/ PER - stans)

MANSONELLA STREPTOCERCA
(MAN - so - NELL - ah/ strep - TOE - sir - kah)

DIROFILARIA IMMITIS
(DI - row - fil- AIR - ree - ah/ im - MI - tis)

LEARNING OBJECTIVES

After reading and studying this chapter, the student should be able to:

- Define the key terms.
- For each organism cited, state the geographic distribution.
- Describe the morphologic characteristics of the parasites cited in this chapter.
- Briefly describe the life cycle of each organism cited, including vector and intermediate host.

- Identify the infective stage of each organism.
- Discuss the clinical presentation of each disease.
- Name the specimen of choice for the diagnosis and/or recovery of each organism.
- Identify means of treatment and prevention for each organism.

KEY TERMS

Amicrofilaremic
(a-micro-fil-air-ee-mik)
Bancroftian filariasis
(ban-kroft-ee-an)
Brugian filariasis
(brew-gee-an)

Calabar swelling
(kal-ah-bar/ swelling)
Copepod (kope-e-pod)
Dirofilariasis
(di-roh-fil-air-ee-eye-ah-sis)

Dracunculiasis
(drah-kunk-u-lie-ah-sis)
Elephantiasis
(el-e-fan-tie-ah-sis)
Filaria (fil-air-ee-ah)

(continued)

KEY TERMS

Knott's technique
  (nots/ TEK-neek)
Loaisis (lo-EYE-ah-sis)
Lymphadenitis
  (lymph-AD-en-EYE-tis)
Lymphangitis (LYMPH-an-JI-
  tis)

Mansonelliasis
  (MAN-so-NEL-eye-AH-sis)
Microfilariae
  (MICRO-fil-AIR-ee-ah)
Onchocerciasis
  (ONK-oh-SIR-ki-ah-sis)
Onchocercoma
  (ONK-oh-SIR-coma)

Sheathed (sheethd)
Skin snip (skin/snip)
Streptocerciasis
  (STREP-toe-SIR-ki-ah-sis)
Sub-periodic (SUB-peri-OD-ik)
Trichinosis (TRIK-i-NO-sis)
Trichinellosis
  (TRIK-i NELL-oh-sis)

INTRODUCTION

In contrast to the intestinal helminths reviewed earlier in the text, tissue nematodes parasitize human blood, skin, or lymphatics (Table 12–1). These organisms produce a variety of pathologies depending on the species and the body site affected. Human filarial infections may be further classified as lymphatic (bancroftian and brugian) and nonlymphatic (loiasis, mansonelliasis, and onchocerciasis). These organisms have complex life cycles, including infective larval stages that are carried by arthropod vectors, adult forms that inhabit the lymphatics or subcutaneous tissues, and **microfilariae** (larval forms) that migrate in the tissues or circulate in the blood.

TRICHINELLA SPIRALIS AND OTHER *TRICHINELLA* SPECIES

Morphology

Trichinella spiralis is the etiologic agent of **trichinosis (trichinellosis)**, one of a number of tissue nematode infections characterized by invasive larval stages. Five species of *Trichinella* are known to cause infection in humans: *Trichinella spiralis, Trichinella nativa, Trichinella nelsoni, Trichinella britoui,* and *Trichinella psuedospiralis*. Of the five species, *T. spiralis* is the most important of the parasites because it lacks host specificity and has a cosmopolitan, worldwide distribution.

Table 12–1 ▶ Classification

Phylum	Class	Blood/ Tissue Species
Nemathelminthes	Nematoda	**Blood Species**
		Wuchereria bancrofti
		Brugia malayi
		Brugia timori
		Loa loa
		Onchocerca volvulus
		Mansonella ozzardi
		Mansonella perstans
		Mansonella streptocerca
		Dirofilaria immitis
		Tissue Species
		Trichinella spiralis
		Dracunculus medinensis

Life Cycle

In nature, *Trichinella spiralis* is an infection of wild and domestic mammals, specifically omnivores and carnivores. The pig, bear, cat, dog and rat are the animals most commonly implicated in infections. Larval forms encyst within the striated muscle of reservoir hosts and are transmitted among hosts by predation.

Human infections with *T. spiralis*, or any of the other four species previously mentioned, are zoonoses, acquired by eating raw or poorly cooked infected meat, usually pork, bear, horse, or walrus. As the muscle tissue is digested, the larvae excyst and penetrate into the intestinal mucosa. There, they undergo four larval molts and develop into adult worms over the next 30 to 40 hours. Mating takes place in the lumen of the gut. The larger female, measuring approximately 5 mm, embeds into the mucosa and produces eggs that are deposited as motile larvae in as few as three days of fertilization. She may produce as many as 1,500 larvae in her lifetime. Males generally die following mating and are passed in the feces.

Larvae penetrate the gut mucosa and are disseminated via the lymphatic and circulatory systems to areas of active striated skeletal muscle, where they encyst. Cyst development occurs in response to the host's immune reaction to larval presence. At maturity, a larva is approximately 1 mm long and coiled within a sheath derived from the muscle fiber. Over time, a granulomatous reaction ensues and cysts become calcified. Larvae may remain viable for years.

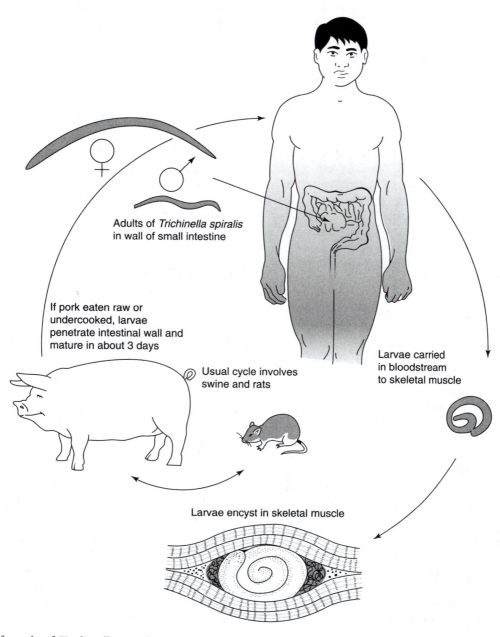

Adults of *Trichinella spiralis*
in wall of small intestine

If pork eaten raw or
undercooked, larvae
penetrate intestinal wall and
mature in about 3 days

Usual cycle involves
swine and rats

Larvae carried
in bloodstream
to skeletal muscle

Larvae encyst in skeletal muscle

FIG 12–1 Life cycle of *Trichinella spiralis*

Man is a dead end host in the life cycle of *Trichinella* and generally, with cannibalism excluded, the cycle ends with larval encystment in the muscle. In nature, cyst-carrying rodents serve as an important reservoir for wild carnivores, as well as for flesh-eating domestic animals, such as pigs. Another common source of swine infection is the use of uncooked garbage and scrap as feed. Governmental legislation regulating the heat treatment of hog food has decreased the incidence of trichinosis in the United States in recent years. The complete life cycle of *Trichinella spiralis* is seen in Figure 12–1.

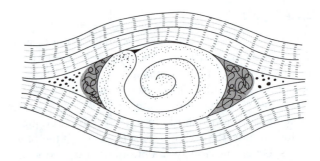

FIG 12–2 Encysted *T. spiralis*

Transmission and Pathogenesis

Trichinosis is acquired by eating raw or undercooked meat containing the *Trichinella* larvae. The organisms are liberated from the muscle following digestion of their capsules and go on to mature and propagate. Symptoms and pathologic changes caused by *Trichinella* infection are dependent on the original number of ingested cysts and the stage of infection: intestinal phase, muscle invasion, and encapsulation.

During the intestinal phases of infection, the ingested larvae develop into adult worms and invade the intestinal muscosa. Symptoms develop within the first 24 hours and the severity of those symptoms relates to the number of worms involved and the amount of tissue damage sustained. Clinical illness mimics influenza, viral infection, or acute food poisoning with diarrhea, nausea, vomiting, malaise, abdominal pain, and fever as the chief complaints.

As the new larvae begin their mass migration and enter into muscle tissue, there may be fever and chills, facial edema (particularly about the eyes: periorbital), aching joints and muscle pains, swelling and weakness. There is a marked eosinophilia, often greater than 50%. Specific symptoms may relate to the muscles affected, leading to difficulty in breathing, eye movement, speech or swallowing. The most severe and life-threatening symptoms involve the heart (myocarditis) and central nervous systems (encephalitis). In severe cases, death may occur.

As the larvae settle into place and encapsulation begins, clinical symptoms begin to subside. The patient enters a period of convalescence during which time the cyst wall forms and larvae calcify (Figure 12–2). Calcified cysts are sufficiently large to be seen on gross examination of exposed muscle fibers.

Laboratory Diagnosis

Symptoms are nonspecific during the intestinal stage of disease. A history of eating raw or poorly cooked pork, bear, walrus, game or ready-to-serve sausage is helpful in diagnosis. Clinical symptoms, including acute gastroenteritis, acute edema of the upper eyelids, and muscle pain are also characteristic signs of trichinosis recognizable to the physician.

Laboratory examination of muscle biopsy specimens revealing encysted larvae provide a confirmation of *Trichinella* infection. Serologic testing procedures, including an ELISA test, are also available but may be falsely negative if performed early in the infection (within two weeks of onset). The parasite is rarely found in patient stool, blood or CSF samples. Other laboratory findings may, however, be indicative of disease. Patients with trichinosis may demonstrate: elevated creatine kinase, aldolase, lactate dehydrogenase and aspartate aminotranferase (transaminase), and elevated serum IgE levels.

Treatment and Prevention

Mebendazole is the drug of choice for the treatment of trichinosis. The clinical response varies. Thiabendazole has also been used as an alternate therapy. Corticosteroids such as prednisone are beneficial in cases with severe symptomology. Steroid use, however, tends to prolong the intestinal phase and suppress the immune response.

Although the incidence of trichinosis was once very common in the United States, infection is now relatively rare. Legislation prohibiting the feeding of uncooked garbage and raw meat scraps to hogs, as well as public education programs about the dangers of eating raw or poorly cooked meat, especially pork, have contributed to the decline in the number of infections.

Pork products, wild game and suspected meats should be thoroughly cooked until the juices run clear or to an internal temperature of 170 degrees. Freezing pork for 20 days at 5 degrees also destroys the parasite. Utensils and meat grinders used to prepare meat should be cleansed thoroughly between usages.

DRACUNCULUS MEDINENSIS

Morphology

The guinea worm *Dracunculus medinensis*, speculated to be the fiery serpent of biblical times, is still an important public health problem in Africa, Iran, India, and Pakistan. Increased incidence rates correspond with areas where standing water sources such as ponds, step wells, or cisterns are used for drinking water. These same water sources may also serve as the breeding sites for the **copepod** (tiny crustacean) vector, and bathing sites for infected individuals. All three factors considered together provide the requirements necessary for the completion of the *Dracunculus medinensis* life cycle.

Because the worms are long and thin, they are often confused with filarial worms. *Dracunculus medinensis* is, however, classified in the order Spirurida, suborder Camallanina, superfamily Dracunculoidea.

Life Cycle

Human infection is initiated through the ingestion of water contaminated with infected copepods, genus *Cyclops*. These tiny crustaceans, also known as water fleas, harbor the infective third stage larvae of *Dracunculus medinensis*. Upon release, the larvae migrate through the duodenum wall, develop, mate, and mature in the loose connective tissue. The entire process takes about a year.

Adult female worms measure 70 to 120 cm (average 1 meter) long by only 2 mm in diameter. The male worm is rarely seen but measures a mere 2 cm long by 0.4 mm in diameter. The gravid female, filled with uteri containing rhabditform larvae, migrates to the subcutaneous tissue (usually of the lower extremity). As the female approaches the skin, a papule forms, then develops into a blister, and ultimately ulcerates, exposing the worm. Upon contact with fresh water, a portion of the worm's uterus prolapses and large numbers of first stage larvae are discharged into the water. The life cycle continues as these larvae are ingested by the appropriate species of *Cyclops*, which serve as the intermediate host. Within the copepod, the larvae take about 8 days to become infective for humans. The complete life cycle is diagrammed in Figure 12–3.

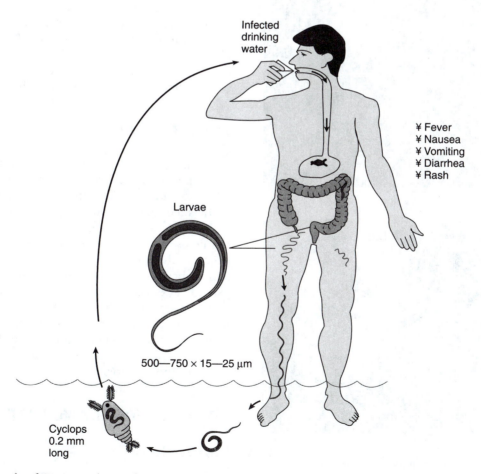

Infected drinking water

¥ Fever
¥ Nausea
¥ Vomiting
¥ Diarrhea
¥ Rash

Larvae

500—750 × 15—25 µm

Cyclops 0.2 mm long

FIG 12–3 Life cycle of *Dracunculus medinensis*

Transmission and Pathogenesis

Following the ingestion of the infected copepod, few or no clinical symptoms occur until just before the blister forms. The gravid female worm's migration to the skin may provoke localized redness and pain. As the blister forms (Figure 12–4A), there is an onset of fever and generalized allergic symptoms, including: urticaria, intense itching, asthma attacks, periorbital edema, nausea and vomiting. There is a relief of symptoms when the blister ruptures, releasing larvae and worm metabolites into the fluid environment. A portion of the worm will continue to protrude from the wound until larval release is complete (Figure 12–4B).

Worms are gradually extracted by winding on a stick, and the ulcer usually heals over in a matter of a few weeks or months. If, however, the worm is damaged or broken during removal, secondary infection, cellulitis, inflammation or abscess formation may result. Occasionally, the adult worm does not erupt through the skin and becomes encapsulated and calcified in the subcutaneous tissue.

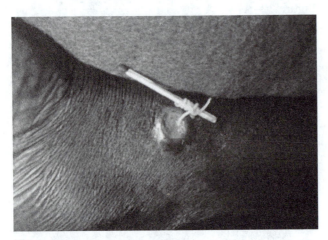

(A)

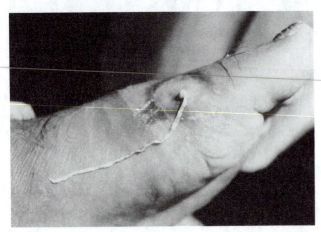

(B)

FIG 12–4 (A) Painful blister induced by the female guinea worm. (B) *D. medinensis* emerges from the ruptured blister. (Image A courtesy of the CDC Image Library)

Laboratory Diganosis

Diagnosis of **dracunculiasis** is typically based on clinical manifestations. In endemic areas, the characteristic worm-containing lesion is easily recognizable. The worm can be stimulated to release first stage larvae for diagnostic purposes by submerging the ulcer in water. On occasion, lesions must be differentiated from carbuncles, deep cellulitis, onchocerciasis, focal myositis, or rheumatism. X-rays may be used to locate dead calcified worms in subcutaneous tissues.

Treatment and Prevention

The traditional method for removal of the adult *D. medinensis* is to slowly wind the worm around a stick at a rate of a few centimeters per day. Although primitive, the method is usually quite successful. If the worm is broken in the extraction procedure, the patient is predisposed to secondary infection.

Medical therapy with agents such as metronidazole or thiabendazole has been limited to the relief of symptoms. These drugs have not been shown to have activity against the worm. Treatment suppresses inflammation and facilitates removal of the worm.

Prevention depends on the provision of properly treated, safe, drinking water. Water suspected of contamination with infected copepods should be boiled, filtered, or chemically treated. Through the efforts of the World Health Organization, the total eradication of the guinea worm may occur in the near future.

THE *FILARIAE*

Human **filarial** nematodes belong to the order Filariata, superfamily Filariodea. They cause infections transmitted by arthropod vectors, primarily biting insects such as flies and mosquitoes. The distribution of specific infections is, therefore, associated with the range of the insect vector. These parasites are long, threadlike, roundworms that live in the host's lymphatic system, subcutaneous, or deep connective tissues for extended periods of time. They produce microfilarial larvae that circulate in the blood and lymphatics and may be responsible for deformity or blindness. The filariae are also masters of adaptation, having developed a periodicity that corresponds to the feeding habits of their vectors.

WUCHERERIA BANCROFTI

Morphology

Wuchereria bancrofti, *Brugia malayi*, and *Brugia timori* are the etiologic agents of lymphatic filariasis, also known as tropical **elephantiasis**. The **bancroftian** form of the disease, caused by *Wuchereria bancrofti*, has an extensive distribution throughout the tropical and subtropical regions of central Africa, Asia, the Pacific Islands, the Caribbean, and Central and South America. The World Health Organization estimates that approximately 107 million people are affected worldwide, many of whom are seriously incapacitated or disfigured by the disease.

Both humans and mosquitoes are needed to complete the life cycle of *Wuchereria bancrofti*. Night-biting mosquitoes of the genera *Anopheles* and *Culex* serve as the vector and intermediate host of the nocturnally periodic *W. bancrofti* strain, while day-biting *Aedes* mosquitoes transmit the sub-periodic strain. Man is the only known reservoir.

Life Cycle

The life cycle of *Wuchereria bancrofti* (Figure 12–5) has historical significance in parasitology as well as clinical significance. *Wuchereria bancrofti* was the first parasitic organism found to have an arthropod vector. Three genera of mosquitoes are known to transmit *Wuchereria bancrofti* in various parts of the world: *Culex*, *Aedes*, and *Anopheles*. Each also serves as the intermediate host. **Microfilariae** are acquired by the mosquito as it takes a blood meal from an infected host. The larvae then penetrate the stomach wall of the mosquito and migrate to the thoracic musculature. There, over the next 10 days, the larvae grow and develop into the infective larval stage. The infective stage, now approximately 1 to 2 mm in length, moves to the proboscis of the mosquito where it can escape as the insect takes its next blood meal.

In the human host, infective larvae make their way into the peripheral lymphatics, undergoing two molts before they mature in the regional lymph nodes and lymphatic vessels. The process takes 6 to 9 months. Adult worms are white and thread-like in appearance and may live up to 7 years. Male worms (2 to 4 cm) and females (5 to 10 cm) mate, and the female begins to periodically deposit **sheathed** (membrane covered) microfilariae into the blood. Microfilariae average 245 to 300 μm in length and have body nuclei that do not extend to the tip of the slightly pointed tail.

In the majority of endemic areas, *Wuchereria bancrofti* microfilariae exhibit a nocturnal periodicity which coincides with the feeding habits of the vector. Microfilariae appear in the peripheral blood in greatest numbers between 10 P.M. and 2 A.M. and are absent during daylight hours. The strain of *Wuchereria bancrofti* recovered most frequently in the Pacific Islands is **sub-periodic**. Infected humans are microfilaremic all the time, with greater concentrations of microfilariae recovered between noon and 8 P.M..

Transmission and Pathogenesis

Man is inoculated with the infective larvae of *W. bancrofti* as the infected mosquito takes a blood meal. The larvae escape from the proboscis of the mosquito and invade the puncture wound. In highly endemic areas, exposure starts in early childhood and many bites are necessary to acquire the disease.

The development of the disease in the human host is a matter of controversy. Although the infection is usually acquired in early childhood, clinical symptoms may not be expressed for years. The clinical manifestations are varied. Some patients appear asymptomatic but harbor large numbers of microfilariae in their circulation and act as a reservoir of infection. In contrast, the most severe clinical manifestations of chronic disease include obstructive lymphatic damage, genital damage, or elephantiasis of the extremities, penis, scrotum, vulva, or the breast. Men are more frequently affected than women.

Early symptoms of **bancroftian filariasis** are fever (known as filarial or elephantoid fever), chills, lymphangitis, lymphadenitis, and eosinophilia. **Lymphangitis** (inflammation of the lymphatic vessels) and **lymphadenitis** (inflammation of the lymph nodes) generally affect the lower extremities, genitals (Figure 12–6A), or the breast. As the infection progresses, the lymph nodes and vessels proximal to the worm exhibit fibrotic changes. Regional lymph nodes become enlarged and the vessels containing the worm become distended, permeable, and painful. The result is lymphedema, with hardening and thickening of the skin known as **elephantiasis** (Figure 12–6B). The inflammation is often accompanied by the formation of abscesses that drain externally. These patients are at risk of secondary bacterial and fungal infections.

Laboratory Diagnosis

Laboratory diagnosis of *W. bancrofti* is made by demonstration of characteristic microfilariae in peripheral blood or lymphatic fluid. Thick smears, stained with Giemsa, are used for the detection of microfilariae. Concentration methods are particularly helpful for the recovery of microfilariae in light infections. Centrifugation of fluid fixed in 2% formalin (**Knott's technique**) or passage of the fluid specimen through a polycarbonate microfilter adds a greater sensitivity to the microscopic examination. Stained microfilariae appear sheathed, measure 245 to 300 μm long, and have numerous body nuclei which do not extend to the tip of the pointed tail (Figure 12–7).

Care should be taken to collect the specimen for optimum recovery of the organism. *Wuchereria bancrofti* exhibits a nocturnal periodicity in the greater part of its endemic area. Specimens should be collected between

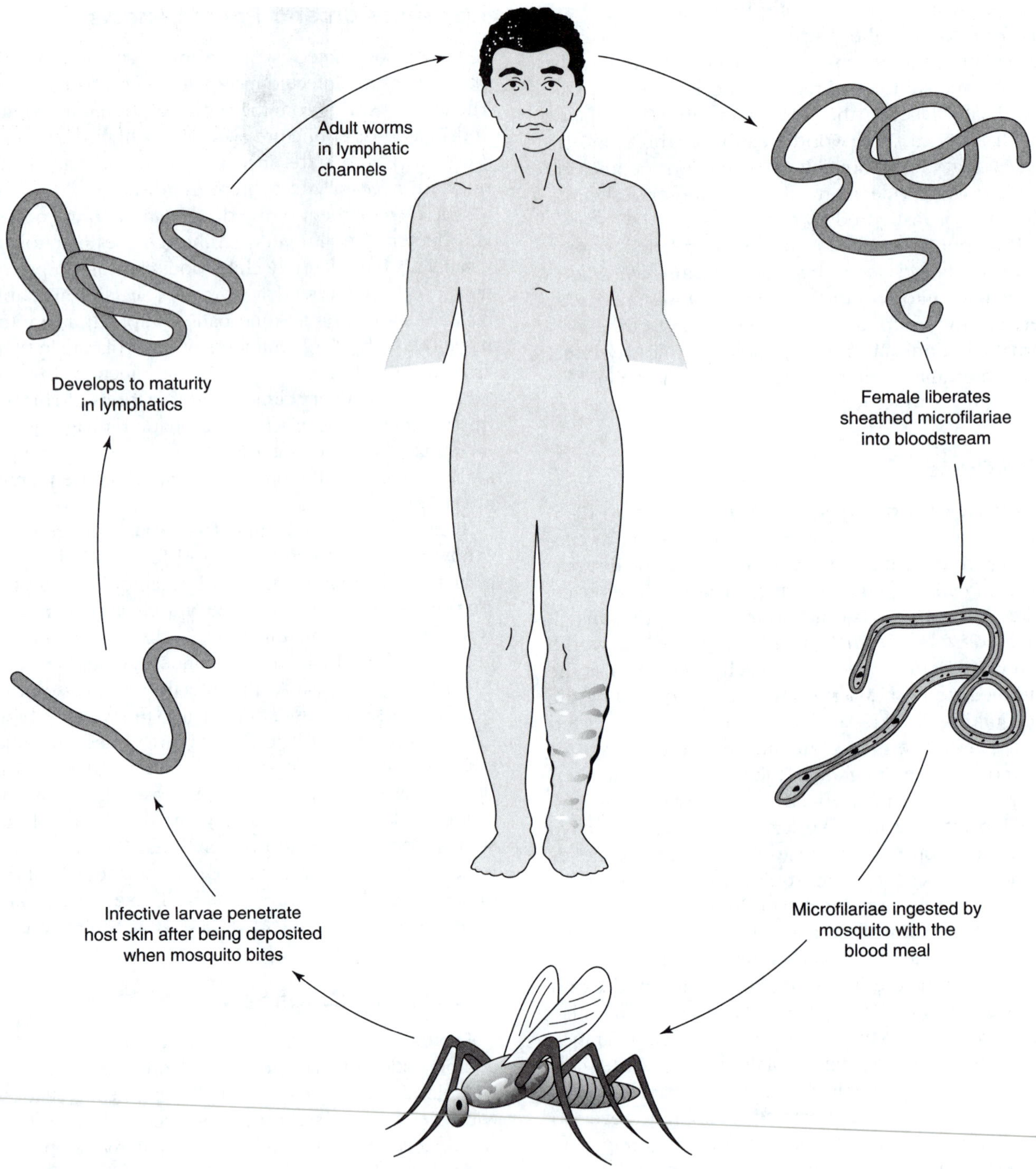

Adult worms
in lymphatic
channels

Develops to maturity
in lymphatics

Female liberates
sheathed microfilariae
into bloodstream

Infective larvae penetrate
host skin after being deposited
when mosquito bites

Microfilariae ingested by
mosquito with the
blood meal

FIG 12–5 Life cycle of *Wuchereria bancrofti* and *Brugia malayi*

the hours of 10 P.M. and 2 A.M. when the microfilariae are at their greatest concentration in the blood.

Serologic testing results, including elevated serum IgE titers and elevated antifilarial antibody, as well as the presence of eosinophilia, support the diagnosis of lymphatic filariasis. In patients who are **amicrofilaremic** (without microfilariae in their blood), diagnosis can be based on assays for circulating antigens of *W. bancrofti* and on clinical grounds. Polymerase chain reaction DNA testing is also available.

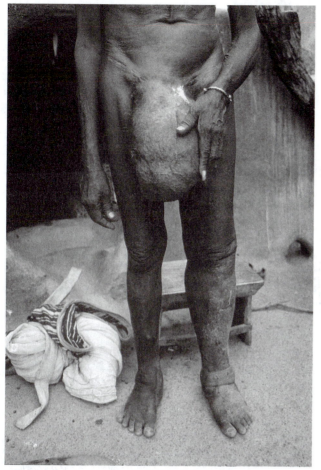

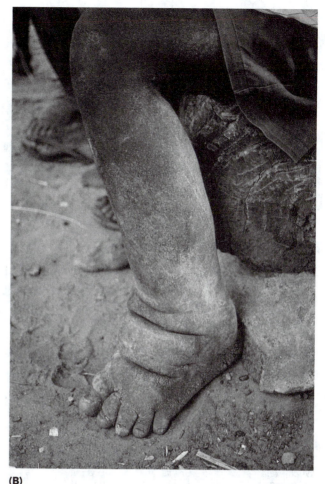

FIG 12–6 (A) An elderly male with hydrocele, elephantiasis of the leg, hanging groin, leopard skin. (B) The legs and feet of a male showing elephantiasis and skin lesions of the left leg. (Image courtesy of the WHO/TDR Image Library. Photographer Andy Crump, 1999, Ghana.)

Treatment and Prevention

The treatment of choice for lymphatic filariasis is diethylcarbamazine (DEC) administered at a rate of 6 mg/kg per day in three divided doses for a period of 3 weeks. DEC is an active microfilaricide but multiple courses may be necessary to eliminate adult worms. Lymphangitis and related inflammatory processes respond to the administration of antihistamines and analgesics. The expression of allergic response to the death of microfilariae correlates to the parasite burden. Side effects, such as fever, chills, headache, nausea, vomiting, arthralgia or urticaria may be diminished by the initial use of small doses of DEC, stepping up to full dose over a period of a few days. Glucocorticosteroids also help control many side effects.

Ivermectin, a drug used with great success in the treatment of river blindness (*Onchocerca volvulus*), also shows promise for the treatment of lymphatic filariasis. Ivermectin is usually given as a single dose of 400 mg/kg of body weight and appears to be as effective as DEC at clearing microfilariae for up to 6 months.

Surgical procedures may be used for the treatment of chronic lymphatic obstruction, particularly hydroceles and scrotal elephantiasis. The use of elastic stockings and pressure bandages may help to eliminate the edema and induration of affected limbs.

All patients treated for filariasis should have repeat testing procedures performed following therapy to confirm the elimination of the parasites.

The use of personal protection in the form of insect repellent, protective clothing and bed netting can reduce the incidence of *W. bancrofti* infection among travelers to endemic regions; however, these measures are not practical for residents. Long-term control of filariasis can only be achieved through vector control programs and mass treatment of infected populations. Since man is the only host for this species,

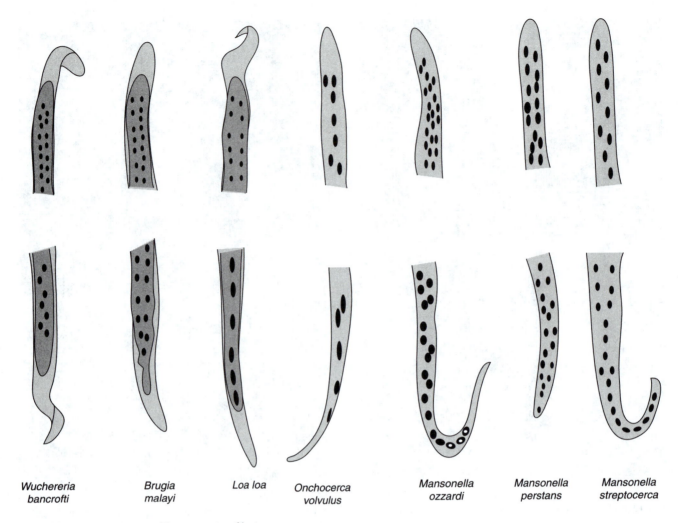

| Wuchereria bancrofti | Brugia malayi | Loa loa | Onchocerca volvulus | Mansonella ozzardi | Mansonella perstans | Mansonella streptocerca |

FIG 12–7 Characteristics of human microfilariae

the transmission of disease may be interrupted by either reducing the population of adult or larval mosquitoes, or by decreasing the number of infected humans within a specific region.

BRUGIA MALAYI AND BRUGIA TIMORI

Morphology

Brugia malayi and *Brugia timori* are the agents of the **brugian** form of lymphatic filariasis (elephantiasis) found throughout Asia. More than 50% of the cases are reported in southern China and India, with the remainder occurring in the Philippines, Thailand, Vietnam, South Korea and parts of Japan. *Brugia timori* exists on the island of Timor and the other islands of the Indonesian archipelago. Similar in nature to bancroftian filariasis and overlapping its geographic distribution, brugian filariasis, is also transmitted by

mosquitoes. In addition to humans, cats, macaques, leaf monkeys and other animals may also serve as reservoir hosts.

Life Cycle

The life cycle of *Brugia* species is similar to that of *Wuchereria bancrofti* (Figure 12–5). The vector and intermediate host for *Brugia* species are the *Mansonia, Anopheles* and *Aedes* mosquitoes, depending on geographic distribution. Upon feeding, the female mosquito ingests microfilariae from an infected host. The microfilariae migrate to the thoracic musculature of the insect where they grow and develop into the infective larval stage. The infective stage, now approximately 1–2 mm in length, moves to the proboscis where it may be released during the mosquito's next blood meal.

In the human host, infective larvae make their way into the peripheral lymphatics, undergoing two molts before they mature in the regional lymph vessels, a process that may take up to 6 to 9 months. Adult male (43–55 mm) and female (13–23 mm) worms mate and then the female begins to periodically deposit sheathed microfilariae into the blood. Microfilariae average 200 to 275 μm in length and have body nuclei that extend to the tip of the tail. The two terminal nuclei are distinctly set apart form the other nuclei (Figure 12–7). Microfilariae of *Brugia malayi* exhibit either a nocturnal periodicity or sub-periodicity depending on geographic distribution. *Brugia timori* microfilariae exhibit only nocturnal periodicity.

Transmission and Pathogenesis

Brugian filariasis is transmitted by a number of genera of predominantly night feeding mosquitoes. Multiple bites or exposures are generally necessary to cause disease. Clinical symptoms may begin within months to years of infection and are similar to those seen in bancroftian infections. The pathologic changes within the host are the result of the immune responses to adult worms and not to the microfilariae. Adult worms living in the lymph nodes and larger lymphatic vessels evoke the inflammatory response that leads to the formation of granulomatous processes with resultant lymphadenitis, lymphangitis and eventual lymphatic obstruction. In contrast to *W. bancrofti*, filarial abscess with ulceration of an affected lymph node is common; however, genital involvement is rare. If elephantiasis occurs, it generally affects the leg below the knee level.

Laboratory Diagnosis

A definitive diagnosis may be made by detecting the microfilariae in the blood or lymphatic aspirate. The time of specimen collection should be considered for optimal parasite recovery, as some strains are nocturnally periodic while others are sub-periodic. Specimen material may be examined microscopically using a Giemsa stain or may be concentrated by centrifugation using Knott's technique. Microfilariae are sheathed, and have body nuclei that extend to the tip of the tail. A distinct pair of terminal nuclei may be seen, separated from the other nuclei in the tail. The microfilariae of *Brugia timori* may be differentiated from those of *Brugia malayi* by size (average size of 310 micrometers versus 250 micrometers for the latter). Also, the sheaths of *B. timori* stain poorly as compared to the sheaths of *B. malayi*.

Serologic testing, including elevated serum IgE titers and elevated antifilarial antibodies, as well as the presence of eosinophilia, support the diagnosis of lymphatic filariasis. Polymerase chain reaction based DNA testing is also available.

Treatment and Prevention

The same treatment regimen used for the elimination of *Wuchereria bancrofti* can be utilized against *Brugia* species. Currently, diethylcarbamazine (DEC) administered in lower dosages in conjunction with anti-inflammatory drugs is the therapy of choice. Allergic reactions in response to the death of microfilariae correlate to the parasite burden and may be diminished with the adjunctive usage of corticosteroids or the "step-dosing" method of administering DEC.

Single dose administration of Ivermectin has been shown to be an effective microfilaricide for up to 6 months and is associated with fewer adverse effects than the DEC regimens.

Visitors to endemic areas are encouraged to avoid mosquito bites by using insect repellants, protective garments and mosquito netting. Garments and netting may be impregnated with insecticide/repellants. Limiting outdoor evening exposure is also prudent.

The interruption of the vector-borne transmission of disease among residents in endemic regions, through vector control programs, must again be combined with the mass treatment of infected individuals. DEC is a useful prophylactic agent at 300 mg per week.

LOA LOA

Morphology

The African eye worm, *Loa loa*, is the etiologic agent of **loiasis** which affects 3 million people in Central Africa. Endemic areas are found throughout the rainforests of Sudan, West Africa, and the basin of the Congo. Adult worms actively migrate throughout the subcutaneous and deep connective tissues and often the diagnosis is made by observation of the worm as it traverses the conjunctiva. The vector is the day-biting mango fly, a member species of *Chrysops*.

Life Cycle

Human loiasis is initiated by the bite of a number of *Chrysops* species, commonly known as mango or deer flies. As the female insect bites, the infective larvae leave the mouth parts of the fly and migrate into the wound site. Following maturation, adult worms (both genders) live and migrate through the subcutaneous and deep connective tissue layers. Adult male worms range in size from 20–35 mm long by 0.5 mm wide. The female adults are slightly longer measuring 50–70 mm in length. Microfilariae, the offspring of the adult worms, make their way into the blood and circulate with a diurnal periodicity that peaks about midday. Microfilariae have a sheath covering and measure

250–300 micrometers in length. One diagnostic feature for this organism is the presence of body nuclei that are continuous to the tip of the microfilarial tail (Figure 12–7).

The mango fly becomes infected as it ingests microfilariae when feeding on a human, the only known reservoir host for *Loa loa*. A developmental cycle takes place within the thoracic muscles of the fly. Within 10–12 days, the infective larvae have migrated to the mouth parts of the fly thus completing the life cycle (Figure 12–8).

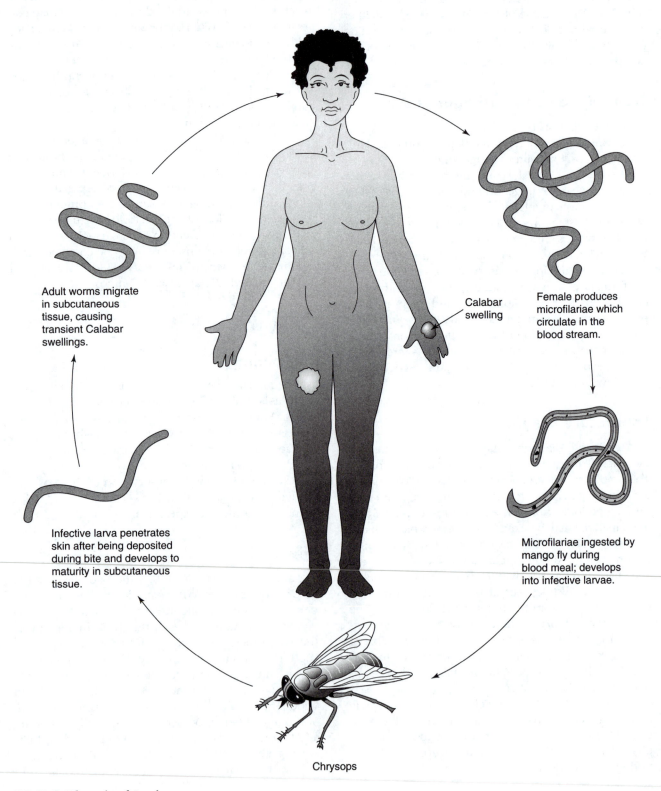

Adult worms migrate in subcutaneous tissue, causing transient Calabar swellings.

Calabar swelling

Female produces microfilariae which circulate in the blood stream.

Infective larva penetrates skin after being deposited during bite and develops to maturity in subcutaneous tissue.

Microfilariae ingested by mango fly during blood meal; develops into infective larvae.

Chrysops

FIG 12–8 Life cycle of *Loa loa*

Transmission and Pathogenesis

Infective larvae of *Loa loa* are transferred to the human host by the *Chrysops* fly. As the fly bites, the larvae enter the wound and migrate through the subcutaneous tissues as immature adult worms. Maturation may take 6 months or more. The worms move rapidly and painlessly through the subcutaneous layer, up to 1 cm per minute; yet among the indigenous population, loiasis is most often an asymptomatic infection. Worms are seldom noticed unless they pass through the conjunctiva of an eye.

One characteristic clinical manifestation of loiasis is the development of episodic angioedema known as **Calabar swellings**. These localized inflammatory reactions are thought to be brought on by a host response to either the worm's metabolic waste or the worm itself. Calabar swellings develop most frequently on the extremities but may be seen anywhere on the body. Lesions develop rapidly and may produce localized pain and itching (pruritus) lasting, on average, one to three days. Patients may also experience lymphadenitis and display a moderate peripheral eosinophilia.

Serious complications of loiasis, although rare, may include encephalopathy, nephropathy and cardiomyopathy as the organism ventures through the central nervous system, kidneys and heart, respectively.

In patients who are not residents of the endemic area, clinical presentation may be more pronounced symptomatically. Allergic symptoms and Calabar swellings may predominate. The presence of microfilariae in the blood is rare with hypereosinophilia and elevated levels of serum IgE. These patients also exhibit increased levels of antifilarial antibodies.

Laboratory Diagnosis

In most cases, the microfilariae of *Loa loa* do not appear in the general circulation for years after infection. Diagnosis of loiasis is typically made on the basis of the patients residence or travel history to endemic regions, combined with a history of episodic angioedema (Calabar swellings) or the presence of conjunctival worms.

The most practical laboratory diagnostic procedure is the examination of blood samples for the identification of microfilariae. Blood collection should be timed for the known diurnal periodicity of the microfilariae. For best recovery, samples should be collected between 10 A.M. to 2 P.M., and thick and thin smears prepared and stained with Giemsa. If necessary, concentration procedures may be utilized. One such method, for example, where the blood sample is lysed in 2% formalin and then centrifuged, is Knott's technique.

Stained microfilariae will appear sheathed, approximately 250–300 micrometers long and will have body nuclei that are continuous to the tip of the tail. A comparison of the characteristic microfilariae is in Figure 12–7.

Other laboratory findings may include eosinophilia, often in the ranges of 50–70%, and a markedly elevated serum IgE.

Treatment and Prevention

Treatment may be surgical or medical. One method involves the surgical removal of the adult worm as it migrates over the bridge of the nose or is seen under the conjunctiva. The procedures involve local anesthesia and simple small incisions. Diethylcarbamazine (DEC) is a therapeutic agent given orally over a period of 3 weeks. It is effective in killing both the microfilariae and adult worms. Antihistamines and anti-inflammatory drugs are often used in concert to reduce the occurrence of adverse affects of DEC. Ivermectin is also an effective microfilaricide.

Protective measures include avoidance of the insect vector through the judicious use of insecticides and personal protective clothing. Public control programs are effective for the clearing and draining of fly breeding grounds. There is no vaccine available but DEC has been used as chemoprophylaxis among travelers. As with other vector-borne diseases, rapid treatment of those individuals who are infected may help reduce the spread of disease.

ONCHOCERCA VOLVULUS

Morphology

Onchocerciasis, also known as river blindness, is caused by the filarial nematode *Onchocerca volvulus*, which infects 18 million people worldwide, 99% of whom live in the equatorial region of Africa. Onchocerciasis is second only to trachoma as the world's leading cause of blindness and presents a major public health problem. More than 120 million people in 37 countries in Africa, Latin America, Yemen and Saudi Arabia are at risk of acquiring the disease. Of those infected, over 6.5 million suffer from severe pruritus, 500,000 are seriously visually impaired, and 270,000 are blind.

In addition to the health consequences, the economic toll is often devastating to the agricultural villages in the endemic areas. River blindness is spread through the bite of the blackfly (*Simulium* spp.), which breeds in fast-flowing streams and rivers. The land along the river bank is usually the most fertile productive farmland, but which must be abandoned to escape the disease. There is currently a global effort, sponsored in part by the World Health Organization, to eliminate river blindness as a public health threat.

Life Cycle

The intermediate host and vector of *Onchocerca volvulus* is the blackfly or buffalo gnat (genus *Simulium*). The infective larvae are transferred to the human host during a bite from the insect. The developing worms migrate through the subcutaneous tissue where they settle and become encapsulated within fibrous tumor-like nodules called **onchocercomas**. The female adult worm may be as long as 50 cm by approximately 0.5 mm in diameter. The adult male averages only 5 cm by 0.5 mm.

About 7 months to 3 years after infection, the female worms begin to actively produce microfilariae which leave the nodule and are found most commonly in the dermis. The microfilariae range in size from 150–350 micrometers in length, are unsheathed and have body nuclei that do not extend into the tail. Adult worms may live as many as 14 years coiled within the nodule and the female may produce millions of microfilariae in her lifetime. The life cycle is completed as the female blackfly take a blood meal and acquires the microfilariae from the skin. The life cycle of *Onchocerca volvulus* is diagrammed in Figure 12–9.

Transmission and Pathogenesis

Following the bite from an infected female blackfly, infective larvae migrate through the subcutaneous

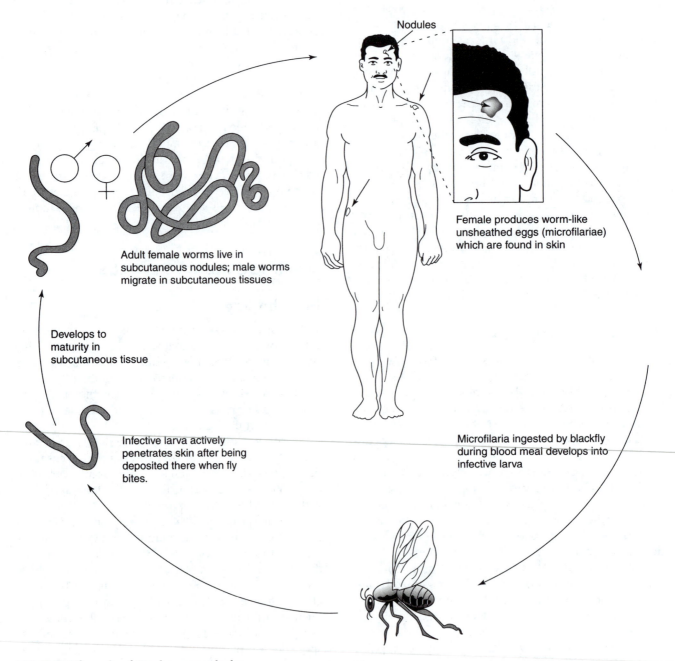

Nodules

Female produces worm-like unsheathed eggs (microfilariae) which are found in skin

Adult female worms live in subcutaneous nodules; male worms migrate in subcutaneous tissues

Develops to maturity in subcutaneous tissue

Infective larva actively penetrates skin after being deposited there when fly bites.

Microfilaria ingested by blackfly during blood meal develops into infective larva

FIG 12–9 Life cycle of *Onchocerca volvulus*

tissues and develop into adult worms. Adult worms may live as long as 14 years in the human host. Within a year of infection, the adults become encapsulated in fibrous tissue nodules that measure a few millimeters to several centimeters in diameter (Figure 12–10). These onchocercomas are not painful, but may be disfiguring. In Africa and Venezuela, the nodules are found more frequently on the trunk while in Guatemala and Mexico, the majority of nodules are seen on the scalp.

In contrast to the filarial nematodes that primarily infect the lymphatics, the pathologic manifestations in onchocerciasis are elicited by the microfilariae and not the adult organisms. Microfilariae migrate from the nodule to the skin, the eyes, and lymph nodes and give rise to the variety of symptoms. Clinical manifestations generally begin to occur one to three years after the initial infection.

The most frequent clinical features of *Onchocerca volvulus* infection are pruritus and rash. The itching may be intense, as the skin becomes swollen, painful and hot. This becomes a condition of chronic inflammation which exaggerates the aging process of the skin. Loss of elasticity occurs and the skin becomes thickened and heavily wrinkled. There may be hyper- or hypopigmentation. Pigmentary changes are more often seen on the extremities.

The most serious complication of this disease is visual impairment. The degree of ocular damage depends on the severity of the infection. Lesions may occur in any part of the eye in response to migrating microfilariae. An acute inflammatory reaction envelops the dying microfilariae and manifests as an opacity on the cornea (Figure 12–11). An accumulation of these lesions leads to bilateral blindness. Mortality rate in adults increases three to fourfold with blindness.

Patients may also experience lymphadenopathy in the inguinal and femoral areas. Enlargement of these lymph nodes coupled with the aforementioned skin changes produces the condition know as hanging groin. These patients are at a heightened risk for inguinal and femoral hernias.

Laboratory Diagnosis

Since microfilariae are found in the skin, the specimen of choice for the diagnosis of onchocerciasis is a skin biopsy or **skin snip**. Tissue samples are placed in saline and teased to reveal the microfilariae or placed into culture medium and examined after four hours of incubation. Microfilariae are unsheathed and have body nuclei that do not extend to the tip of the tail. They need to be differentiated from larval forms of *Mansonella streptocerca* which may also be found in skin specimen preparations. Adult forms may be surgically removed from infected nodules.

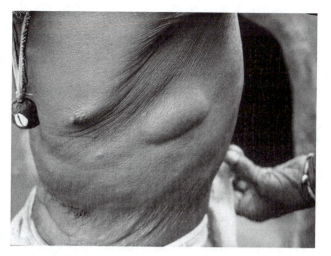

FIG 12–10 An elderly village chief undresses prior to bathing. He has an onchocerciasis nodule clearly visible on his torso. (Image courtesy of the WHO/TDR Image Library, photograph by Andy Crump, Ghana, 1999.)

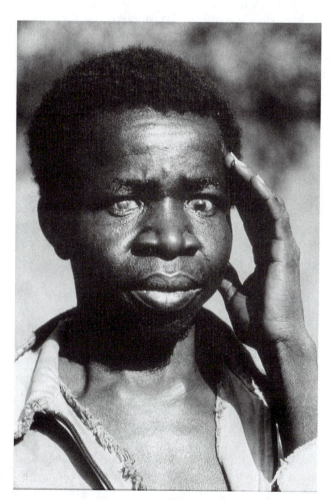

FIG 12–11 An adult male blinded by onchocerciasis (river blindness). (Image coutesy of the WHO/TDR Image Library, taken in West Africa, 1991, by Tony Ward.)

Patient travel history and clinical symptoms, as well as the presence of eosinophilia and elevated IgE levels, aid the diagnosis of river blindness.

Treatment and Prevention

Ivermectin is the treatment of choice for river blindness. In 1987, Merck licensed the drug Ivermectin (Mectizan) for the treatment of onchocerciasis and began a major effort to eliminate the disease with a pledge to deliver the drug at no cost for as long as necessary. Ivermectin is administered as a single yearly oral dose of 150 mcg/kg of body weight. Ivermectin is highly active as a microfilaricide. It does not kill the adult worms; however, it reduces the fertility of the mature female worm. Ivermectin is safe during pregnancy. If the eye is involved, prednisone at 1 mg/kg/day is started for several days before initiating therapy with Ivermectin to minimize the inflammatory response to dying microfilariae. Diethylcarbamazine (DEC) is also effective at killing the microfilariae but may lead to severe side effects, particularly in heavy infections. Surgical excision of adult worms is recommended when nodules appear on the head. Removal of adult worms reduces the risk of ocular damage by the migrating larvae.

Vector control programs have successfully reduced or eliminated transmission of onchocerciasis in many endemic regions. *Simulium* larvae are easily destroyed by aerial spraying of breeding sites with selected insecticides. Wearing protective clothing may also help to prevent blackfly bites. The key to breaking the cycle of transmission in any given area is the elimination of the blackfly vector for a period of not less than 14 years, so that the reservoir of adult worms dies out within the human population. In conjunction with vector control activities, Ivermectin is administered to infected individuals to kill microfilariae and reduce clinical manifestations.

MANSONELLA OZZARDI

Morphology

Mansonella ozzardi is the only filarial nematode that is strictly confined to the New World, with a distribution throughout Central and South America and the Caribbean islands. The adult worms inhabit the body cavities and visceral fat. The microfilariae of *M. ozzardi* circulate in the bloodstream without periodicity and the infection is generally asymptomatic.

Life Cycle

The adult worms inhabit the visceral fat, which surrounds organs, and the mesentery. The mature female measures 65 to 80 mm while the male usually ranges only 24 to 28 mm in length. The unsheathed microfilariae migrate through dermal tissue making their way into the blood circulation without exhibiting a periodicity. They may be found within the intravascular spaces such as capillaries. The larval forms (microfilariae), averaging 88 micrometers, are ingested by midge flies (*Culicoides*) or in some geographic regions by blackflies (*Simulium*). Within the insect, the infective larvae develop further and are passed on to the next host when the insect feeds again. Humans are the only known reservoir hosts.

Transmission and Pathogenesis

Throughout most of its geographic distribution, *Mansonella ozzardi* is transmitted by midges of the genus *Culicoides*, except in the Amazon river basin where blackflies contribute as a vector. The infection is generally asymptomatic in the native population. Neither the adult nor larval worms evoke inflammatory changes in the human host. As with other filarial infections, symptoms may be more pronounced and severe in non-residents. Only on rare occasions have lymphadenopathy, pruritus, fever, skin lesions or marked eosinophilia been reported.

Laboratory Diagnosis

Diagnosis of *Mansonella ozzardi* infection is based on the recovery and identification of the unsheathed, non-periodic microfilariae from a peripheral blood specimen or skin biopsy sample. Greater success is obtained by using thick smears or employing Knott's concentration technique. Microfilariae have body nuclei that do not extend to the tip of the tail and therefore must be differentiated from other blood-borne microfilariae (Figure 12–7).

Treatment and Prevention

Asymptomatic patients do not require therapy. DEC, given in large doses (6 mg/kg) three times daily for 10 days has proven effective in the elimination of the larval microfilariae in patients with more severe clinical manifestations.

Mansonella ozzardi infection may be prevented by the use of insect repellents to discourage fly bites. The use of netting and screens is insignificant because the insects are small enough to pass through the finest grade of mesh. Eradication or control of the insect's swampy breeding habitats and other vector control measures are not practical.

MANSONELLA PERSTANS

Morphology

Mansonella perstans, formerly known as *Dipetalonema perstans*, causes a filarial infection common among man and apes in large areas of the central portion of Africa and in the northeastern region of South America. These areas are also endemic for the tiny midges (*Culicoides*) that serve as vector for this organism.

Life Cycle

The adult worms are similar in size to *M. ozzardi* and reside in the serous cavities (pleural, peritoneal and pericardial). Their microfilariae are also unsheathed but larger, measuring around 190–200 micrometers long. They are found in the blood and therefore may be ingested by a feeding insect vector, *Culicoides* spp. The larvae are non-periodic and have body nuclei that extend to the tip of the tail. The terminal nucleus may appear to be slightly removed from the rest.

Transmission and Pathogenesis

Although the prevalence of *Mansonella perstans* is high in areas where the vector is endemic, the clinical and pathologic manifestations of the disease are poorly documented in the medical literature. The majority of the cases appear to be asymptomatic or benign. In some instances, transient Calabar-like swellings have been reported. Mature worms living in the various serous cavities appear to produce minimal inflammatory changes within the host.

Laboratory Diagnosis

Microfilariae may be recovered from the blood or serosal effusions. Blood samples may be taken at any time and prepared in the same manner as for the identification of other filarial infections. Larvae must be differentiated from the other blood-borne microfilariae. (Figure 12–7). Even though the disease is mild or asymptomatic the only clues may be an eosinophilia or an elevated antifilarial antibody titer.

Treatment and Prevention

There is little evidence to support that DEC is effective in treating disease caused by *M. perstans*; however, it remains the standard therapeutic option. Ivermectin has no activity against this organism. Mebendazole has been shown to be successful and is given for thirty days at 100 mg orally twice daily.

As with *M. ozzardi* infection, there are no vector control measures in place to prevent the spread of *M. perstans*. Travelers to endemic areas are advised to apply insect repellent generously to all exposed surfaces and to impregnate garments with permethrins to deter insect bites and exposure.

MANSONELLA STREPTOCERCA

Morphology

Mansonella streptocerca (formerly *Dipetalonema streptocerca*) is found in the same regions as *M. perstans* in the Congo basin of West Africa. The infection, known as **streptocerciasis,** is transmitted by tiny midges of the genus *Culicoides* and is found in both man and monkeys.

Life Cycle

The adult worms of *Mansonella streptocerca* live in the dermis, just below the surface of the skin. Microfilariae measuring 180 to 240 μm in length, may be found in the skin and also in the blood. Here they can be acquired by biting midges (genus *Culicoides*). The microfilariae are unsheathed and have body nuclei that extend to the tip of the tail, which ends in a characteristic partial coil known as a shepherd's crook.

Transmission and Pathogenesis

Streptocerciasis is acquired through the bite of an infected midge. Infection in many individuals is characterized by a pruritic dermatitis with the development of hypopigmented macules. Streptocerciasis must be differentiated from onchocerciasis, which causes pruritic dermatitis, and leprosy, which is characterized by hypopigmented macules. Many infected individuals also have inguinal adenopathy.

Laboratory Diagnosis

Mansonella streptocerca infection should be suspected in patients from endemic areas who present with characteristic symptoms: pruritis and hypopigmented macules. A specific diagnosis may be made by demonstration of representative microfilariae from skin snip samples soaked in saline. Microfilariae are unsheathed, measure 180 to 240 μm, and have body nuclei that extend in a single column to the tip of its crooked tail (Figure 12–7).

Treatment and Prevention

Diethylcarbamazine (DEC) is the drug of choice for the treatment of *Mansonella streptocerca* infection. Ivermectin has also shown promise as a treatment. A common side effect of both drugs is intense pruritis.

Vector control programs are non-existent in endemic areas. Travelers are best protected by using insect repellent to protect against insect bites. The use of bed netting or protective screens is ineffective because the insects (midges) are small enough to pass through.

DIROFILARIA IMMITIS

Morphology

Dirofilaria immitis, the dog heartworm, is a common zoonotic filarial infection of domestic and wild canines in the greater part of the tropical, subtropical, and warm temperate regions of the world. Although human infection is still relatively rare, human pulmonary **dirofilariasis** has been reported with increasing frequency since first reported in 1941.

Life Cycle

The adult worms live in the right heart of dogs and other canines. Adult females measure 25 to 30 cm in length by 1 mm in diameter. Unsheathed microfilariae measuring 300 to 325 μm long by 7 μm in diameter are found in the dog's circulation, where they can be ingested by the mosquito vector. Following development in the mosquito, the infective larvae may be transmitted as the insect takes a blood meal. Within the dog, the developmental cycle takes approximately 6 months.

Man is an accidental host in *Dirofilaria immitis* infections. Worms do not grow to maturity in the human host and, subsequently, microfilariae are not found in the circulation.

Transmission and Pathogenesis

Human infection is acquired through the bite of an infected mosquito. Parasites typically migrate to the lung resulting in the production of a well-defined solitary nodule called a coin lesion. Many patients remain asymptomatic and the nodule is found coincidently on routine X-ray or autopsy. Symptomatic patients may complain of persistent cough, chest discomfort, hemoptysis, or other symptoms that may warrant a chest examination. Eosinophilia may also be present. In many cases, a single worm may occlude a branch of the pulmonary artery causing an infarct.

Laboratory Diagnosis

Diagnosis of *Dirofilaria immitis* infection is made by the histologic examination of pulmonary nodule sections. Patients may exhibit a moderate eosinophilia, but no microfilariae are found in the blood.

Treatment and Prevention

The only known treatment for dirofilarial infection is surgical removal of the worm. Chemotherapy is ineffective.

Very little information is known about the transmission of human infection with *Dirofilaria immitis*. Preventive measures are undetermined.

SUMMARY

The tissue nematodes parasitize human skin, blood or lymphatics and produce a variety of pathologies depending on the species and the body site affected. These organisms have complex life cycles including larval stages and intermediate hosts. In some cases, as with *Trichinella spiralis* or *Dirofilaria immitis*, man is a dead end host for the parasite.

Human filarial nematodes are transmitted by arthropod vectors, primarily biting insects such as flies and mosquitoes. They produce microfilarial larvae that circulate in the blood and lymphatics and may be responsible for deformity or blindness. Many of these organisms have developed a periodicity that corresponds to the feeding habits of their vector. Human filarial infections may be classified into those that affect the lymphatics (bancroftian and brugian filariasis) and those that are nonlymphatic (loiasis, mansonelliasis, and onchocerciasis).

The type of specimen required for the recovery and identification of the parasite varies with the species suspected. Care should be taken to make note of patient symptoms and place of residence or travel history. Many microfilariae exhibit a periodicity in the blood that should be considered when specimens are collected. The identification of microfilariae may be made by comparison of specific characteristics: presence or absence of a sheath; nuclear arrangement in the tail of the microfilariae; and organism size.

REVIEW QUESTIONS

1. Sheathed microfilariae are recovered from a peripheral blood sample of a patient from the Philippines. These larvae, described as having two discrete nuclei in the tip of a pointed tail, are characteristic of:

   a. *Wuchereria bancrofti*

   b. *Brugia malayi*

   c. *Loa loa*

   d. *Onchocerca volvulus*

2. The microfilariae of this nematode are sheathed and have pointed tails that are devoid of nuclei:

   a. *Brugia malayi*

   b. *Loa loa*

   c. *Wuchereria bancrofti*

   d. *Dracunculus medinensis*

3. The etiologic agent of river blindness is:

   a. *Dracunculus medinensis*

   b. *Mansonella streptocerca*

   c. *Loa loa*

   d. *Onchocerca volvulus*

4. The common name for this tissue nematode is the guinea worm:

   a. *Dirofilaria immitis*

   b. *Loa loa*

   c. *Mansonella ozzardi*

   d. *Dracunculus medinensis*

5. These sheathed microfilariae are obtained from peripheral blood specimens with diurnal periodicity. They have body nuclei that are continuous to the tip of the rounded tail:

   a. *Loa loa*

   b. *Wuchereria bancrofti*

   c. *Brugia malayi*

   d. *Mansonella perstans*

6. Trichinella spiralis is commonly acquired by:

   a. the bite of an infected mosquito

   b. ingesting water containing infected copepods

   c. eating raw or poorly cooked infected meat

   d. the bite of an infected blackfly

7. The skin snip is the specimen of choice for the recovery of:

   a. *Dracunculus medinensis*

   b. *Onchocerca volvulus*

   c. *Brugia timori*

   d. *Loa loa*

Match the organism with the appropriate vector.

8. _____ *Wuchereria bancrofti*   a. *Chrysops* (mango fly)

9. _____ *Loa loa*   b. *Culicoides* (midge)

10. _____ *Onchocerca volvulus*   c. *Anopheles* (mosquito)

11. _____ *Mansonella perstans*   d. *Simulium* (blackfly)

Match the clinical manifestation with the appropriate organism.

12. _____ River blindness   a. *Trichinella spiralis*

13. _____ Muscle cysts   b. *Onchocerca volvulus*

14. _____ Elephantiasis   c. *Loa loa*

15. _____ Calabar swelling   d. *Wuchereria bancrofti*

CASE STUDY

You are a clinical laboratory scientist in a large metropolitan hospital. A 32-year old man comes into the emergency room with vague complaints of visual impairment and rash. A complete patient history is difficult because the patient has only recently immigrated from Guatemala and speaks English poorly. Physical examination reveals a subcutaneous nodule on the patient's scalp and pinpoint opacities on the man's left cornea. Blood tests show an elevated serum IgE titer and eosinophilia.

Questions

1. What parasitic infection/organism should the physician suspect?

2. What is the specimen of choice for diagnosis?

3. What form of the parasite is most frequently recovered?

4. List the characteristic features of the parasite.

5. What is the treatment of choice?

▶ BIBLIOGRAPHY

Beaver, P. C., Jung, R. C., & Cupp, E. W. (1984). *Clinical parasitology* (9th ed.). Philadelphia: Lea & Febiger.

Beers, M. H. & Berkow, R. (1999). *The Merck manual of diagnosis and therapy.* (17th ed.). Whitehouse Station, NJ: Merck Research Laboratories.

Centers for Disease Control and Prevention. (1991). Trichinosis surveillance, United States, 1987–1990. *Morbidity and Mortality Weekly Report, 40*(ss-3), 35–42.

Fauci, A. S. (1998). *Harrison's principles of internal medicine* (14th ed.). New York: McGraw-Hill.

Faust, E. C., Thomas, E. P., & Jones, J. (1941). Discovery of human heartworm infection in New Orleans. *Parasitology, 27*, 115–122.

Garcia, L. S. & Bruckner, D. A. (1993). *Diagnostic medical parasitology* (2nd ed.). Washington, DC: American Society of Microbiology.

Kean, B. H., Mott, K. E. & Russell, A. J. (1978). *Tropical medicine and parasitology: Classic investigations* (Vol. 2), (pp. 374–412, 444–457). Ithaca, NY: Cornell University Press.

Lightner, L. K., Ewert, A., Corredor, A., & Sabogat, E. (1980). A parasitologic survey for *Mansonella ozzardi* in the Comisaria del Vaupes, Columbia. *American Journal of Tropical Medicine and Hygiene, 29*, 42–45.

Markell, E. K., John, D. K., & Krotoski, W. A. (1999). *Medical parasitology* (8th ed.). Philadelphia: W. B. Saunders.

Moorhead, A., Grunewald, P. E., Dietz, V. J., & Schantz, P. M. (1999). Trichinellosis in the United States, 1991–1996: Declining but not gone. *American Journal of Tropical Medicine and Hygiene, 60*, 66–69.

Nutman, T. B., Nash, T. E., & Ottesen, E. A. (1987). Ivermectin and the successful treatment of the patient with *Mansonella ozzardi* infection. *Journal of Infectious Diseases, 156*, 662–665.

Plaisier, A. P., van Oortmarsen, G. J., Remme, J., and Habbema, J. D. F. (1991). The reproductive lifespan of *Onchocerca volvulus* in West African savanna. *Acta. Trop.* 48, 271–284.

Pozio, E. et al. (1992). Taxonomic revision of the genus *Trichinella. Journal of Parasitology, 78*, 654–659.

Shenoy, R. K., Kumarswami, V., Rajan, K., Thankom, S., & Jalajokumari. (1992). Ivermectin for the treatment of periodic Malayan filariasis: A study of efficacy and side effects following single oral dose and retreatment at six months. *Annals of Tropical Medicine and Parasitology, 86*, 271–278.

Shimeld, L. A. (1999). *Essentials of diagnostic microbiology*.Albany, NY: Delmar Publishers.

Talaro, K. P., & Talaro, A. (1999). *Foundations in microbiology* (3rd ed.). Boston: WBC McGraw-Hill.

Wahlgren, M. (1982). The successful treatment of *Diptalonema perstans* filariasis with mebendazole. *Annals of Tropical Medicine and Parasitology, 76*, 557–559.

CHAPTER THIRTEEN
Trematodes

LEARNING OBJECTIVES

After reading and studying this chapter, the student should be able to:

- List the clinically significant trematodes which cause human disease.

- List and describe the characteristics used to identify trematodes.

- Describe and compare life cycles of trematodes, and identify the stage of development which is infective for man; identify and characterize intermediate and definitive hosts.

- Compare the morphological characteristics of trematode ova, larvae and adult forms; determine which stage of development is usually diagnostic for human infection.

- Describe the transmission and pathogenesis of human intestinal trematode infections.

- Describe the treatment and prevention of infection with trematodes.

KEY TERMS

Boss (BOS)
Cercariae (sir-KAR-ee-ay)
Fluke (FLOOK)
Hermaphroditic (her-MA-fro-DI-tik)

Metacercariae (MET-a-sir-KAR-ee-ay)
Miracidium (MIR-a-SID-ee-um)
Operculum (o-PER-ku-lum)
Schistosomulum (SHIS-toe-SOM-u-lum)

Tegument (TEG-u-ment)
Trematode (TREM-a-toad)

INTRODUCTION

Trematodes are members of the phylum Platyhelminthes (flatworms) and the class Trematoda, and are called **flukes**. The outer covering of the flatworms is called the **tegument**, which allows absorption of nutrients. Most trematodes are **hermaphroditic**, with male and female reproductive organs present in a single fluke; schistosomes are trematodes which have separate sexes. Flukes have complex life cycles, usually involving two intermediate hosts. Snails are important as first intermediate hosts. The ciliated larval stage of a fluke, which develops within the ovum, is called a **miracidium**. In the life cycle of a trematode, the miracidium infects the snail. The egg of a trematode may or may not contain a miracidium when passed in feces. Unembryonated eggs undergo a developmental phase during which the miracidium is formed.

Reproduction of the miracidium in the snail gives rise to a large number of **cercariae**. The cercariae are released into water, and swim around until the next host is encountered. Cercariae of the schistosomes directly penetrate the skin of humans, leading to infection. Other cercariae encyst, after penetrating the flesh of vertebrates (fish) or invertebrates (crayfish), or on vegetation, producing **metacercariae**.

The ova of all trematodes (except schistosomes) have a structure known as an **operculum**. This structure acts as an "escape hatch" for the miracidium, and varies in shape among species. A thickening called a knob or a **boss**, may be found at the opposite end of the shell from the operculum. Spines are present on the eggs of some trematodes, namely, the schistosomes.

The diagnosis of human infection with trematodes is usually made by the identification of characteristic eggs. Characteristic features of trematode eggs are illustrated in Figure 13–1 and 13–2. The larvae of flukes are rarely encountered, since they usually occur outside the human host. The adult flukes, leaflike in structure, also are rarely seen.

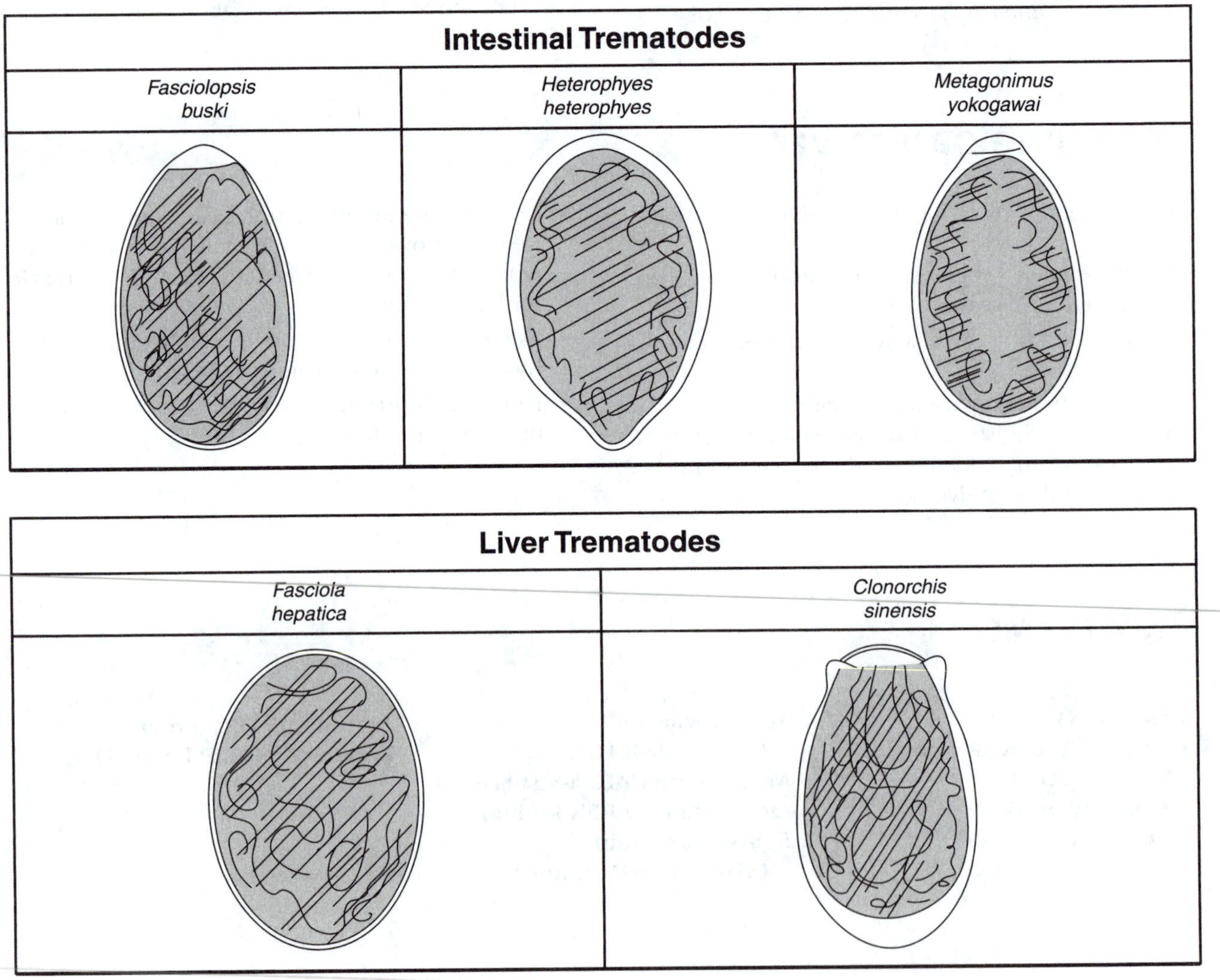

Intestinal Trematodes

Fasciolopsis buski	Heterophyes heterophyes	Metagonimus yokogawai

Liver Trematodes

Fasciola hepatica	Clonorchis sinensis

FIG 13–1 Ova of intestinal and liver trematodes

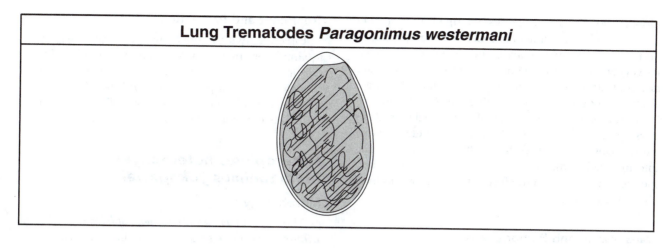

Lung Trematodes *Paragonimus westermani*

Blood Trematodes (schistosomes)

Schistosoma mansoni	*Schistosoma haematobium*	*Schistosoma japonicum*

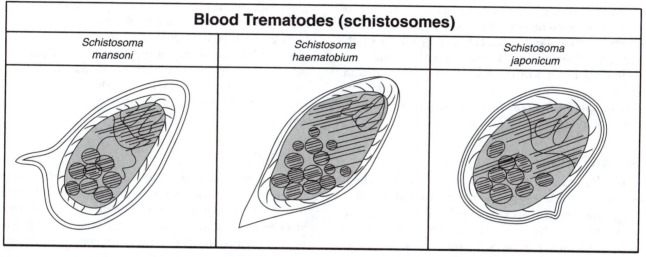

FIG 13–2 Ova of lung and blood trematodes

INTESTINAL TREMATODES

These flukes inhabit the small intestines of humans, where the adult worms deposit eggs which are passed in the feces. They require a freshwater snail to act as the first intermediate host.

Fasciolopsis buski

Morphology

Fasciolopsis buski is called the giant intestinal fluke. It is the largest fluke inhabiting humans (approximately 2–7 cm long), and lives in the small intestine. The broadly ellipsoidal egg is 130–140 μm long and 80–85 μm wide (Figure 13–3). The egg has a small operculum at the pointed end of the transparent eggshell, and is unembryonated when passed.

Life Cycle

The life cycles of trematodes are similar, but differ in intermediate hosts and stage of development of the

eggs passed in feces (Figure 13–4). The primary reservoir for the giant intestinal fluke is the pig, although the dog may harbor the parasite. After passage of the unembryonated egg in the feces, development of the miracidium occurs in water in approximately one

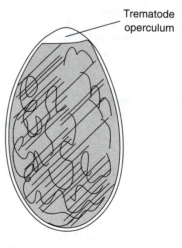

Trematode operculum

FIG 13–3 *Fasciolopsis buski* (130–140 μm × 80–85 μm)

month. The snail acts as the first intermediate host, after penetration by the miracidium. Cercariae are produced and released from the snail, and encyst on freshwater vegetation (second intermediate host), such as water chestnuts and bamboo shoots, forming metacercariae. Humans acquire infection with *F. buski* after ingesting metacercariae encysted on infected vegetation. After passing into the intestinal tract, the metacercariae excyst. Development to the adult form occurs in the intestine. Self-fertilization occurs in the intestine, and the eggs are passed in the feces. The adult worm lives about six months.

Transmission and Pathogenesis

Transmission of infection occurs by ingestion of metacercariae on raw or undercooked vegetation. The infection is prevalent in the Far East, including southeast Asia, Thailand, and Vietnam. Local inflammation occurs when the worms attach to the mucosal wall. Diarrhea and abdominal pain may be present. Eosinophilia is common. Bowel obstruction may occur in heavy infections.

Laboratory Diagnosis

The diagnosis of infection with *F. buski* is made by examination of stool specimens for ova and parasites. The characteristic eggs are passed in feces. They may be confused with the eggs of *Fasciola hepatica*, because of similarities in size and structure.

Treatment and Prevention

Infections with *F. buski* may be treated with praziquantel or niclosamide. Prevention of infection requires proper human fecal waste disposal, efforts at reducing the snail population, and the elimination of the practice of eating raw vegetation. The use of human fecal waste as fertilizer should be prohibited.

Heterophyes heterophyes/ Metagonimus yokogawai

Morphology

The eggs of *Heterophyes heterophyes* and *Metagonimus yokogawai*, small flukes collectively called heterophyids, are tiny (approximately 30 by 15 μm), and are virtually indistinguishable (Figure 13–5); however, the eggshells of the latter eggs are thinner. The egg has shoulders, and may or may not have a small boss opposite the operculum. The embryonated egg contains a formed miracidium. The adult forms of both flukes are tiny and measure approximately 1–2 mm long.

Life Cycle

The egg containing a fully developed miracidium is ingested by a freshwater snail. The miracidium is released after ingestion. The miracidium penetrates the snail tissue, and undergoes developmental stages to produce cercariae. The mature cercariae are released

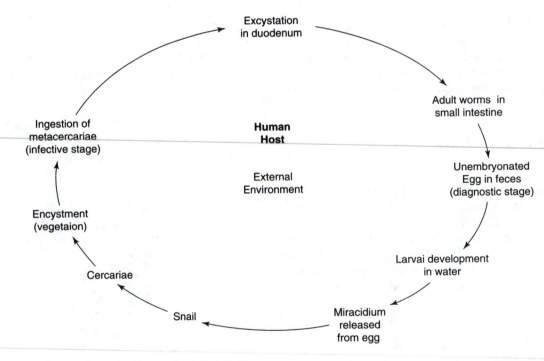

FIG 13–4 Life cycle of *Fasciolopsis buski* and *Fasciola hepatica*

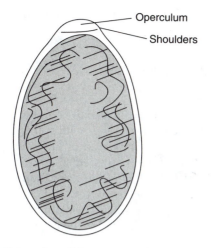

FIG 13–5 *Heterophyes/Metagonimus* (30 μm × 15 μm)

into the water, where they find freshwater fish to act as the second intermediate hosts. Cercariae encyst in the flesh of the fish to form metacercariae. After ingestion by the definitive host, metacercariae excyst, and develop into adult worms in the small intestine. Eggs are produced and the cycle continues (Figure 13–6).

Transmission and Pathogenesis

Transmission of infection occurs by ingestion of uncooked or inadequately cooked fish. Although light infections are usually asymptomatic, heavy infections with both species may cause diarrhea, abdominal pain and eosinophilia. Granulomas may result from penetration of the intestinal wall by the eggs, with resulting migration in the capillaries and lymphatics. Infection is common in the Far East, especially in Japan and the Philippines. The helminth has been found in sushi. Mammals and birds may harbor the parasites.

Laboratory Diagnosis

The diagnosis of heterophyiasis or metagonimiasis is usually made by finding the characteristic ova during a routine examination of stool for ova and parasites. Care must be taken to distinguish the ova from those of the liver fluke, *Clonorchis sinensis*. Adult worms are rarely found.

Treatment and Prevention

Praziquantel is the treatment of choice for infections with *H. heterophyes* and *M. yokogawai*. Prevention of infection is accomplished by proper cooking of fish, especially of fish from endemic areas. Proper disposal of human fecal waste is also important in controlling the spread of infection.

LIVER TREMATODES

These flukes parasitize the biliary tracts of humans.

Fasciola hepatica
Morphology

The ova of *Fasciola hepatica*, known as the sheep liver fluke, are considered to be indistinguishable from those of *F. buski* (see Figure 13–3). The eggs of each

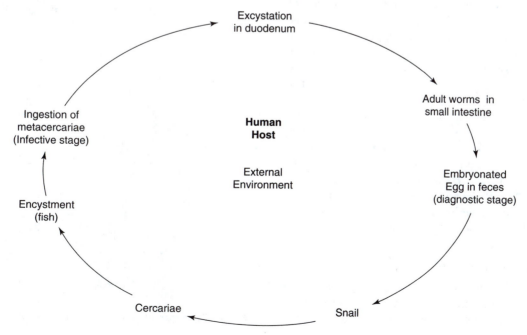

FIG 13–6 Life cycle of *Heterophyes/Metagonimus*

species are similar in size, and have an undeveloped miracidium and a distinct operculum. The adult worm is 2–3 cm long.

Life Cycle

The life cycle of *F. hepatica* is similar to that of *F. buski* (see Figure 13–4), with the passage of unembryonated eggs in feces. The miracidium develops within two weeks, escapes from the egg and infects the snail, which acts as the first intermediate host. Cercariae develop in the snail and are released in the water, where they encyst, forming metacercariae on vegetation. Human infection follows ingestion of contaminated vegetation. The metacercariae excyst in the duodenum, and larvae pass through the intestinal wall and into the liver and bile ducts. The adult worms of this helminth reside in the large bile ducts and gallbladder in humans, rather than in the intestine, although eggs are passed in the feces.

Transmission and Pathogenesis

The infection is transmitted by ingestion of raw water vegetation, such as watercress, harboring infective metacercariae. Symptoms of infection include abdominal pain, diarrhea, and indigestion. Migration through the liver may result in damage, depending on the number of worms. In the bile ducts, mechanical irritation is common. Obstruction of the biliary tract may occur. Unlike *F. buski*, found primarily in the Far East, distribution of *F. hepatica* is worldwide.

Laboratory Diagnosis

The diagnosis of infection caused by *F. hepatica* is based on the finding of characteristic eggs in human feces. Since the eggs of this parasite and *F. buski* are indistinguishable, clinical history may be essential in making the proper diagnosis. The Entero-test may also be used to diagnose infection. Eggs recovered from duodenal aspirate specimens (containing bile fluid) may help to differentiate these two parasitic infections.

Serological methods, using enzyme immunoassay (EIA) or immunoblot techniques, may be helpful for the early diagnosis of fascioliasis (see Chapter 3), since antibodies my be detectable within three weeks, while the eggs may not appear in the stool until six weeks following infection. Serological assays may also be used as a test of cure following therapy.

Treatment and Prevention

A halogenated phenol, bithinol, is the drug of choice for treatment of infection. Triclabendazole has also been effective. Prevention of infection lies in the avoidance of ingestion of raw vegetation, and adherence to good sanitary practices.

Clonorchis sinensis

Morphology

The eggs of the Chinese liver fluke, *Clonorchis sinensis* are delicate-looking, with a thick, brownish shell, and prominent shoulders around the operculum (Figure 13–7). A comma-shaped structure may be present at the opposite end. The flask-shaped egg, similar to that of *H. heterophyes* and *M. yokogawai*, measures 30 by 15 μm, and contains a fully formed miracidium. The adult fluke averages 1–2.5 cm in length.

Life Cycle

The life cycle of *C. sinensis* resembles that of *H. heterophyes/M. yokogawai* (see Figure 13–6). The miracidium is released from the embryonated egg in freshwater, or after ingestion by a snail. Cercariae develop, and encyst as metacercariae in freshwater fish. Humans are infected by eating raw or undercooked fish. Metacercariae excyst in the duodenum, and pass through the common bile duct into the bile capillaries. The adult worms mature and deposit eggs in the small bile ducts. The embryonated eggs pass in bile fluid to the feces, where they leave the host.

Transmission and Pathogenesis

The infection is transmitted by ingestion of metacercariae in raw or undercooked fish. Light infections are usually asymptomatic, with little change in the liver. Heavier infections may result in an inflammatory

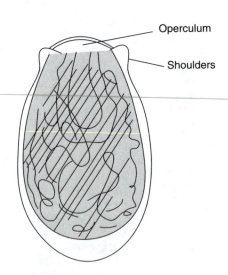

FIG 13–7 *Clonorchis sinensis* (30 μm × 15 μm)

response in the biliary epithelium, and abdominal pain, fever, and eosinophilia. Obstructive jaundice may occur.

Laboratory Diagnosis

Infection is detected by identification of characteristic ova in stool specimens or duodenal aspirates. The adult worm is rarely found.

Treatment and Prevention

Praziquantel is the treatment of choice. Prevention of infection requires good sanitary practices, as well as ingestion of only properly cooked fish.

LUNG TREMATODES

These flukes reside in the lung. Infection may mimic symptoms of tuberculosis.

Paragonimus westermani

Morphology

The oval egg of the oriental lung fluke, *Paragonimus westermani*, measures 100 by 55 μm on average (Figure 13–8) and is unembryonated when passed. The operculated egg resembles the egg of the tapeworm *Diphyllobothrium latum* in size and appearance; however, the lung fluke ovum is characterized by the presence of opercular shoulders, and has a thickened shell at the opposite end. The oval, brownish adult worm measures about 10 by 8 mm.

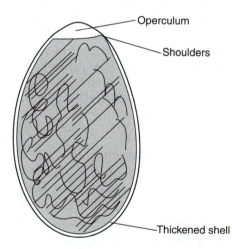

FIG 13–8 *Paragonimus westermani* (100 μm × 55 μm)

Life Cycle

Unembryonated eggs are passed in the feces or sputum. After larval development in water for about two weeks, a miridicium is released, which then infects a snail host (Figure 13–9). Cercariae are produced, and released to infect crayfish or crabs through ingestion of the snail, or through the gill chamber of the second intermediate host. Humans are infected after ingesting the metacercariae in uncooked crabs or crayfish. Excystation of the metacercariae occurs in the duodenum, followed by migration through the intestinal wall into the abdominal cavity, through the diaphragm into the pleural cavity and lungs. In the bronchiolar area, larvae develop into adults; eggs are released into the bronchial secretions. Eggs may be coughed up and swallowed. They may, therefore, also be passed in feces.

Transmission and Pathogenesis

Infection is transmitted by ingestion of encysted metacercariae in raw or undercooked crustaceans. Symptoms of paragonimiasis are related to the worm burden; light infections are often asymptomatic. Pulmonary symptoms include cough, chest pain, hemoptysis and bronchitis, often accompanied by eosinophilia. A serious complication of infection is caused by migration of larvae to the brain, resulting in neurological symptoms.

Laboratory Diagnosis

Infection is diagnosed by finding characteristic ova in pulmonary secretions, such as sputum, and occasionally, in feces. Flecks of blood in sputum resembling iron filings, are suggestive of infection with *P. westermani*. Immunoassays for antibodies in serum or pleural effusions may also be used to detect pulmonary and extra-pulmonary infections, and may be useful in monitoring therapy (see Chapter 3).

Treatment and Prevention

The treatment of choice is praziquantel. Prevention of infection requires avoidance of ingestion of undercooked crabs and crayfish, and good sanitary practices.

BLOOD TREMATODES

These adult flukes reside in the blood vessels surrounding the intestinal tract, liver, and urinary bladder. Infection occurs following direct skin penetration by free-living cercariae, after release from a snail, without the presence of a second intermediate host. Unlike

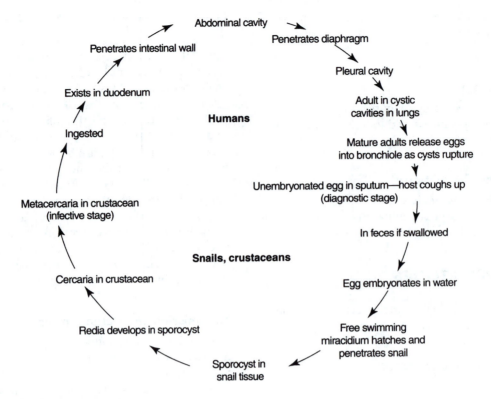

FIG 13-9 Life cycle of *P. westermani*

the previously discussed trematodes, sexes are separate, requiring the presence of male and female worms for the mating process, and the subsequent production of eggs. Although the schistosomes are considered to be blood flukes, they are not isolated from the blood.

Schistosoma mansoni/S. japonicum/ S. haematobium

Morphology

The adult blood flukes measure on average 1.5 to 2 cm, with the female being the larger of the two. The eggs of *Schistosoma mansoni* are oval and are approximately 115–180 by 40–80 μm in size; those of *S. haematobium* are just slightly smaller (Figure 13–10). The smallest eggs are those of *S. japonicum*; these eggs are rounder and measure 50–80 by 40–60 μm. Schistosome eggs lack the operculum present in the eggs of other trematodes. A characteristic feature of schistosome eggs is the presence of a spine. The well-developed spine of *S. mansoni* is located laterally; that of *S. haematobium* is prominent and terminal. The spine of *S. japonicum* is small and lateral, and often unrecognizable.

Life Cycle

Actively swimming cercariae penetrate human skin. After skin penetration, the schistosome cercariae lose their tails. The organism is now called a **schistoso-mulum**. These forms enter the circulation, mature in the portal blood, and reside in the blood vessels around the intestinal tract and liver (*S. mansoni* and *S. japonicum*) and urinary bladder (*S. haematobium*) (Figure 13–11). After mating of male and female worms, eggs are produced and make their way to the intestine or the lumen of the urinary bladder; they then leave the body in feces (*S. mansoni* and *S. japonicum*) or urine (*S. haematobium*). The mature miracidium is released from the egg in water. It finds and penetrates a suitable snail host. Cercariae are produced and released from the snail into the water.

Transmission and Pathogenesis

Humans are infected by skin penetration of schistosome cercariae while swimming or bathing in contaminated water. Chronic cases of schistosomiasis are usually asymptomtic. In symptomatic cases, inflammation often occurs at the site where the cercariae enter the skin (swimmer's itch). Other symptoms include abdominal pain, weight loss, bloody diarrhea,

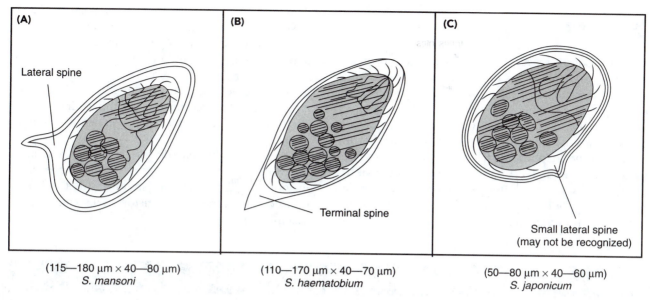

(A)

Lateral spine

(115—180 μm × 40—80 μm)
S. mansoni

(B)

Terminal spine

(110—170 μm × 40—70 μm)
S. haematobium

(C)

Small lateral spine
(may not be recognized)

(50—80 μm × 40—60 μm)
S. japonicum

FIG 13–10 Schistosome ova

eosinophilia, hepatosplenomegaly, and possible cirrhosis. Painful urination, hematuria and dysuria may develop in cases of *S. haematobium* infection.

Laboratory Diagnosis

The recovery of characteristic eggs in stool specimens (*S. mansoni* and *S. japonicum*), or in urine specimens (*S. haematobium*) is diagnostic for schistosomiasis. Travel history may be helpful in diagnosing this infection. Although several serologic assays have been developed for the diagnosis of schistosomiasis (see Chapter 3), their usefulness is limited by the frequency of cross-reactions with other helminthic infections.

Treatment and Prevention

Praziquantel is the drug of choice for treating schistosomiasis. Oxamniquine provides a cost-effective treatment for schistosomiasis caused by *S. mansoni* infection only. Prevention of infection requires good sanitation practices, control of the snail population, and the avoidance of freshwater skin exposure in endemic areas. Niclosamide may be applied to the skin as a protective barrier to penetration by schistosome cercariae.

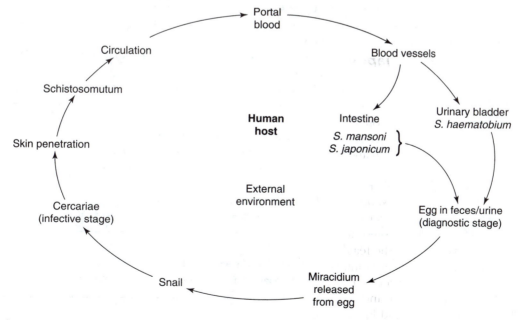

FIG 13–11 Life cycle of a schistosome

SUMMARY

Trematodes cause human diseases ranging from asymptomatic infections to chronic debilitating and serious infections. The characteristic features of trematodes are summarized in Table 13–1. These parasites may be classified as intestinal, liver, lung, and blood flukes. All the trematodes, except for the blood flukes, are hermaphroditic. Flukes have complex life cycles, each requiring a particular species of snail to act as the first intermediate host. Cercariae develop in the snail host, and are released into freshwater. Intestinal, liver, and lung flukes require a second intermediate host. Cercariae often encyst as metacercariae on freshwater vegetation, in fish, or crustaceans, such as crabs and crayfish. After ingestion, metacercariae excyst in the intestinal tract, and migrate to the intestines, the bile ducts, or the lung.

Schistosomes are unique among flukes, having separate sexes; they require no secondary intermediate host, and the cercarie directly penetrate the skin of the definitive host.

Diagnosis of trematode infection is based on the recovery of characteristic eggs from clinical specimens, including feces, urine, and sputum. Adult flukes are occasionally found. Travel history is also important in making a diagnosis.

Table 13–1 ► Key Characteristics of Trematodes

TREMATODE	CHARACTERISTIC FEATURES
Fasciolopsis buski	Giant intestinal fluke; largest fluke inhabiting humans Large, operculated eggs found in feces Transmission is by ingestion of metacercariae encysted on vegetation
Heterophyes, Metagonimus	Small, virtually indistinguishable intestinal flukes Small, operculated eggs found in feces Transmission is by ingestion of metacercariae encysted in freshwater fish
Fasciola hepatica	Sheep liver fluke Large, operculated eggs (indistinguishable from those of *F. buski*) found in feces Transmission is by ingestion of metacercariae encysted on vegetation
Clonorchis sinensis	Chinese liver fluke Small, delicate, operculated eggs with prominent shoulders found in feces Transmission is by ingestion of metacercariae encysted in fish
Paragonimus westermani	Oriental lung fluke Large, operculated eggs resembling those of the tapeworm, *Diphyllobothrium latum*, found in sputum or feces Transmission is by ingestion of metacercariae encysted on vegetation
Schistosoma mansoni	Blood fluke Oval egg with a large lateral spine found in feces Transmission by skin penetration of cercariae from freshwater snail
Schistosoma japonicum	Blood fluke Round egg with a small lateral spine found in feces Transmission by skin penetration of cercariae from freshwater snail
Schistosoma haematobium	Blood fluke Oval egg with a large terminal spine found in urine Transmission by skin penetration of cercariae from freshwater snail

REVIEW QUESTIONS

1. Which group of trematodes includes adult worms having separate sexes?
   a. intestinal flukes
   b. liver flukes
   c. lung flukes
   d. blood flukes

2. Which parasite forms metacercariae on freshwater vegetation?
   a. *Fasciola hepatica*
   b. *Clonorchis sinensis*
   c. *Paragonimus westermani*
   d. *Heterophyes heterophyes*

3. The ciliated larval stage of a trematode is called a/an
   a. oncosphere
   b. trophozoite
   c. miracidium
   d. cercaria

4. The chinese liver fluke is
   a. *Fasciola hepatica*
   b.. *Clonorchis sinensis*
   c. *Paragonimus westermani*
   d. *Heterophyes heterophyes*

5. The largest fluke which inhabits humans is
   a. *Paragonimus westermani*
   b. *Heterophyes heterophyes*
   c. *Schistosoma haematobium*
   d. *Fasciolopsis buski*

6. A risk of eating undercooked crabs or crayfish is infection with which parasite?
   a. *Paragonimus westermani*
   b. *Heterophyes heterophyes*
   c. *Schistosoma haematobium*
   d. *Fasciolopsis buski*

7. Eggs of which parasite would be expected to be recovered from a urine specimen?
   a. *Paragonimus westermani*
   b. *Heterophyes heterophyes*
   c. *Schistosoma haematobium*
   d. *Fasciolopsis buski*

8. Infection with which group of parasites is asociated with swimming or bathing in comtaminated water?
   a. intestinal flukes
   b. liver flukes
   c. lung flukes
   d. blood flukes

9. Which parasite is most apt to be diagnosed by examination of sputum specimens?
   a. *Schistosoma mansoni*
   b. *Schistosoma japonicum*
   c. *Metagonimus yokogawai*
   d. *Paragonimus westermani*

10. The eggs of *Fasciolopsis buski* and which other parasite are virtually indistinguishable?
    a. *Paragonimus westermani*
    b. *Fasciola hepatica*
    c. *Clonorchis sinensis*
    d. *Paragonimus westermani*

CASE STUDY

A 68-year old male presented to the emergency room, suffering from cough, chest pain, some difficulty breathing, and blood-tinged sputum. Sputum specimens were sent for routine microbiological culture, culture for tuberculosis, and an examination for parasites. Hematology studies showed moderate eosinophilia. The patient's history was unremarkable, except for a meal of "slightly-steamed" crabs eaten 1–2 weeks earlier.

The sputum cultures were negative for pathogens. Examination of sputum for parasites revealed operculated helminth ova, measuring 100 by 50 μm.

Questions

1. What is the name of the parasite which is causing this patient's symptoms?

2. How would you relate the life cycle of this parasite to the patient's illness.

3. What is the relationship between the steamed crab dinner and the patient's illness?

4. What is the recommended treatment for this infection?

5. What other helminth produces eggs which could be confused with this parasite? Explain.

▶ **BIBLIOGRAPHY**

Ash, L. R. & Orihel, C. (1999). Intestinal helminths. In Murray, P. R., Baron, S. J., Pfaller, M. A., Tenover, F. C., & Yolken, R. H.(Eds.). *Manual of clinical microbiology* (7th ed.). (pp. 1421–1435). Washington, DC: ASM Press.

Garcia, L. S. & Bruckner, D. A. (1997). *Diagnostic medical parasitology* (3rd ed.). Washington, DC: ASM Press.

Koneman, E. W., Allen, S. D., Janda, W. M., Schreckenberger, P. C., & Winn, Jr, W. C. (1997). *Color atlas and textbook of diagnostic microbiology* (5th ed.). Philadelphia: Lippincott.

Shimeld, L. & Rodgers, A. T (1999). Intestinal helminths. In Shimeld, L. (Ed.). *Essentials of diagnostic microbiology*. (pp. 603–615). Albany, NY: Delmar Publishers.

Zeibig, E. A. (1997). *Clinical parasitology*. Philadelphia: W. B. Saunders.

CHAPTER FOURTEEN
Cestodes

OUTLINE

INTESTINAL CESTODES

Diphyllobothrium latum
(di-FIL-o-BOTH-ree-um LAY-tum)

TAENIA SAGINATA

(TEE-nee-a SA-jin-AH-ta)/***Taenia solium*** (TEE-nee-a SO-lee-um)

HYMENOLEPIS NANA

(HI-men-OL-ep-is NAY-na)

Hymenolepis diminuta
(HI-men-OL-ep-is dim-in-U-ta)

Dipylidium caninum
(dip-ee-LID-ee-um kay-NIN-um)

TISSUE CESTODES

Echinococcus granulosus
(ee-KIN-o-KOK-us GRAN-u-LO-sus)

Multiceps species (MUL-tee-seps)

LEARNING OBJECTIVES

After reading and studying this chapter, the student should be able to:

- List the clinically significant cestodes which cause human disease.
- Give the common names for the tapeworms.
- List and describe characteristics used to identify cestodes.
- Describe and compare life cycles of cestodes, identifying the stage of development which is diagnostic, as well as infective, for humans; iden-

tify and characterize intermediate and definitive hosts.

- Compare the morphological characteristics of cestode ova and the proglottids of adult forms.
- Describe the transmission and pathogenesis of human cestode infections.
- Describe the treatment and prevention of infection with cestodes.

KEY TERMS

Bothria (BOTH-ree-a)
Brood capsule
  (BROOD kap-sul)
Calcareus corpuscles (cal-SAR-ee-us KOR-pus-els)
Cestode (SES-toad)
Coenurus (ko-NUR-is)

Coracidium (KOR-a-SID-ee-um)
Cysticercoid (SIS-ti-SIR-koyd)
Cysticercus (SIS-ti-SIR-cus)
Hydatid cyst (hi-DA-tid SIST)
Oncosphere (ON-ko-sfer)
Plerocercoid
  (PLER-o-SIR-koyd)

Procercoid (pro-SIR-koyd)
Proglottid (pro-GLO-tid)
Rostellum (ro-STEL-um)
Scolex (SKO-leks)
Sparganum (spar-GAN-um)
Strobila (stro-BIL-a)
Tapeworm (TAPE-worm)

INTRODUCTION

Cestodes are members of the phylum Platyhelminthes (flatworms) and the class Cestoda, and are called **tapeworms**. Humans may be infected with adult or larval forms of tapeworms. An adult tapeworm has a long, flattened, whitish, ribbon-like body. It consists of a **scolex**, an organ of attachment, usually bearing suckers or hooks, located at the anterior end; a neck, from which the tapeworm grows; and **proglottids** (a segment that grows from the neck). The characteristic features of cestode proglottids are illustrated in Figure 14–1.The scolex may have a structure called a **rostellum**, a crown-like structure, which may or may not bear hooks. The outer covering of the cestode is the tegument. This absorptive structure, also found in the trematodes (Chapter 13), allows materials to enter and waste products to be excreted from the body of the tapeworm. The proglottids are segments which progress from immature to mature and gravid forms distally. The entire body of a tapeworm is known as a **strobila.**

Although eggs are usually the diagnostic stage found in feces, gravid proglottids may be found. A six-hooked embryo, called an oncosphere, develops in most cestode eggs. Eggs passed in feces may be embryonated, or the oncosphere may develop after passage of eggs in feces. The characteristic features of cestode ova are illustrated in Figure 14–2.

Tapeworm larvae are not found in feces. The cysticercus larva of *Taenia* species, having a single scolex invaginated into a fluid-filled cyst, develops in the intermediate host (cow or pig), and is the infective form for man. The cysticercoid larva of *Hymenolepis* species, and *Dipylidium caninum*, develops in the intermediate host (beetle, flea). The hydatid cyst larval stage of the only intestinal tissue tapeworm species, *Echinococcus granulosus*, consists of multiple scolices, daughter cysts, brood capsules (each containing several inverted scolices), and fluid, and is found in human tissues. Procercoid and plerocercoid larvae of *Diphyllobothrium latum* develop in the first (copepod) and second (freshwater fish) intermediate hosts, respectively. Spherical structures called calcareous corpuscles are found in both larval and adult stages of

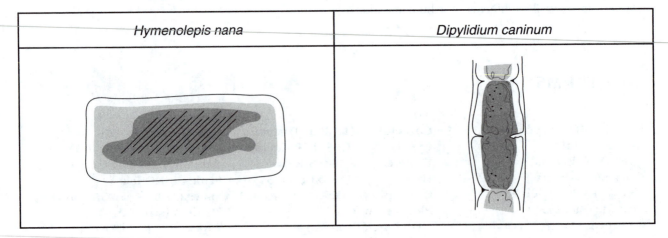

FIG 14–1 Proglottids of intestinal cestodes

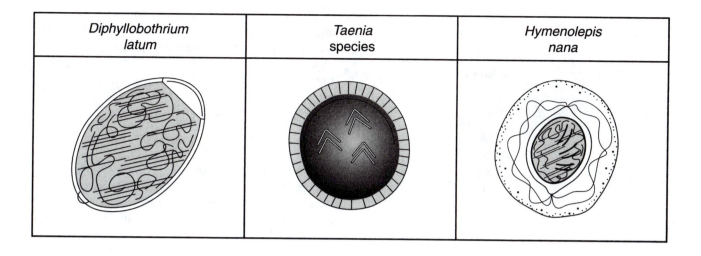

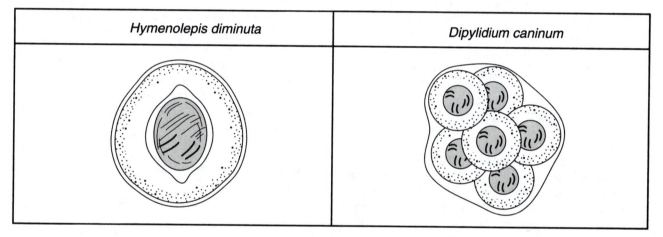

FIG 14–2 Ova of intestinal cestodes

tapeworms. These bodies consist of concentric layers of calcium carbonate. Most tapeworms require at least one intermediate host during their life cycles.

INTESTINAL CESTODES

Diphyllobothrium latum

Morphology

Diphyllobothrium latum, the broad fish tapeworm, is the largest tapeworm found in humans, with the strobila often measuring more than 10 m.

In place of the suckers or hooks found on most tapeworm scolices, this tapeworm has two shallow sucking grooves, called **bothria** (Figure 14–3).

The wide proglottid has a central rosette-shaped uterus (Figure 14–4). Unembryonated eggs are released from gravid proglottids, and may be recovered from feces. *D. latum* is the only tapeworm that can lay eggs.

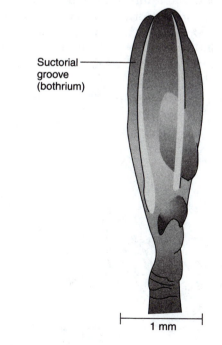

Suctorial groove (bothrium)

1 mm

FIG 14–3 The scolex of *D. latum*

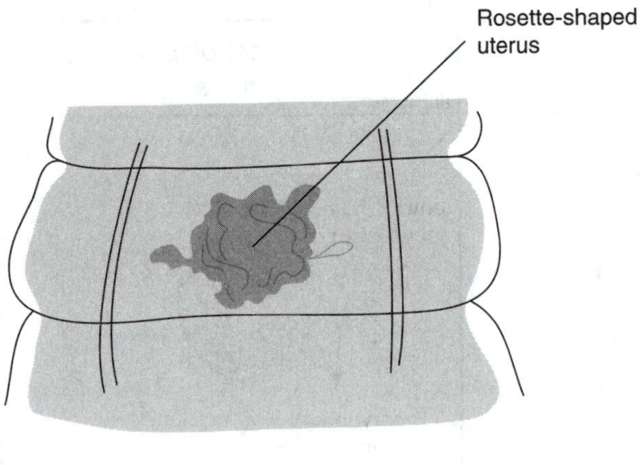

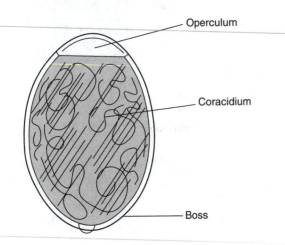

Rosette-shaped uterus

FIG 14–4 *Diphyllobothrium latum* proglottid

The operculated eggs measure 56–75 μm by 40–52 μm (Figure 14–5). *D. latum* is the only tapeworm that produces operculated eggs. A boss is present at the end opposite the operculum. Eggs may be confused with the eggs of the lung fluke *Paragonimus westermani*; however, the tapeworm eggs lack opercular shoulders present on the fluke eggs.

Life Cycle

The life cycle of *D. latum* is complex, involving two intermediate hosts (Figure 14–6). The adult tapeworm resides in the small intestine. After self-fertilization occurs (the cestodes are hermaphroditic), eggs are produced, and the unembryonated eggs leave the human host in the feces. When contact with fresh water occurs, the egg disintegrates, and a ciliated embryo known as a **coracidium** is released into the water to infect the first intermediate host, a crustacean known as a copepod, in the genus *Cyclops*. The procercoid larva develops in the copepod. The infected copepod is ingested by the second intermediate host, a freshwater fish. Ingestion of the infective plerocercoid larvae in raw or undercooked freshwater fish, such as

Operculum

Coracidium

Boss

FIG 14–5 *Diphyllobothrium latum* egg

pike, results in human infection. The scolex emerges, and attaches to the intestinal wall. The tapeworm matures in the small intestine. Sparganosis develops when a human acts as an intermediate host, by ingesting infected copepods.

Transmission and Pathogenesis

Diphyllobothriasis is endemic in parts of the United States (Alaska and the Great Lakes area), as well as in Scandinavia, Latin America, Asia and Africa, and is acquired by ingestion of tapeworm larvae in raw or undercooked freshwater fish. Although this fish is usually the second intermediate host, harboring the plerocercoid larva, the infected fish may itself be eaten by a larger fish, which acts as a vehicle to deliver the larvae to the human host. Most individuals with tapeworm infection are asymptomatic. Digestive disturbances, such as abdominal pain and weight loss may occur. A deficiency in vitamin B-12 may also develop, resulting in a macrocytic type of anemia.

If the first intermediate host (copepod) of *Diphyllobothrium* species is ingested by humans, as in contaminated water, the procercoid larva may develop into a **sparganum,** which migrates into the body's subcutaneous tissue.

Laboratory Diagnosis

The diagnosis of *D. latum* infection is made by the recovery of characteristic eggs in human feces. Proglottids and, rarely, the scolex may be found.

Treatment and Prevention

Praziquantel and niclosamide are recommended for the treatment of *D. latum* infection. Praziquantel is sometimes effective for treatment of a sparganum, although surgical removal may be necessary. Prevention of infection requires avoidance of the ingestion of raw or undercooked fish, as well as the proper disposal of human waste.

Taenia saginata/Taenia solium

Morphology

The two species of *Taenia* are *T. saginata*, the beef tapeworm, and *T. solium*, the pork tapeworm. These parasites measure approximately 5 cm and 3 cm, respectively, and are similar in many ways but have different clinical implications.

The scolex of *T. saginata* has four suckers, but no hooks, while the scolex of *T. solium* has a rostellum with two rows of hooks plus four suckers.

The proglottids differ in appearance and number, as well as in the number of uterine branches within each proglottid (Figure 14–7). *T. saginata* usually has

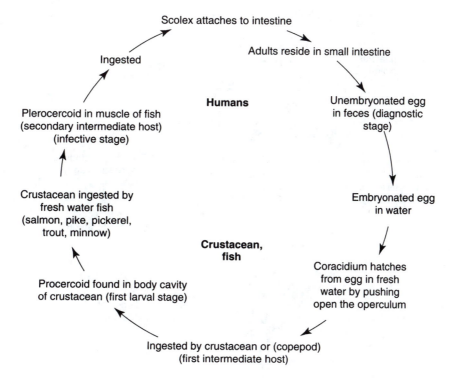

FIG 14–6 Life cycle of *D. latum*

greater than 1,000 proglottids, while *T. solium* has fewer than 1,000 proglottids in an adult worm. The beef tapeworm proglottid measures approximately 17 × 5 mm, and has 15–25 lateral uterine branches on each side of the uterus; the pork tapeworm proglottid is somewhat shorter, and has 7–14 lateral uterine branches.

The indistinguishable spherical to oval eggs of the two *Taenia* species are radially striated, with a yellowish, brown shell (Figure 14–7), and measure 30–40 μm. A six-hooked oncosphere is present in embryonated eggs.

Life Cycle

Human infection with *T. saginata* or *T. solium* is acquired by ingestion of uncooked beef or pork, respectively, containing the cysticercus larvae of the parasite (Figure 14–8). The larva is digested out of the meat in the stomach. The scolex of the larva attaches to the mucosa of the small intestine; development of the adult tapeworm follows. Eggs are produced, and are passed in human feces. Eggs are ingested by cows or pigs, respectively, acting as intermediate hosts. The oncosphere hatches from the egg, and develops into the cysticercus larva in the animal's tissue.

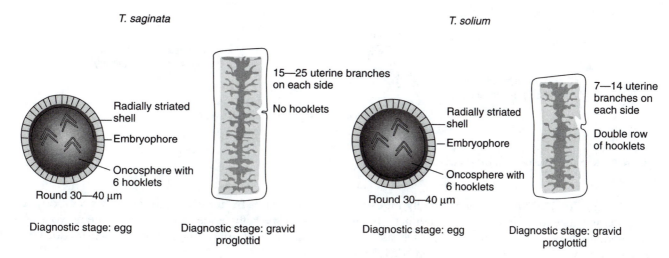

FIG 14–7 A comparison of *T. saginata* and *T. solium*, showing eggs and proglottids.

(A)

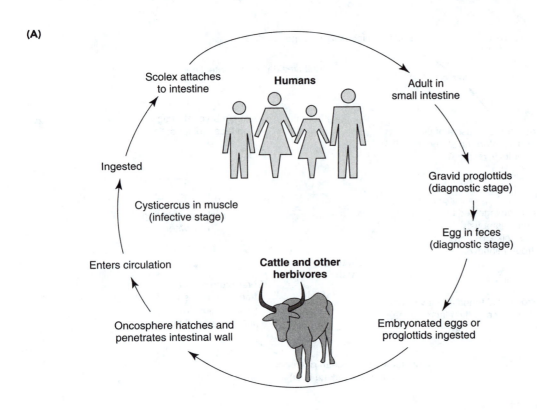

(B)

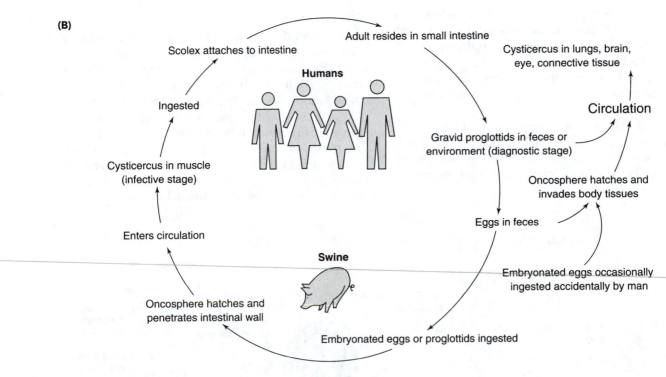

FIG 14–8 (A) Life cycle of *T. saginata* (B) Life cycle of *T. solium*

If the eggs of *T. solium* are accidentally ingested by humans (instead of pigs), the human acts as an intermediate host, and a condition known as cysticercosis may develop. The oncosphere develops and escapes from the egg, and invades the body tissues, especially tissues and organs of the nervous system. Maturation of the adult tapeworm does not occur.

Transmission and Pathogenesis

Beef and pork tapeworm infection occurs worldwide, especially in areas having poor sanitary conditions. Ingestion of raw or undercooked beef or pork contaminated with beef or pork tapeworm larvae leads to tapeworm infection. Most cases of taeniasis are asymptomatic. Mild symptoms, such as diarrhea, indigestion or abdominal pain may occur. Slight eosinophilia may be present.

Human ingestion of the eggs of *T. solium* may be a result of contamination of food or water with feces containing tapeworm eggs. Cysticercosis is common in developing countries where pigs are raised. This illness is particularly prevalent in Mexico, Peru, and other Latin American countries with poor sanitation. Symptoms of cysticercosis depend on the location of the cysticerci. This condition may be serious, particularly when the cysticercus larva migrates to the brain, causing a condition called neurocysticercosis. This infection is the most frequently occurring parasitic infection of the central nervous system. Neurological symptoms may result from invasion of brain tissue by the larvae, and include headache, and seizures. Tissue reactions may also be caused by death of the larvae in the brain.

Laboratory Diagnosis

The diagnosis of *Taenia* infection is made by recovery of gravid proglottids or eggs in human feces, after rupture of proglottids. Eggs are usually not found in large numbers, and the scolex is infrequently present.

Cysticercosis is diagnosed by radiographical findings such as computed tomographic (CT) scans, or magnetic resonance imaging (MRI) studies of multiple intracranial lesions. Serologic studies may be used to confirm the diagnosis. An immunoblot assay using purified *T. solium* antigens appears to be the test of choice for the diagnsis of cysticercosis, having a specificity of 100%, and a high sensitivity (see Chapter 3).

Treatment and Prevention

Praziquantel and niclosamide are effective treatments for taeniasis. Although antihelminthic agents hasten the disappearance of the active parenchymal lesions characteristic of cysticercosis, surgical removal of cysticercus larvae is often necessary. A serious inflammatory reaction may occur following destruction of the cysts in the brain.

Prevention of infection requires thorough cooking of beef and pork, as well as good sanitary practices. A promising porcine vaccine is under development.

Hymenolepis nana

Morphology

Hymenolepis nana, called the dwarf tapeworm, is the smallest tapeworm that infects humans, with the adult worm measuring 25–40 mm in length. It is the most common tapeworm found in the United States, and is frequently found in mice and other rodents. This cestode is unusual among tapeworms, in that no intermediate host is required to complete the life cycle.

The scolex of *H. nana* bears a short rostellum with one row of hooks, along with four suckers, similar to those found in *T. saginata*.

H. nana proglottids are approximately 2 mm wide and 1 mm long. The sac-like gravid uterus is usually full of eggs, and fills up most of the uterine cavity (Figure 14–9) However, the uterus is not seen, since it disintegrates, and releases the ova.

The round to oval thin-shelled egg of *H. nana* measures approximately 30 by 45 μm, and contains an inner envelope with two polar thickenings, each having four to eight polar filaments, which extend into the space within the shell (Figure 14–10). The six-hooked oncosphere with three pairs of hooklets is often very active.

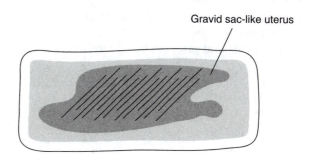

FIG 14–9 *Hymenolepis nana* proglottid

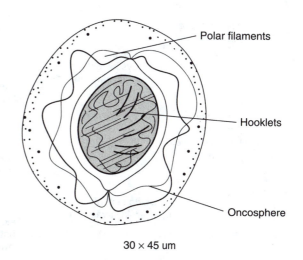

30 × 45 um

FIG 14–10 *Hymenolepis nana* egg

Life Cycle

Infection with *H. nana* is usually acquired by ingestion of infective eggs. Although no intermediate host is required to complete the life cycle, larvae may develop in intermediate hosts, such as beetles or fleas. Ingestion of beetles found in grain or cereals will transport the larvae into the human host. After maturation of the cysticercoid larva in the small intestine, the scolex attaches to the mucosa, where the adult tapeworm resides and reproduces (Figure 14–11). Eggs are discharged when the gravid proglottids disintegrate, and are pased from the body in feces. Eggs are infective when passed. They may be ingested by humans or by other animal hosts, which become infected when cysticercoid larvae develop. Eggs may also hatch in the intestine. The resulting cysticercoid larvae may develop to adulthood, resulting in autoinfection.

Transmission and Pathogenesis

Infection is usually transmitted by ingestion of infective eggs. Although most cases are asymptomatic, mild gastrointestinal symptoms, such as diarrhea, abdominal pain, and weight loss may occur.

Laboratory Diagnosis

Diagnosis of infection is made by recovery of characteristic eggs in human feces.

Adult worms and proglottids are rarely seen in the stool.

Treatment and Prevention

Praziquantel is the treatment of choice for infection with *H. nana*. Niclosamide is also effective. Good sanitary practices are essential in the prevention of infection.

Hymenolepis diminuta

Morphology

Hymenolepis diminuta resembles *H. nana* in several ways. The parasite is common in rats, and also infects humans. The adult worm is larger than the dwarf tapeworm, measuring 20 to 60 cm in length.

The scolex of *H. diminuta* resembles that of *H. nana,* bearing a small rostellum, but lacking the hooks found in *H. nana.*

The proglottids of *H. diminuta* are virtually indistinguishable from those of *H. nana* (see Figure 14–9), containing a sac-like uterus full of eggs. These normally disintegrate, and are not seen.

The eggs of *H. diminuta* resemble those of *H. nana* without the polar filaments (see Figure 14–10), but are somewhat larger in size (60–80 μm.)

Life Cycle

Rats act as definitive hosts for *H. diminuta.* Eggs are passed in rat feces, and may be ingested by an intermediate host, such as a grain beetle or flea. Cysticercoid larvae develop in the intermediate hosts.

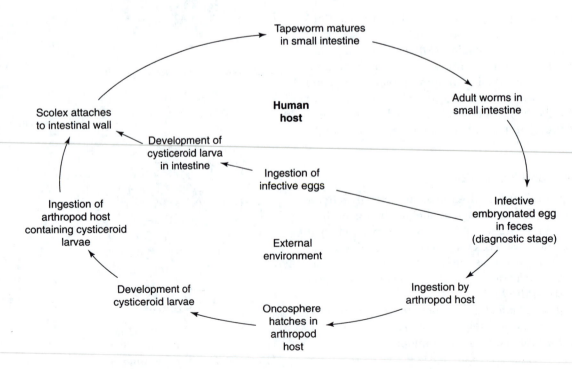

FIG 14–11 Life cycle of *Hymenolepis nana*

Ingestion of infected beetles, present in grain or cereals, may lead to infection in man, as well as in rats. The adult worm develops in the human intestine, and the life cycle is much like the life cycle of *H. nana* (see Figure 14–11).

Transmission and Pathogenesis

Transmission of infection occurs by ingestion of infected beetles or other arthropods, usually in grains and cereals. Symptoms, if any, are mild, and usually include diarrhea, nausea, and slight abdominal pain.

Laboratory Diagnosis

The diagnosis of infection with *H. diminuta*, like *H. nana*, is made by the recovery of characteristic eggs in feces. Neither proglottids, nor the scolex are usually found in stool specimens.

Treatment and Prevention

Niclosamide is the recommended treatment for *H. diminuta* infection, although praziquantel is also effective. Prevention of infection requires sanitary practices which limit exposure of grains and cereals to rats and insects. Careful examination of such foods for the presence of insects, or rodent droppings is necessary to avoid human exposure to the parasites.

Dipylidium caninum

Morphology

Dipylidium caninum is a tapeworm commonly found in dogs and cats. The tapeworm may cause infection in humans, especially in children. The adult tapeworm is 10 to 50 cm in length.

The scolex has the four suckers typical of cestode scolices. In addition, several rows of tiny hooklike spines are present on the cone-shaped rostellum of the scolex.

The uterus in the gravid proglottid contains numerous packets of eggs, each packet containing 5 to 20 eggs.

The colorless eggs of *D. caninum* measure approximately 30 to 60 μm in diameter, with a six-hooked oncosphere present in each egg (Figure 14–12). The eggs are enclosed in membrane-bound packets.

Life Cycle

The dog or cat is the usual definitive host. Gravid proglottids and packets of eggs are passed in the feces of the animal (Figure 14–13). The dog or cat flea, acting as the intermediate host, ingests the eggs, continuing the life cycle. Cysticercoid larvae develop in the flea. Humans (especially children) are infected after

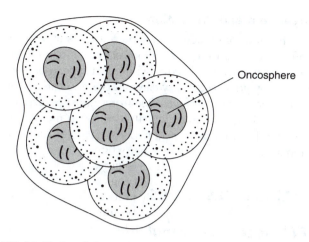

FIG 14–12 *Dipylidium caninum* egg packet

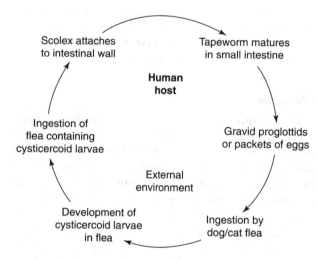

FIG 14–13 Life cycle of *Dipylidium caninum*

accidentally ingesting the fleas. The larvae mature to adulthood in the intestine.

Transmission and Pathogenesis

Infection is initiated after ingestion of *D. caninum* cysticercoid larvae. This is usually a result of hand-to-mouth delivery of fleas from infected cats or dogs. Most infected individuals are asymptomatic, although some patients with a heavy worm burden may experience mild gastrointestinal symptoms, such as nausea, diarrhea, indigestion, and slight abdominal pain.

Laboratory Diagnosis

The diagnosis of infection with *D. caninum* is made by the recovery of characteristic gravid proglottids and egg packets (following rupture of proglottids) in human feces.

Treatment and Prevention

The drug of choice for treatment of this tapeworm infection is niclosamide, although praziquantel has been shown to be effective. The infection can be prevented by good veterinary care of dogs and cats, especially keeping the animals free from parasites, as well as fleas. Good personal hygiene is critical to preventing the hand-to-mouth transmission of infected fleas to humans.

TISSUE CESTODES

Echinococcus granulosus

Morphology

Echinococcus granulosus is known as the minute tapeworm of dogs, or the hydatid tapeworm. The worm is about 4 mm in length, and consists of a scolex bearing four suckers, numerous hooks, and three proglottids. Although not found, the eggs of *E. granulosus* are identical to those of *Taenia* species.

Life Cycle

Dogs acquire the infection by the ingestion of infective cysts in the tissues of herbivorous animals, such as sheep, which act as intermediate hosts. Each cyst contains a scolex, which develops into an adult tapeworm (Figure 14–14). The adult tapeworm, which does not infect humans, resides in the small intestines of dogs and other canines. In humans, who act as intermediate rather than definitive hosts, this parasite causes unilocular hydatid cyst disease, an illness characterized by the presence of one or more cysts in a variety of tissues and organs of the body.

A hydatid cyst, which may reach the size of a grapefruit, has a laminated outer layer, and an inner layer of germinal tissue from which the daughter cysts and brood capsules (smaller cysts containing several developing inverted scolices) bud (Figure 14–15). The cyst also contains loose pieces of germinal tissue and scolices. This is known as hydatid sand. In addition, there is a great deal of fluid inside the cyst.

Humans acquire the infection by accidentally ingesting the eggs of *E. granulosus,* usually by hand-to-mouth contact with infected dog feces. The ingested eggs migrate to the various body tissues, and produce hydatid cysts. The life cycle is terminated at this point. Herbivores ingest the ova from pastures contaminated with dog feces.

Transmission and Pathogenesis

Humans contract hydatid cyst disease by ingestion of *E. granulosus* eggs, usually by hand-to-mouth contact with infected dog feces. Symptoms vary, depending on the location of the cyst in tissue. Although cysts may form in many areas of the body, the lung and the liver are most commonly affected. Pulmonary symptoms, such as cough and chest pain, may develop with lung infection. One serious complication of hydatid cyst disease is the risk of anaphylactic shock, following rupture of the cyst.

Laboratory Diagnosis

The eggs of *E. granulosus* are not found in human feces. The diagnosis of hydatid cyst disease may be made by radiographic and serologic studies (see Chapter 3). A combination of assays, including enzyme immunoassay and immunoblot techniques, has been suggested to diagnose hydatid cyst disease. The demonstration of hydatid sand is also diagnostic.

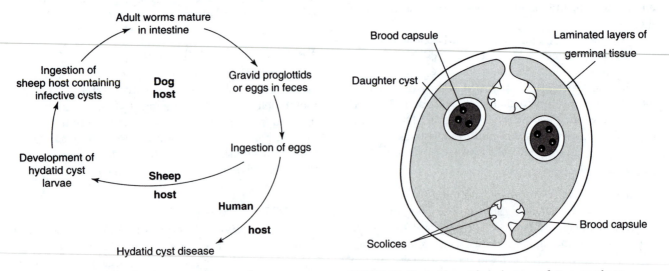

FIG 14–14 Life cycle of *Echinococcus grarnulosus*

FIG 14–15 Hydatid cyst larval stage of *E. granulosus*

Treatment and Prevention

Although surgical removal of hydatid cysts has long been considered the treatment of choice, several anti-helminthic agents are now available. These include praziquantel and mebendazole. Infection is prevented by good personal hygiene to prevent hand-to mouth transmission of eggs from dogs to humans, avoidance of ingestion of sheep viscera by dogs, and anti-helminthic treatment of dogs, as necessary.

Multiceps species

Morphology

Species of *Multiceps,* which are almost impossible to separate, parasitize dogs, foxes and wolves. The eggs of *Multiceps* and *Taenia* species cannot be distinguished. The larval form of *Multiceps* species is a cyst form called a **coenurus**, and is considered to be an intermediate form between a cysticercus, having a single scolex, and a hydatid cyst, having brood capsules (and daughter cysts) and multiple scolices.

Life Cycle

The adult tapeworm resides in the intestine of the canine definitive host, and eggs are passed in the feces. Ingestion of the eggs by herbivorous animals, such as sheep and goats, results in infection. Ingestion of the meat of these animals, harboring coenurus cysts, and acting as intermediate hosts, leads to infection in the canine definitive host. The human accidentally becomes an intermediate host, after ingestion of *Multiceps* eggs. After hatching, the larvae migrate through the intestinal wall, into the bloodstream, and into the tissues. The coenurus, which contains multiple invaginated scolices, develops in the tissues. Cysts are most apt to develop in the central nervous system of the intermediate host.

Transmission and Pathogenesis

Humans accidentally acquire infection with *Multiceps* species by ingestion of eggs passed in the feces of canine hosts. Symptoms are dependent on the location of coenurus cysts. Neurological symptoms, such as headache and seizures, may accompany cysts located in the central nervous system.

Laboratory Diagnosis

A space-occupying lesion seen by radiographic examination of the brain or spinal cord may be suggestive of infection. Histologic examination of a dissected coenurus confirms the diagnosis.

Treatment and Prevention

Surgical removal of cysts is the recommended treatment. Infection is prevented by good hygiene to prevent hand-to mouth transmission from dogs, as well as the proper disposal of animal carcasses.

SUMMARY

Cestodes cause human diseases ranging from asymptomatic infections, to serious life-threatening illnesses. Intestinal and tissue cestodes were discussed in this chapter. Characteristic features of cestodes are summarized in Table 14–1.

Cestodes are hermaphroditic and have complex life cycles. With the exception of *H. nana,* all intestinal tapeworms require one or more intermediate hosts. Except for *D. latum,* all intestinal tapeworms produce eggs containing six-hooked oncospheres, and have scolices bearing four suckers, with or without hooks, which are used for attachment to the intestinal epithelium. Although infections with the adult beef and pork tapeworms are similar, ingestion of eggs of the latter tapeworm (*T. solium*), may lead to the serious illness, neurocysticercosis. Diagnosis of intestinal cestode infection is usually based on the recovery of eggs or gravid proglottids from human feces. Packets of eggs are characteristic of *D. caninum.*

Ingestion of eggs of tissue cestodes leads to infections characterized by the formation of larval cysts in body tissues. *E. granulosus* causes unilocular hydatid cyst disease, especially in the lung and liver. *Multiceps* species lead to development of cysts, especially in the central nervous system. Surgical removal of cysts may be necessary.

Table 14–1 ▶ Key Characteristics of Cestodes

CESTODE	CHARACTERISTIC FEATURES
Diphyllobothrium latum	Broad fish tapeworm Scolex has lateral sucking grooves (bothria) Operculated eggs Embryo is a ciliated coracidium Gravid proglottid wider than long; rosette-shaped uterus Procercoid and plerocercoid larvae Transmission by ingestion of poorly cooked fish Ingestion of first intermediate host may result in sparganosis
Taenia saginata	Beef tapeworm Scolex has 4 suckers, but no hooks Spherical to oval, striated eggs, typical of *Taenia* species Embryo is a 6-hooked oncosphere Greater than 1,000 proglottids Lateral uterine branches number 15-25 Cysticercus larvae Transmission by ingestion of poorly cooked beef
Taenia solium	Pork tapeworm Scolex has 4 suckers with 2 rows of hooks Spherical to oval, striated eggs, typical of *Taenia* species Embryo is a 6-hooked oncosphere Fewer than 1,000 proglottids Lateral uterine branches number 7–14 Cysticercus larvae Transmission by ingestion of poorly cooked pork Ingestion of eggs may result in cysticercosis
Hymenolepis nana	Dwarf tapeworm Scolex bears a short rostellum with 4 suckers and 1 row of hooks Thin-shelled round to oval egg contains oncosphere and polar filaments Embryo is a 6-hooked oncosphere Proglottid contains sac-like gravid uterus full of eggs Cysticercoid larvae Transmission by ingestion of infective eggs
Hymenolepis diminuta	Rat tapeworm Scolex bears rostellum, but lacks hooks seen in *H. nana* Eggs resemble those of *H. nana* without polar filaments Embryo is a 6-hooked oncosphere Proglottids indistinguishable from those of *H. nana* Cysticercoid larvae Transmission by ingestion of infected arthropods
Dipylidium caninum	Dog and cat tapeworm Scolex has 4 suckers, and rows of tiny, hooklike spines Eggs enclosed in membrane-bound packets Embryo is 6-hooked oncosphere Proglottid contains uterus with packets of eggs Cysticercoid larvae Transmission by ingestion of cysticercoid larvae

Echinococcus granulosus	Hydatid tapeworm
	Scolex has 4 suckers and numerous hooks
	Eggs identical to *Taenia* species
	Hydatid cyst larvae
	Transmission by accidental ingestion of eggs
	Hydatid cysts develop in tissues
Multiceps species	Parasitizes dogs, foxes, and wolves
	Coenurus larvae, intermediate between cysticercus and hydatid cyst
	Transmission by accidental ingestion of eggs

REVIEW QUESTIONS

1. The organ of attachment of a tapeworm is called a:
   a. rostellum
   b. scolex
   c. proglottid
   d. strobila

2. The segment of a tapeworm, which forms distally from the neck region is called a:
   a. rostellum
   b. scolex
   c. proglottid
   d. strobila

3. The tapeworm which has two shallow suckers on its scolex, in place of suckers, is:
   a. *H. nana*
   b. *T. solium*
   c. *T. saginata*
   d. *D. latum*

4. The tapeworm associated with the condition neurocysticercosis is:
   a. *H. nana*
   b. *T. solium*
   c. *T. saginata*
   d. *D. latum*

5. The procercoid larva of *D. latum* develops in a:
   a. copepod
   b. freshwater fish
   c. beetle
   d. rodent

6. The _____ acts as an intermediate host in the life cycle of *H. diminuta*.
   a. copepod
   b. freshwater fish
   c. beetle
   d. rodent

7. Which cestode requires no intermediate host?
   a. *H. nana*
   b. *T. solium*
   c. *H. diminuta*
   d. *D. latum*

8. Packets of eggs are characteristic for which tapeworm?
   a. *T. solium*
   b. *H. diminuta*
   c. *E. granulosus*
   d. *D. caninum*

9. Hydatid cyst disease is associated with the tapeworm:
   a. *E. granulosus*
   b. *D. caninum*
   c. *Multiceps* species
   d. *T. solium*

10. A coenuris cyst is characteristic of:
    a. *E. granulosus*
    b. *D. caninum*
    c. *Multiceps* species
    d. *T. solium*

CASE STUDY

A previously healthy 39-year old medical student was seen in the emergency room, after having a seizure. He was a student at a medical school in Mexico, and was home in the United States on vacation. His history was otherwise unremarkable, although he reported that he had been suffering from severe headaches for several weeks. His neurological examination showed no focal abnormalities. A computerized tomography scan (CT scan) of the head revealed multiple calcified lesions in both cerebral hemispheres.

Questions

1. What parasite would you consider to be responsible for the patient's condition? What is the name of this illness?

2. How does man acquire this infection? How does it differ from intestinal tapeworm infection?

3. What factor in the patient's history might predispose him to this infection?

4. Why is it important to distinguish between the beef tapeworm and the pork tapeworm?

5. What danger lies in the treatment of the patient, and the subsequent destruction of the parasite?

▶ BIBLIOGRAPHY

Bern, C., Garcia, H. H., Evans, C., Gonzalez, A. E., Verastegui, M., Tsang, V. C. W., & Gilman, R. H. (1999). Magnitude of the disease burden from neurocysticercosis in a developing country. *Clinical Infectious Diseases, 29,* 1203–1209.

Garcia, L. S. & Bruckner, D. A. (1997). *Diagnostic medical parasitology* (3rd ed.). Washington, DC: ASM Press.

Koneman, E. W., Allen, S. D., Janda, W. M., Schreckenberger, P. C., & Winn, Jr, W. C. (1997). *Color atlas and textbook of diagnostic microbiology* (5th ed.). Philadelphia: Lippincott.

Shimeld, L. & Rodgers, A. T. (1999). Intestinal helminths. In Shimeld, L. (Ed.). *Essentials of diagnostic microbiology.* (pp. 603–615). Albany, NY: Delmar Publishers.

Zeibig, E. A. (1997). *Clinical parasitology.* Philadelphia: W. B. Saunders.

GLOSSARY

Acanthopodia Spiny cytoplasmic projections that characterize the trophozoite stage of *Acanthamoeba* species.

Accolé Early trophozoite forms of *P. falciparum* found at the edges of red blood cells; also called appliqué forms.

Agglutination (a-GLU-tin-AY-shun) A chemical reaction involving the binding of antibodies to particulate antigens. When these antigens react with specific antibodies, visible agglutination, or clumping of the particles occurs.

Amastigote Nonflagellate, intracellular morphologic stage found in some of the hemoflagellates.

Amebic keratitis A chronic infection of the cornea, characterized by ulcerative lesions caused by *Acanthamoeba* species.

Ameboflagellate Having both an ameboid and flagellate stage in its life cycle.

Amicrofilaremic Void of microfilariae (larval forms) in the blood.

Anergic The impaired ability to elicit an adequate immune response.

Aphasia The inability to speak coherently.

Apicomplexa (APE-ee-com-PLEKS-a) The phylum containing protozoan parasites which have complex life cycles and which are pathogenic for humans; includes *Cryptosporidium, Isospora, Cyclospora, Toxoplasma,* and *Pneumocystis* species.

Aschelminthes (ASH-hel-min-thes) The phylum containing the nematodes.

Axoneme (AKS-o-neem) The portion of a flagellum located intracellularly.

Axostyle (AKS-o-stil) A rodlike structure consisting of a pair of axonemes that provides rigidity to certain flagellate cells.

Bancroftian filariasis Parasitic infection caused by the filarial nematode *Wuchereria bancrofti.*

Benign tertian malaria *Plasmodium vivax* malaria (48-hour periodicity).

Bentonite flocculation (BF) (BEN-toe-nite flok-u-LAY-shun) An agglutination method involving the use of particles of bentonite coated with antigen.

Binary fission (BI-na-ree FI-shun) Multiplication of a parasite, involving splitting of the parent cell into two equal cells, after duplication of cytoplasm and genetic material.

Biological safety hood An enclosure in which work can be done on potentially dangerous organisms without risk of acquiring or spreading infection.

Blackwater fever A complication of *P. falciparum* malaria characterized by the passage of reddish to black colored urine resulting from massive intravascular hemolysis.

Boss (BOS) A thickening or a knob which may be found in trematodes at the opposite end of the shell from the operculum.

Bothria (BOTH-ree-a) Shallow sucking grooves found in place of suckers or hooks, on the scolices of *Diphyllobothrium latum.*

Bradyzoite Another name for the slow growing trophozoite of *Toxoplasma gondii* which are found within tissue cysts.

Brood capsule (BROOD kap-sul) Hydatid cysts consisting of many smaller cysts which contain several developing inverted scolices.

Brugian filariasis Parasitic infection caused by the filarial nematode *Brugia* species.

Buccal capsule (BUK-al kap-sul) Primitive mouth, found in some helminths.

Buccal cavity (BUK-al CAV-it-e) Primitive but prominent mouth.

Cardiomegaly Enlargement of the heart.

Calabar swelling A transient swelling of the subcutaneous tissues seen in infections with the filarial nematode *Loa loa.*

Calcareus corpuscles (cal-SAR-ee-us KOR-pus-els) Structures found in both larval and adult stages of tapeworms, which consist of concentric layers of calcium carbonate.

Central body (SEN-trul BOD-ee) A clear, transparent area resembling a vacuole, which is usually observed in stool specimens, in individuals harboring the intestinal parasite, *Blastocystis hominis.*

Cercariae (sir-KAR-ee-ay) Result from reproduction of the miracidium in the snail. The cercariae are released into water, and generally swim around in the water until the next host is encountered.

Cestode (SES-toad) A member of the phylum Platyhelminthes (flatworms) and the class Cestoda.

Chagoma An erythematous primary lesion of Chagas' disease.

Chancre A painful ulcerative lesion.

Chiclero ulcer A cutaneous lesion caused by *Leishmania mexicana* infection.

Chromatin (KRO-ma-tin) Genetic material, consisting of DNA, found in the nucleus. When present along the inner nuclear membrane (peripheral nuclear chromatin), it is characteristic of the genus *Entamoeba.*

Chromatoidal bar (KRO-ma-TOY-dal bar) A rod-shaped mass of RNA, characteristically found in the cysts of amebae.

Chromatoid bodies (KRO-ma-toyd BOD-ees)   Rod-shaped masses of RNA, characteristically found in the cytoplasm of amebic cysts.

Cilia (SIL-ee-a)   Short, thread-like extensions of cytoplasm, which act as organelles of locomotion for protozoan ciliates.

Ciliophora (SIL-ee-OF-o-ra)   The phylum containing the ciliates.

Coenurus (ko-NUR-is)   The larval form of *Multiceps* species, having multiple invaginated scolices and no daughter cysts.

Commensals (ko-MEN-sals)   Parasites not known to cause disease in humans.

Complement fixation (CF) (KOM-ple-ment fiks-AY-shun)   The binding of serum complement which occurs during an antigen-antibody reaction. This "fixation " of complement prevents the complement from reacting with cells sensitized with other antigen-antibody complexes. To indicate the presence of "unfixed" complement, red blood cells are sensitized with specific antibodies. Cell lysis indicates the presence of "unfixed" complement; the absence of hemolysis indicates that the complement has been bound in the test antigen-antibody complex, and is unavailable to react with sensitized blood cells.

Congenital transmission   The passage of disease from pregnant mother to fetus.

Copepod   Tiny crustaceans, also known as water fleas, that act as the intermediate host for *Dracunculus medinensis*.

Coracidium (KOR-a-SID-ee-um)   The ciliated embryo which develops in the eggs of *Diphyllobothrium latum*, and which is released into the water to infect the first intermediate host, a crustacean known as a copepod, in the genus *Cyclops*.

Costa (KOSS-ta)   A rodlike structure which connects the undulating membrane to the trophozoite in certain protozoan flagellates.

Counterimmunoelectrophoresis (CIE) (KOUN-ter-IM-u-no-ee-LEK-tro-for-EE-sis)   An immunoassay similar to, but more sensitive than, immunodiffusion, involving the movement of antigen and antibody toward each other through a gel medium, when an electric current is passed through a buffer solution.

Cribriform plate   Perforated portion of the ethmoid bone.

Cutaneous   Pertaining to the skin.

Cyst (SIST)   The dormant, resistant stage of a protozoan, which is the infective stage for humans and is significant in the transmission of disease.

Cysticercoid (SIS-ti-SIR-koyd)   The tapeworm larval form of *Hymenolepis* species and *Dipylidium caninum*, developing in the arthropod intermediate host.

Cysticercus (SIS-ti-SIR-cus)   The tapeworm larval form of *Taenia* species, having a single scolex invaginated into a fluid-filled cyst, which develops in the porcine (*T. solium*) or bovine (*T. saginata*) intermediate host.

Cytopyge (SI-toe-pige)   The excretory pore found opposite the cytostome in *Balantidium coli*.

Cytostome (SI-toe-stom)   An oral groove found in certain types of protozoan flagellates.

Decorticated (dee-KOR-ti-ka-ted)   Description of the egg of *Ascaris lumbricoides*, after loss of the characteristic mamillated outer covering.

Definitive host (dee-FIN-i-tiv HOST)   The host in which the parasite reaches sexual maturity and where the adult form of the parasite usually resides, or in which sexual stages of reproduction occur.

Direct fluorescent antibody (DFA) (di-REKT floor-ES-ent AN-ti-bod-ee)   Immunoassay generally used to detect antigen, using a fluorescein-labeled monoclonal antibody produced *in vitro* against the parasite. When the labeled antibodies are applied to a slide containing the parasite, the organism fluoresces when viewed by fluorescence microscopy.

Dirofilariasis   Human infection with the filarial nematode *Dirofilaria immitis* (dog heartworm).

Diurnal periodicity   Pertaining to the daylight portion of a 24-hour day.

Dracunculiasis   Human tissue infection with the guinea worm *Dracunculus medinensis*.

Dysentery (DIS-in-te-ree)   A gastrointestinal illness characterized by diarrhea, with blood and mucus in the stools. Amebic dysentery is caused by the intestinal parasite, *Entamoeba histolytica*.

Dyspnea   Shortness of breath.

Edema   Swelling.

Elephantiasis   Lymphedema of the subcutaneous tissues, with hardening and thickening of the skin, brought about by the presence of filaria (*Wuchereria bancrofti* or *Brugia* species) which obstruct the lymphatic vessels.

Embryonated (EM-bree-o-na-ted)   An egg containing a developing embryo.

Encephalomyelitis   An acute inflammation of the brain and spinal cord.

Endemic (en-DEM-ik)   The presence of a parasite in an area at all times.

Enzyme immunoassay (EIA) (EN-zime IM-u-no-ASS-ay)   An immunoassay involving the use of enzyme-labeled antigens and antibodies, which is analogous to the fluorescent antibody method, with an enzyme used as a label in place of the fluorescein dye. After binding of antigen and antibody takes place, a colorimetric substrate is added. A color change resulting from the enzyme-substrate interaction indicates a positive reaction. The intensity of the color is proportional to the concentration of the antigen-antibody complex.

Enzyme-linked immunosorbent assay (ELISA) (EN-zime-linkt IM-u-no-SOR-bent ASS-ay)   See enzyme immunoassay.

Erythema   Redness.

Erythrocytic cycle   The portion of the asexual malarial reproduction cycle that takes place within red blood cells.

Espundia   *L. braziliensis* infection, the principal cause of mucocutaneous disease in Central and South America.

Excystation (EGGS-sis-TA-SHUN)   The process whereby the cyst develops into the trophozoite form.

Exoerythrocytic cycle   Part of the life cycle for malaria that occurs outside the red blood cells.

Febrile   Having a fever, an elevated body temperature.

Filariae   A group of human filarial (blood/tissue) nematodes that are transmitted by arthropod vectors, primarily biting insects such as flies and mosquitos.

Filariform larva (fil-AR-i-form LAR-va)   The infective third stage larva of certain helminths, such as the hookworms, and *Strongyloides stercoralis*. This form is not capable of living independently and must find a host.

Flagella (fluh-JEL-a)   Whiplike appendages, which act as organelles of locomotion and are characteristic of protozoan flagellates.

Fluke (FLOOK)   A member of the helminth class Trematoda.

Fluorescent antibody (FA) (floor-ES-ent AN-ti-bod-ee)   The use of a fluorescent dye (fluorescein isocyanate) linked (conjugated) to serum antibody (or antigen) which fluoresces under ultraviolet light. The observation of this fluorescent tag suggests the presence of an antigen-antibody complex.

Formalin   An aqueous solution of formaldehyde, used in the recovery and long-term preservation of protozoan cysts, helminth eggs, and larvae.

Formalin-ethyl acetate sedimentation technique   A widely used method of obtaining a large concentration of parasites in a sample.

Free-living   A large and diverse group of protozoan organisms that inhabit fresh and salt water, decaying organic matter and damp soil.

Gametocytogenesis   The formation of male and female sex cells (gametocytes).

Glomerulonephritis   Inflammation of the glomeruli of the kidney.

Glycogen mass (GLI-ko-jen mass)   A mass of food stored as glycogen, which may be present in the cysts of certain species of amebae.

Granulomatous amebic encephalitis (GAE)   A subacute, chronic condition of the central nervous system caused by *Acanthamoeba* species.

Gravid (GRA-vid)   Egg-bearing female.

Helminth (HELL-minth)   Worm.

Hemoglobinuria   The presence of hemoglobin in urine.

Hermaphroditic (her-MAF-ro-DIT-ik)   Having both male and female reproductive structures.

Hemoflagellate   Flagellated protozoa that parasitize the blood and tissues of the human host: genus *Leishmania* and genus *Trypanosoma*

Hermaphroditic (her-MA-fro-DI-tik)   The presence of male and female reproductive organs present in a single organism.

Histiocyte   Phagocytic cells of the reticuloendothelial system.

Hyaline knob (HI-a-lin nob)   Lemon shaped structure resembling a nipple, located at the anterior end of the protozoan parasite, *Chilomastix mesnili*.

Hydatid cyst (hi-DA-tid SIST)   The larval stage of the only intestinal tissue tapeworm, *Echinococcus granulosus*. These cysts develop following accidental ingestion of the eggs of this cestode, and consist of a laminated outer layer and an inner layer of germinal tissue, plus multiple scolices, daughter cysts, brood capsules, and fluid. Hydatid cyst disease is characterized by the presence of one or more cysts in a variety of tissues and organs of the body.

Hypnozoite   The resting stage of a parasite.

Immunoassay (IM-un-o-ASS-ay)   A method for detection of antigen or antibody; also known as **immunodiagnostic assay**.

Immunoblot (IB) (IM-u-no-blot)   A technique whereby antigens are separated by electrophoresis and blotted onto a nitrocellulose membrane. After binding to the membrane, antigens are subsequently identified by staining with labeled antibodies; also known as the Western Blot assay.

Immunodiffusion (ID) (IM-u-no-di-FU-shun) (gel diffusion)   A technique used to visualize precipitation reactions between antigens and antibodies in a gel. The double-diffusion assay, known as the Ouchterlony method, uses two wells cut in an agar gel medium, one filled with antibody, and one with antigen. Following diffusion of reactants, lines of precipitation occur when the ratio of antigen and antibody is in optimal proportions.

Immunoelectrophoresis (IE) (IM-u-no-e-LEK-tro-for-EE-sis)   An immunoassay involving the electrophoretic separation of antigens in a gel, followed by diffusion of antibodies from serum placed in a trough extending parallel to the electrophoretic path. Lines of precipitation form, depending on the antibodies present in the serum.

Indirect fluorescent antibody (IFA) (IN-di-rekt floor-ES-ent AN-ti-bod-ee)   Immunoassay that uses a fluorescein-labeled parasite antigen to detect antibody in human serum. Unlabeled parasite antigens may also be used. After applying known antigens to a slide, patient serum is added. After binding between antigen and antibody has occurred, the slides are washed to remove excess serum, then are covered with a fluorescent dye conjugated to anti-human globulin. Binding of the fluorescent dye indicates the presence of the appropriate antibody in the patient's serum.

Indirect hemagglutination (IHA) (IN-di-rekt HEEM-a-GLU-tin-AY-shun)   An agglutination reaction for antibody detection involving the use of protein antigens bound to red blood cells.

Intermediate host (in-ter-MEE-dee-at HOST)   The host in which the immature or larval form usually resides, or in which the parasite undergoes asexual reproduction.

Intrathecal   Into the spinal canal.

Ischemia   Insufficient blood supply.

Kala azar   Visceral leishmaniasis, the most severe of the *Leishmania* infections.

Karyosome (KAR-ee-o-som)   A clump of chromatin material found within the nuclei of amebae. The size, configuration and location of the karyosome is distinctive for each ameba and is helpful in identification.

Kerandel's sign   Delayed sensation to pain associated with trypanosomiasis.

Kinetoplast   A structure consisting of a blepharoplast and a parabasal body.

Kissing bug   The common name for the vector for *Trypanosoma cruzi*.

Knott's technique   A concentration method for the recovery of parasitic organisms in blood and body fluids which involves the centrifugation of the sample fixed in 2% formalin.

Larva (LAR-va)   An immature form of a helminth.

Latex agglutination (LA) (LAY-teks a-GLU-tin-AY-shun)   An agglutination method utilizing latex particles to suspend the antigen.

Leishmaniasis   Infections caused by members of the genus *Leishmania*.

Loaisis   Human infection with the filarial nematode *Loa loa*.

Lymphadenitis   Inflammation of the lymph nodes.

Lymphadenopathy   Enlargement of the lymph nodes.

Lymphangitis   Inflammation of the lymphatic vessels.

Macrogamete (MA-kro-GAM-eet)   Female sex cell.

Macrogametocyte   The female sex cell of the malarial parasite.

Malarial paroxysm   A periodic episode characterized by fever, chills, headache, sweats and fatigue.

Malarial pigment   Brownish colored pigment found in red cells infected with *Plasmodium* spp. made up of the waste products of hemoglobin metabolism.

Malignant jaundice An infection in dogs caused by species of *Babesia*.

Malignant tertian malaria *Plasmodium falciparum* malaria (48-hour periodicity).

Mansonelliasis Human infection with the filarial nematode *Mansonella* species.

Mastigophora (MAS-tig-OF-or-a) Flagellates.

Maurer's dots or clefts Irregular, dark red, rod or wedge shaped markings in red blood cells infected with *P. falciparum*.

Median bodies (MEE-dee-in BOD-ees) Structures which cross the axonemes in *Giardia lamblia* at an oblique angle, giving the appearance of a "mouth." They are thought to be involved in metabolism; also known as parabasal bodies.

Merozoite (MER-o-ZO-ite) Cells produced within shizonts during shizogony, or asexual reproduction; malarial form produced within liver cells during the asexual pre-erythrocytic cycle and in the red blood cells (erythrocytic cycle)

Metacercariae (MET-a-sir-KAR-ee-ay) Formed when cercariae encyst in the flesh of vertebrates (fish) or invertebrates (crayfish), or on freshwater vegetation.

Microfilariae The larval stage of the filarial parasite.

Microgamete (MY-kro-GAM-eet) Male sex cell.

Microgametocyte The male sex cell of the malarial parasite.

Microspora (MY-kro-SPOR-a) The phylum containing tiny intracellular parasites which cause infections in a variety of vertebrates and invertebrates. Human infections frequently occur in immunocompromised individuals, especially in HIV-infected patients.

Miracidium (MIR-a-SID-ee-um) The ciliated larval stage of a fluke, which develops within the ovum.

Montenegro (leishmanin) skin test A delayed hypersensitivity reaction provoked by a suspension of killed leishmanial promastigotes administered intradermally.

Mucocutaneous Pertaining to the mucous membranes and the skin.

Myalgia Muscle aches.

Myocarditis Inflammation of the myocardium.

Nematode (NEM-a-toad) A roundworm having a complete digestive system, including a mouth and an anus. Separate sexes exist, with the females typically being larger than the males. Roundworms, members of the phylum Aschelminthes and the class Nematoda, are the most common helminths which infect humans.

Nocturnal periodicity Pertaining to the night time portion of a 24-hour day.

Non-periodic Without period, occurring randomly.

Nuchal rigidity Stiff neck.

Nucleic acid probe (nu-KLEE-ik A-sid PROBE) Small pieces of DNA or RNA complementary to the nucleic acid of the parasite, which can be used to detect parasites by forming hybrids with parasite nucleic acid.

Occult blood Blood that is present in such small amounts that it can only be detected microscopically or by chemical testing.

Occupational Safety and Health Administration (OSHA) A federal agency established to monitor and reduce the occurrence of occupational hazards, injuries, and illnesses.

Ocular micrometer A measuring scale within the eyepiece of the microscope.

Onchocerciasis Human infection with the filarial nematode *Onchocerca volvulus*, also known as river blindness.

Onchocercoma Fibrous tumor-like nodules which encapsulate the filarial nematode *Onchocerca volvulus* in the subcutaneous tissues.

[[Author — next 2 terms same; which def. should be used?]]

Oncosphere (ON-ko-sfer) The six-hooked embryo found in most cestode eggs.

Oncosphere (ON-ko-sfer) A six-hooked larva found in a cestode egg.

Oocyst (O-o-sist) The encysted form of the zygote, formed during sexual reproduction, and often infective for humans; the infective form of *Toxoplasma gondii* shed in cat feces.

Ookinete A developmental form of the malarial parasite within the mosquito.

Operculum (o-PER-ku-lum) A structure which acts as an "escape hatch" for the miracidium present in the ova of all trematodes (except schistosomes).

Oriental sore Infection caused by the organisms of the *Leishmania tropica* complex; Old World cutaneous leishmaniasis.

Pain bois Infection caused by *L. guyanensis* (forest yaws) in the Guianas and parts of Brazil and Venezuela.

Parasite (PAR-a-site) A live organism living in, or on, and exhibiting some metabolic dependence on another organism known as a host.

Parasitemia The parasites gain entry to the bloodstream and lymphatic system.

Parthenogenic (PAR-then-o-JEN-ik) Self-fertilizing.

Pathogen (PATH-o-jen) A disease-causing microbe.

Platyhelminthes (PLAY-tee-hel MIN-thees) The phylum containing flatworms, including trematodes (flukes) and cestodes (tapeworms).

Plerocercoid (PLER-o-SIR-koyd) The infective tapeworm larva of *Diphllobothrium latum* which develops in the second intermediate host, a freshwater fish. Ingestion results in human tapeworm infection.

***Pneumocystis carinii* pneumonia (PCP)** An acute interstitial plasma cell pneumonia caused by *Pneumocystis carinii*.

Pneumocystosis An acute interstitial plasma cell pneumonia caused by *Pneumocystis carinii*.

Polar tubule (PO-lar TOO-bul) The organelle which acts as an extrusion mechanism to introduce sporoplasm into a new host cell, and found within the spore produced by members of the microsporidia.

Polymerase chain reaction (PCR) (po-LIM-er-ase CHAYN ree-AK-shun) An amplification procedure which greatly increases the quantity of target-specific DNA to enhance the sensitivity of nucleic acid probes in the detection of parasites.

Primary amebic meningoencephalitis (PAM) A rapidly progressive, fatal infection of the central nervous system caused by *Naegleria fowleri*.

Procercoid (pro-SIR-koyd) This tapeworm larva of *Diphyllobothrium latum* develops in the copepod, which acts as the first intermediate host. The infected copepod is ingested by the second intermediate host, a freshwater fish.

Proglottid (pro-GLO-tid) A segment which develops from the neck of a tapeworm. A proglottid may be immature, mature, or gravid, filled with eggs.

Promastigote A long, slender morphologic form in hemoflagellate development, containing a free flagellum that extends anteriorly from the axoneme.

Pruritus Severe itching.

Pseudopods (SOO-doe-pods)   Cytoplasmic protrusions, found on amebae, which act as organelles of locomotion.

PVA   polyvinyl alcohol; a water soluble synthetic resin combined with Schaudinn's fixative to make a stool preservative for the recovery of intestinal parasites.

Quartan malaria   Malaria characterized by a 72-hour periodicity of fever (*P. malariae*)

Recrudescence   a recurrence of malarial symptoms in patients with previously low grade, asymptomatic parasitemia.

Reduviid bug   The common name for the vector for *Trypanosoma cruzi.*

Retinochoroiditis   An inflammation of the retina which extends to the choroid/vascular coat of the eye.

Rhabditiform larva (rab-DIT-i-form LAR-va)   The free-living first stage larva of certain helminths, such as the hookworms, and *Strongyloides stercoralis.* This form is non-infective.

Rigor   Shaking chills.

Romana's sign   Conjunctivitis and unilateral edema of the face and eyelids associated with Chagas' disease.

Rostellum (ro-STEL-um)   A crown-like structure which may be present on a tapeworm scolex, and which may or may not bear hooks.

Sandfly   One of a variety of species of tiny phlebotomine flies (genera *Phlebotomus, Lutzomyia, Psychodopygus*) that are the vector for *Leishmania* species.

Sarcocyst (SAR-ko-sist)   The cyst form of *Sarcocystis* species, found in muscle.

Sarcodina (SAR-ko-DI-na)   Amebae.

Sarcomastigophora (SAR-ko-MAS-tig-OF-or-a)   The phylum containing the amebae (Sarcodina) and the flagellates (Mastigophora).

Schistosomulum (SHIS-toe-SOM-u-lum)   The form which develops after skin penetration by schistosome cercariae, when the cercariae lose their tails.

Schizogony (skiz-OG-o-nee)   A stage in the asexual cycle of the malarial parasite that takes place within the red blood cell; asexual reproduction among the Sporozoa.

Schizont (SKY-zont)   Developmental form produced during schizogony, or asexual reproduction.

Schüffner's dots   Tiny, red staining granules (Giemsa stained) found in the cytoplasm of red blood cells infected with *P. vivax* or *P. ovale.*

Scolex (SKO-leks)   The organ found on a tapeworm which attaches to the intestinal epithelium. It usually bears suckers or hooks, and is located at the anterior end of the worm.

Sheathed   An outer membrane covering that surrounds the microfilariae at birth and may either be retained or lost depending on the genus.

Sheather's sugar flotation   A technique for obtaining a concentration of parasites useful in identifying *Cryptosporidium* and *Isospora* oocysts.

Skin snip   A bloodless skin biopsy used for the recovery and identification of tissue nematodes.

Sodium acetate-formalin (SAF)   A stool preservative used for the recovery of intestinal parasites.

Somnolence   Excessive sleepiness.

Sparganum (spar-GAN-um)   If the first intermediate host (copepod) of *Diphyllobothrium* species is ingested by humans, as in contaminated water, the procercoid larva may develop into a sparganum, which migrates into the body's subcutaneous tissue.

Spore (SPOR)   Tiny developmental structures formed during the reproductive cycle of members of the microsporidia.

Sporoblast (SPOR-o-blast)   The immature precursor to the sporocyst found in protozoan oocysts.

Sporocyst (SPOR-o-sist)   A sac formed during the reproductive cycle within the oocyst of certain coccidia, and which gives rise to a characteristic number of sporozoites; the developmental structures contained within the oocyst of *Toxoplasma gondii.*

Sporogony (spor-OG-o-nee)   Sexual reproduction among the Sporozoa; a stage in the sexual cycle of the malarial parasite that takes place in the mosquito.

Sporozoite (SPOR-o-ZO-ite)   Formed within oocysts of coccidian parasites; spindle-shaped infective stage of the malarial parasite, found in the mosquito.

Stage micrometer   A slide that has lines inscribed on it that are exactly 0.01 mm apart, used for calibration of the ocular micrometer.

Standard precautions   The standard for reducing worker exposure to blood-borne pathogens which assumes that all human blood and body fluids are potentially infectious for HIV, HBV, and other blood-borne pathogens.

Streptocerciasis   Human infection with the filarial nematode *Mansonella streptocerca.*

Strobila (stro-BIL-a)   The entire body of a tapeworm.

Sub-periodic   Describes those microfilariae that can be detected in the blood throughout the day but are present in greater numbers during the night.

Sucking disc (SUHK-ing disk)   A prominent concave area located on the ventral side of the cells of *Giardia lamblia.* This structure allows attachment of the parasite to the intestinal mucosa.

Tachyzoite   Actively proliferating trophozoite.

Tapeworm (TAPE-worm)   A cestode, which has a long, flattened whitish ribbonlike body. It consists of a scolex, a neck, from which the tapeworm grows, and proglottids.

Tegument (TEG-u-ment)   The absorptive outer covering of a flatworm.

Tertian   Within 48 hours.

Texas cattle fever   An infection in cattle caused by species of *Babesia.*

Tissue cyst   Resting form of *Toxoplasma gondii* found within muscle tissue.

Toxoplasmosis   A generally benign disease caused by infection with the protozoan *Toxoplasma gondii.* Immunocompromised patients and the developing fetus are at greatest risk of clinical disease.

Trematode (TREM-a-toad)   A helminth belonging to the class Trematoda.

Triatomid bug   The common name for the vector for *Trypanosoma cruzi.*

Trichinellosis   Human infection with the tissue nematode *Trichinella spiralis.*

Trichinosis   Human infection with the tissue nematode *Trichinella spiralis.*

Trophozoite (TRO-fo-ZO-ite)   The motile, actively multiplying form of a protozoan, susceptible to destruction outside the host, which usually lives in the large intestine causing tissue damage.

Tsetse fly (*Glossina*)   Serves as the intermediate host and vector for both forms of African sleeping sickness.

Undulating membrane (UN-du-la-ting MEM-brain)   The wavy membranous structure attached to the outer portion of some flagellates.

Uta Disease caused by *L. peruviana* in the Peruvian Andes.

Visceral Pertaining to the internal organs enclosed within the body cavity.

Winterbottom's sign The enlargement of the postcervical chain of lymph nodes associated with African sleeping sickness.

Ziemann's dots Dust-fine, pink staining dots (Giemsa stained) found in the cytoplasm of red blood cells infected with *P. malariae*.

Zinc sulfate flotation technique A flotation method of obtaining concentrations of parasites in a sample.

Zoonosis Disease communicable from animals.

Zygote A fertilized stage formed by the union of male and female sex cells.

INDEX